Clinical Procedures for Ocular Examination

THIRD EDITION

Clinical Procedures for Ocular Examination

THIRD EDITION

Nancy B. Carlson, OD
Professor of Optometry
New England College of Optometry
Boston, Massachusetts

Daniel Kurtz, OD, PhD
Professor of Optometry
New England College of Optometry
Boston, Massachusetts

McGraw-Hill
Medical Publishing Division
New York   Chicago   San Francisco   Lisbon   London   Madrid   Mexico City
Milan   New Delhi   San Juan   Seoul   Singapore   Sydney   Toronto

Clinical Procedures for Ocular Examination, 3/e

Previous editions copyright © 1996 and 1991 by Appleton & Lange

1234567890 DOC DOC 09876543

ISBN-0-07-137078-1

This book was set in Times Roman by Binghamton Valley Composition.
The editors were Darlene Cooke, Michelle Watt, and Regina Brown.
The production supervisor was Rick Ruzycka.
The index was prepared by Herr's Indexing Service.
R. R. Donnelley was the printer and binder.

This book was printed on acid-free paper.

Library of Congress Cataloging-in-Publication Data

Clinical procedures for ocular examination / edited by Nancy B. Carlson, Daniel Kurtz—
    3rd ed.
        p. ; cm.
    Includes bibliographical references and index.
    ISBN 0-07-137078-1
      1. Eye—Examination. 2. Eye—Diseases—Diagnosis. I. Carlson, Nancy B. II. Kurtz,
    Daniel.
      [DNLM: 1. Eye Diseases—diagnosis. 2. Optometry—instrumentation. 3. Vision
    Tests—methods.   WW 141 C641 2004]
    RE75.C474   2004
    617.7'15—dc21

                                                                                    2003051047

CONTENTS

CONTRIBUTORS

Robert C. Capone, OD
Associate Professor of Optometry
New England College of Optometry
Boston, Massachusetts
Staff Optometrist, East Boston Neighborhood Health Center
East Boston, Massachusetts

Ronald K. Watanabe, OD
Associate Professor of Optometry
New England College of Optometry
Boston, Massachusetts

David A. Heath, OD, MEd
Vice President and Dean for Academic Affairs
New England College of Optometry
Boston, Massachusetts

Catherine Hines, OD
Stanley, North Carolina

PREFACE TO THE THIRD EDITION

More than 7 years have passed since the publication of the second edition of **Clinical Procedures for Ocular Examination**. During that period, the optometric profession achieved several significant milestones: all the states have passed laws enabling optometrists to use therapeutic pharmaceutical agents (TPAs) to treat a wide variety of ocular diseases and most optometrists are now privileged to treat open angle glaucoma. The movement to standardize optometry on a national level continues. The intellectual foundations of optometric practice have been strengthened by an ever-growing body of scientific literature. Consequently, we have updated the reference sections with recent citations and added or modified procedures in accordance with contemporary concepts and knowledge.

One of the key motivations for the 1990 edition of this book was the lack of standardization for many clinical procedures. Books such as this one have alleviated the problem to some degree. Nevertheless, it remains true now as it did at the time of the first and second editions: there is still more than one acceptable way to perform many of the procedures. In some of these instances we have added variations in the step-by-step procedures, clearly indicating that there is a valid, alternate way to perform that step or procedure.

This edition continues the practice of earlier editions of not including highly technical or equipment-specific techniques. To learn to operate these tools, one must refer to the manual that comes with the instrument. We remain true to our primary mission: to describe how to perform a wide variety of useful tests without a large body of theory.

INTRODUCTION

The purpose of **Clinical Procedure for Ocular Examination** is to provide students and practitioners with detailed step-by-step procedures for a comprehensive battery of techniques used in the examination of the eye. These procedures include tests for assessing the refractive error, the accommodative function, the binocular coordination, and the health of the eyes, monitoring the fit and condition of contact lenses, and screening tests for neurological and systemic health conditions. The book contains detailed, step-by-step instructions on how to perform each technique. For each procedure, the reader is provided with complete information on what equipment is needed, how to set up the equipment and the patient properly, and how to record the findings. Expected findings are listed for most tests. The text includes diagrams and photographs to reinforce the descriptions of the techniques.

The emphasis in this book is technical. It provides little in the way of the theory or the background of the tests. Removal of the theoretical discussion leaves a pure, concise description of the techniques and allows the reader to concentrate on the mechanics of the procedures. Readers who are unfamiliar with the techniques can use the descriptions in this manual to learn the test procedures with little or no supervision. Readers who are already familiar with the techniques can use this manual to review a test procedure to ensure that they or someone under their supervision is performing it correctly. Mastery of the techniques and interpretation of the findings, however, cannot be obtained solely through the use of this book, but requires supervised clinical practice as well as a thorough understanding of the theoretical basis for each technique. Included in the References section at the end of the book are sources that will provide the reader with the necessary theory and background for each of the procedures.

The first chapter of the book deals with the case history, which is a critical phase of the examination and marks the beginning of the diagnostic thought process. The patient's reason(s) for seeking an eye examination are established in the case history. The examiner can now begin to develop his examination strategy. Based on the patient's chief complaints and routine background information gathered in the case history, the examiner can decide which phases of the examination to concentrate on and which problem-specific testing should be done.

The second chapter describes the entrance tests. These techniques are the first procedures performed following the case history. They are relatively simple procedures that use minimal, primarily hand-held equipment. They screen for problems in each of the three major problem areas: refraction, visual function, and health. Most of the entrance tests actually screen for problems in more than one of these three areas. Thoughtful interpretation of the results of the entrance tests can greatly increase the efficiency of the examination. Augmented by the information gathered in the case history, these data aid the examiner in pinpointing the patient's problem areas and appropriately directing the examination strategy.

Chapters 3 to 5 correspond to the problem areas of refraction, visual function, and ocular health. Traditionally, a complete ocular examination consisted of comprehensive testing in each of these three areas. The information thus obtained was referred to as the "minimum defined data base." If a problem was discovered through these procedures, additional problem-specific tests were performed to enhance further evaluation. In this age of managed health care, providers no longer have the luxury of performing a battery of procedures on every patient simply to collect data. It is important to detect problems quickly, with a minimum number of tests, allowing time to probe each problem with more specific testing.

In Chapters 3 to 5 we have defined tests that can be considered "core" tests. Core tests can be viewed as providing the center or nucleus of the exam. They supply the examiner with enough information to detect but not to diagnose the vast majority of ocular, neurological, or visual anomalies, even in the absence of patient symptoms. The examiner's philosophy and the demographic characteristics of the patient will influence what tests will be included in the core tests. The traditional minimum defined data-base of the past included more tests than those currently defined as core tests. This reduction in the number of procedures included in a complete examination is reasonable, since the minimum defined data-base already contained some redundancy. For this reason, excluding certain tests will not affect the quality of information obtained. However, examiners must be aware of the increased importance of screening for unexpected problems, and diligently follow up with problem-specific testing in the case of any abnormal test results.

Each of these three chapters also describes a wide variety of problem-specific tests, by which the examiner explores a specific area of concern in detail. These tests are not done on a routine basis, but are selected on the basis of the patient's case history and the results of other testing. Problem-specific tests are not placed in a separate chapter. They are included in the chapter corresponding to their problem area.

Included within these chapters are flowcharts that illustrate how tests might be grouped or sequenced in order to promote examination efficiency. These charts do not represent the only appropriate sequencing of the techniques, but they do illustrate one sequence for efficiently combining the procedures.

Separate flowcharts are presented for the most commonly applied core entrance tests, refractive tests, and ocular health assessment tests. Since functional testing and problem-specific testing are almost always customized to the patient and depend strongly on the individual's problem or complaint, there is no standard flowchart for these parts of the ocular examination.

Individual flowcharts could not possibly work for all patients. Rather, they are intended to provide a standard sequence of testing for the majority of patients seen in most examiners' practices. This standard test order can be compared to the itinerary of a trip. The traveler plans the trip from start to finish along a standard pathway, or "main route." Similarly, the flowcharts depict a standard itinerary of optometric tests that lead from the beginning to the end of the routine exam.

However, many patients need problem-specific tests, which can be compared to points of interest along the main route. When indicated, the examiner takes a "side trip." That is, he performs certain tests that are supplemental to the main route. The flowcharts and text show when side trips are indicated. Once the necessary side trip is completed, the examiner should usually return to the main route and continue the examination from there. For the sake of examination efficiency, however, some side trips may be postponed.

Chapter 6 concentrates on the procedures necessary for basic fitting and monitoring of contact lenses. These procedures are considered problem-specific since they are useful only for contact lens patients. It is possible to quickly and efficiently incorporate these procedures into a comprehensive ocular examination.

Chapter 7 deals with procedures used to screen a patient's systemic health. The eye care professional is often the patient's entry point into the health care system. Optometrists therefore have the responsibility to evaluate the overall health of the patient. The examiner may select to perform certain procedures based on the patient's age, medical history, or presenting symptoms or as the result of information gathered during the comprehensive examination. Alternately, the examiner may prefer to perform these screening procedures routinely on all patients. Patients with abnormal results should be referred to the appropriate health care provider for more thorough evaluation and diagnosis.

Chapter 8 concentrates on procedures used to assess the cranial nerves when screening for neurological disorders. These techniques are rarely used for routine screening, but they are particularly helpful when a problem is suspected on the basis of the patient's case history or ocular examination findings. Many of these screening procedures should be performed as side-trips from certain entrance tests.

Throughout the text, the masculine form of the third person singular pronoun is used. This form is used for the sake of simplicity, and applies equally to men and women without prejudice.

ACKNOWLEDGMENTS

We wish to thank our students who have used the numerous outlines, flowcharts, and handouts that are the foundation of this book. Through their questions they helped us to determine the appropriate level of detail needed to describe each procedure. We owe a special debt to Dr. David Heath and Dr. Catherine Hines, who invested countless hours and drafted much of the text for the first two editions. We also wish to thank Mr. Ed MacKinnon and Dr. Terrence Knisely for photography; Dr. Susan Baylus for her work on many of the computer graphics; and Dr. Patti Augeri and Dr. Maureen Hanley, who were involved in developing the laboratory manual that was the foundation for Chapter 5. We extend special thanks to Dr. Alysha Jacobs, Dr. Tina Parker, Ms. Megan Lind and Ms. Rosanne LaBollita for typing, research assistance, and general help in the preparation of this book.

We would also like to acknowledge the sacrifices, support, and contributions of our significant others: Tom Corwin, Brian Carlson, Adam, Esther, and Nathan Kurtz, and Kyra and Lynne Silvers.

CASE HISTORY

Nancy B. Carlson, OD

Case history is the most important procedure in the entire repertoire of examination procedures and it is one of the most difficult to learn. History-taking can be mastered only after the acquisition of a broad base of knowledge and after years of clinical experience. An experienced and knowledgeable clinician often can determine the diagnosis from the history alone. Conversely, the novice is frequently overwhelmed by the information gathered in the case history and is rarely able to effectively use the information in the diagnostic process. It is beyond the scope of this book to provide sufficient information for a novice clinician to conduct a proficient, comprehensive case history. Rather, a script is presented illustrating the main components of a case history for a typical primary care examination. The main components of a typical follow-up examination are also presented.

The case history is usually conducted at the beginning of the examination, and is the time for the clinician and patient to become acquainted. The clinician must present himself to the patient as a caring and empathetic individual if he expects the patient to comply with his advice. At the same time, the clinician begins the diagnostic thought process by asking the patient appropriate questions to determine the potential causes for the patient's symptoms. The information is then used in deciding which procedures the clinician will use to confirm or rule out each potential diagnosis. During the case history the clinician also has an opportunity to begin educating the patient about his visual function and about his ocular and general health.

The case history for a typical primary care examination is divided into three main parts: the Interview, the Questionnaire, and the Summary. In the interview portion, the clinician asks open-ended questions to assess the patient's reason for seeking care (the chief complaint) and to ascertain the visual needs of the patient's daily life (visual demands). If the patient does not initially volunteer a complaint, it is wise to ask key, probing questions about his vision and visual function (visual efficiency).

The second portion of the case history, the questionnaire, consists of a series of questions to determine if the patient is at risk for any of a variety of ocular or neurological disorders. During the questionnaire the clinician asks about the patient's previous ocular history, his medical history, and his family's ocular and medical history. The clinician also gives the patient a list of symptoms of common eye problems to find out if the patient has ever experienced any of them. Some clinicians gather this information in a written questionnaire that the patient fills out prior to the examination. Although this is an efficient method of data collection, many clinicians prefer to speak directly with the patient about these concerns. If a written questionnaire is used, it must be followed by a conversation between the clinician and the patient to establish a doctor–patient relationship.

Finally, the case history concludes with a brief recapitulation, or summary, of the patient's chief complaint or complaints, but this time in the clinician's words. This summary assures both the clinician and the patient that the clinician understands the patient's concerns, and gives the patient an opportunity to add anything that may have been missed.

The case history can be modified for a problem-focused examination for a previously seen patient by omitting the information that has been gathered in the previous primary care examination and by asking only the questions that are relevant to the patient's reason for the visit. A problem-focused case history should include the patient's reason for visit, questions about the symptoms that will help the clinician in the differential diagnosis process, and a summary of the patient's complaints in the clinician's words.

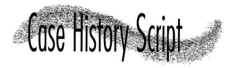

PURPOSE   To gather information about the patient's chief complaint, visual function, ocular and systemic health, and lifestyle. To establish a caring relationship with the patient. To begin the process of differential diagnosis and the process of patient education.

Case History Components for a Primary Care Examination

- **Interview**
    1. Chief complaint.
        a. Initiation: "Why did you come in today?" or "Are you having any problems with your eyes?"
        b. Elaboration of the chief complaint (FOLDARQ).
           For each complaint, the clinician asks about:
           Frequency: How often does this occur?
           Onset: When did the problem begin?
           Location: Where is the problem located?
           Duration: How long do your symptoms last?
           Associated factors: What other symptoms do you experience with this problem?
           Relief: What seems to make your symptoms go away?
           Quality: How would you rate the severity of your symptoms?
    2. Patient's visual demands.
       "What kind of work do you do?"
       "What are your hobbies?"
       "Do you drive?"
    3. Visual efficiency, if not already covered in the chief complaint.
       "Can you see clearly and comfortably both far away and close up?"
- **Questionnaire**
    1. Patient's eye history.
        a. "When was your last eye exam? By whom? What was the outcome of that examination?"
        b. Corrective lenses history.
           If the patient wears glasses, ask: "How long have you been wearing glasses? Are they for distance, near, or both? Can you see clearly and comfortably with them? When were your glasses last changed?" If the patient does not currently wear glasses, ask "Have you ever worn

glasses? What were they for? When did you wear them? When and why did you stop wearing them?"

"Do you wear contact lenses?" (for further contact lens history, see Chapter 6).

2. Patient's medical history.

"Have you ever had any medical attention to your eyes? Any surgery, injuries, or serious infections?"

"Have you ever worn an eye patch?"

"Have you ever used any medication for your eyes?"

"Have you ever been told that you have an eye turn or a lazy eye?"

"Have you ever been told that you have cataracts, glaucoma, or any other eye disease?"

"How is your general health?"

"When was your last physical examination? By whom?"

"Are you currently under the care of a physician for any health condition?"

"Have you ever been told that you have diabetes, high blood pressure, thyroid disease, heart disease, or any infectious disease?"

"Are you taking any medications? If yes, what medication, how long have you been taking the medication, what is it for, and what is the dosage?"

"Do you have any allergies? If yes, to what, what are your symptoms, and how are your allergies treated?"

3. Symptoms of common eye problems.

"Have you experienced any of the following: flashes of light, floaters, halos around lights, double vision, frequent or severe headaches, eye pain, redness, tearing, or a sandy, gritty feeling in your eyes?"

4. Family history.

"Has anyone in your family had cataracts, glaucoma, or blindness? If yes, who, when, for how long, and what was the treatment?"

"Has anyone in your family had diabetes, high blood pressure, thyroid disease, heart disease, or any infectious disease? If yes, who, when, for how long, and what was the treatment?"

- **Summary**

"Is there anything else about your eyes, your general health, or your family's eyes or health that you would like to tell me about?"

"The reason for your visit today is . . . and you have concerns about . . . ?"

Case History Components for a Problem-Focused Exam
- **Establish the reason for the patient's visit.**

Ask, "What is the reason for your visit today?" or "I see that you are here for a dilated exam.

Are there any other problems you are having that I can take care of for you today?"

- **Probe the patient's symptoms.**
    1. Use the questions from the Interview, section 1b above to elaborate on the patient's reason for this visit.
    2. If you will be using diagnostic pharmaceutical agents during the examination, always ask the patient about his medical history, the medications he is currently taking, and any allergies he has, particularly to medications.

- **Summary**
    Summarize what the patient has told you by saying, "The reason for your visit today is . . . and you have concerns about . . . ?"

RECORDING

- Record all information, including the negatives.

ENTRANCE TESTS

2

Nancy B. Carlson, OD

CHAPTER AT A GLANCE

INTRODUCTION TO THE ENTRANCE TESTS

The entrance tests are the first procedures performed following the case history. The intelligent selection of the procedures to be included in this sequence and the ongoing interpretation of the data gathered can make the difference in whether or not an efficient and accurate differential diagnosis is obtained at this point in the examination.

With the increasing pressures of health care economics, providers are adapting examination strategies that are primarily directed by symptomatology or positive test findings to maximize the efficiency of care and minimize the costs of delivery. The resulting decrease in the overall number of examination procedures performed on any given patient increases the importance of entrance test selection and their role of screening for visual disorders.

The entrance test sequence is usually composed of 8 to 12 procedures that have a low cost/benefit ratio, can be performed quickly, and do not depend on technologically sophisticated equipment. Typically, these tests have been used to elicit information that helps to define the status of each of the primary problem areas: health, refraction, and functional vision. Frequently, entrance tests apply across categories and screen for problems in more than one area (Table 2–1).

The entrance tests, considered a part of the minimum defined database, provide valuable information by screening for the presence of ocular anomalies in the absence of patient symptoms. Examples include neurological deficits as revealed by pupillary testing and visual field screenings, accommodative insufficiency identified by accommodative amplitude testing, or a muscle imbalance as noted by cover test. The information obtained from this testing sequence also provides baseline diagnostic information for future comparison. The entrance tests are often performed by technicians before the doctor sees the patient.

It is critical to emphasize that there is no one right set of entrance tests. Ask a number of eye care providers what they include in this sequence and you are likely to get a variety of answers. In fact, it is reasonable, and probably desirable, to expect that a given provider will have two or three lists that are age referenced. A test such as amplitude of accommodation serves a valuable role among children, young adults, and early presbyopes, yet provides little useful information for the elderly. For the elderly, it may be far more useful to include an Amsler grid test to evaluate macular function as a part

TABLE 2–1. MATRIX INDICATING THE PRIMARY AND SECONDARY AREAS OF DIAGNOSTIC SIGNIFICANCE FOR EACH OF THE ENTRANCE TESTS

Entrance Tests	Area of Diagnostic Significance		
	Refraction	Functional	Health
Externals		+	*
Visual acuity	*	+	*
Pinhole visual acuity	*	+	*
Amplitude of accommodation	+	*	+
Color vision			*
Cover test	+	*	+
Stereopsis	+	*	
Worth 4 Dot		*	+
Near point of convergence		*	
Hirschberg		*	+
Brückner test		*	+
Extraocular muscle testing		+	*
Pupils			*
Screening visual fields			*
Finger counting fields			*
Interpupillary distance	*		*

*, primary; +, secondary.

of the preliminary exam. The selection of tests for inclusion in the entrance test sequence must be based on a careful consideration of the cost of performing the test in terms of practitioner time and the return in terms of the usefulness of the information.

In this text, 19 procedures are included under the entrance tests section. Two of these, screening visual fields and finger counting fields, serve the same function. They are offered as alternatives. Pinhole acuity is measured only in the event of decreased visual acuity. Three variations of visual acuity are included: the standard Snellen test, which is used in most primary care examinations; the LogMAR Visual Acuity, a method used widely in low vision and in clinical research; and the Massachusetts Visual Acuity Test with Lea Symbols, which is used for screening or VA measurement in young children. The Worth 4 Dot is usually done only if there is a significant decrease in a patient's stereoacuity. The Brückner test is included as an alternative to the Hirschberg test, and can be invaluable in screening infants and young children for strabismus and anisometropia.

There are tests included in other chapters that could be considered for inclusion as entrance tests. One of these, blood pressure measurement, is included as an entrance test with increasing frequency as optometrists assume

responsibility for the detection of systemic diseases with related ocular manifestations. Other procedures to consider include the Amsler grid test, accommodative facility, associated phoria, and the dominance sighting test.

Once the decision as to what constitutes the entrance tests is made,
thought must be given to the testing sequence. The entrance tests sequence
is intended to be efficient. Factors that affect the sequencing include the
equipment needed (many of the entrance tests use common equipment) and
whether the test is done with or without the patient's correction. The flowchart in Figure 2–1 illustrates a recommended sequence of entrance tests for
a primary care examination on an adult patient.

Flow of the Entrance Tests

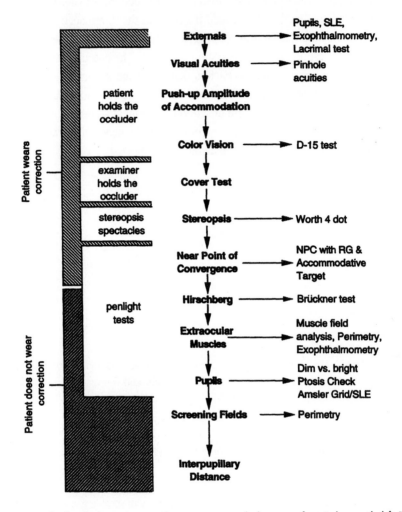

Figure 2–1. Flowchart for the entrance tests. The main route or standard sequence of tests is shown on the left. Recommended side trips or secondary tests are represented to the right. Tests are grouped according to the need for correction and equipment.

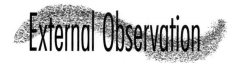

External Observation

PURPOSE To identify gross abnormalities in the patient.

EQUIPMENT

- No specific equipment is called for. A penlight may facilitate certain observations.

SET-UP

- There is no specific set-up.

STEP-BY-STEP PROCEDURE

1. Be observant.
2. In general, look for anything odd or unusual about the patient and any asymmetries between one side of the body and the other, paying particular attention to the face.
3. Observation includes certain specific points of reference:
   a. The patient's posture, including head tilts, gait, and carriage
   b. The patient's head, face, and accessory ocular structures
   c. The patient's eyes: their placement in his head, the conjunctiva, cornea, iris, and lens.
4. Compare the patient's features to your concept of an expected normal appearance. Compare one side of his body and face to the other to note any asymmetries.

RECORDING

- If in your professional judgment the patient is normal in areas observed, record WNL, which means "within normal limits."
- Describe any abnormalities or asymmetries you observe.

EXAMPLES

- Ext: WNL
- Ext: OD larger than OS and lower in face by 1 cm

Visual Acuity (VA): Minimum Legible

 PURPOSE To measure the clarity of vision or the ability of the visual system to resolve detail. A patient's visual acuity depends on the accuracy of the retinal focus, the integrity of the eye's neural elements, and the interpretive faculty of the brain.

INDICATIONS

Visual acuity should be done on all patients as the first procedure following the case history.

Note: It is important to understand that there are a number of ways by which a patient's visual function may be measured. The procedure described below, although the most common clinically, may not be applicable in certain circumstances (eg, infants, low-vision patients, and illiterate patients).

EQUIPMENT

- Projector with visual acuity slide or wall-mounted acuity chart.
- Near point visual acuity card.
- Occluder.
- Lamp.

SET-UP

- The patient wears his habitual correction for the distance being tested. When the examiner wants to measure the patient's VA both with (cc) and without (sc) correction, the acuity should be measured without correction first.
- The patient holds the occluder.
- An acuity chart, with lines from 20/50 to 20/15 exposed, is shown.

STEP-BY-STEP PROCEDURE

1. Always observe the patient, not the chart. The examiner should memorize the letters on the chart so he is able to observe the patient throughout the procedure.

2. Instruct the patient to cover his left eye and not to squint.
3. Instruct the patient to read the smallest line of letters he can. If using an acuity slide in a projected chart and the patient is unable to read 20/50, reposition the chart so the 20/60 line becomes the lowest line.
4. Encourage the patient to read the letters on the next smaller line, even if he has to guess. Stop the patient when more than half the letters on a line have been missed.
5. Have the patient cover the right eye and repeat steps 2, 3, and 4.
6. Sometimes the patient will be unable to read even the largest letter on the chart. In this event, have the patient walk toward the chart until he can just make out the largest letter (usually a big E). Note the distance at which this occurs.
7. If the patient cannot see the letters at any distance, initiate the following testing sequence, stopping at the level at which the patient can accurately respond.
   a. *Counting fingers* (CF): At a distance of approximately 1 foot, expose a selected number of fingers. Ask the patient to tell you how many fingers you are holding up. Increase the distance from the patient until his responses are no longer accurate. Move back toward the patient until he can reliably report the number of fingers presented.
   b. *Hand motion* (HM): Using a moving hand as the target, ask the patient if he can see the hand moving. Begin at approximately 1 foot and increase the distance until the patient reports he no longer detects the motion. Then move back toward the patient until he detects the motion once again.
   c. *Light projection* (LProj): Holding a penlight or transilluminator at a distance of approximately 20 inches from the patient, position the light in different areas of the patient's visual field. Each time ask the patient to point at the light and note the areas of the field in which the patient has vision.
   d. *Light perception* (LP): Direct a penlight or transilluminator at the patient and ask if he can see the light.
8. Now test near visual acuity. Repeat steps 1 through 5 at near using the following set-up:
   a. Provide high illumination on the near point card. The light source should be either above or slightly behind the patient. Care should be taken that the light is not directed at the patient's eyes.
   b. Instruct the patient to hold the card at the appropriate distance.
      (1) 16 in (40 cm) for a reduced Snellen Acuity Card
      (2) 14 in for a Jaeger Acuity Card

RECORDING

- Write Vcc or VAcc: cc means "with correction." If the VA is taken without correction, use sc instead of cc. If the patient's acuity is taken through contact lenses, use CL.
- Record each eye separately and then both eyes together. Use the abbreviation of OD for the right eye, OS for the left eye, and OU for the two eyes together.
- Record the patient's distance acuity first, followed by the near acuity.
- For each eye, record the Snellen fraction or print size for smallest (lowest) line in which more than half the letters were correctly identified. (See the additional techniques described in this section if the patient could not see any of the letters at the 20-foot testing distance.)
- If the patient read additional letters on the next line, follow the fraction or print size with a + (plus) sign and the number of letters read.
- If letters were missed, follow the fraction or print size with a—(minus) sign and the number of letters missed.
- When recording, + and—signs may be used simultaneously.
- Record the quality of the patient's response if it was abnormal, eg, slow.
- If the patient had to walk toward the chart to discern the largest letter, record the distance at which he could first read the letter as the numerator and the letter size (usually 400) as the denominator.
- If the patient's distance vision is so poor that a Snellen acuity could not be obtained, measure using the sequence of techniques listed below and record the acuity that applies:

    1. Counting fingers (CF) _____ (distance)
    2. Hand motion (HM) _____ (distance)
    3. Light projection (LProj). Record the areas of the visual field for which this was true.
    4. Light perception (LP)
    5. No light perception (NLP)

EXAMPLES

- VAcc   OD $20/40^{+1}$,   20/30 @ 16"
         OS $20/25^{-2}$, $20/30^{-2/+2}$ @ 16"
- VAcc   OD $20/25^{-2}$,   20/25 @ 16"
         OS $20/30^{+2}$, $20/40^{+2}$ @ 16" (read very slowly)
- Vsc   OD   8/400,   J-16 @ 14"
         OS   20/200, $J-3^{-1}$ @ 14"
- Vcc   OD   FC   @ 4 ft
         OS   LProj all quadrants

VISUAL ACUITY *at a glance*

1. Distance VA setup
   - Patient wears habitual correction
   - Patient holds occluder
   - Dim room illumination
   - Project appropriate chart

2. Test distance vision
   - Test right eye at distance
   - Test left eye at distance
   - Test both eyes at distance

3. Near VA setup
   - Use habitual correction
   - Place card at appropriate distance
   - Illuminate card
   - Patient holds occluder

4. Test near vision
   - Test right eye at near
   - Test left eye at near
   - Test both eyes at near

5. If the patient cannot read the largest letter on chart, proceed through
   - Finger counting
   - Hand motion
   - Light projection
   - Light perception

EXPECTED FINDINGS

- A visual acuity of 20/20 or better is considered normal.
- The difference between the two eyes should be no greater than one line.
- Any abnormality in VA must be addressed in the course of the examination and explained in the problem and plan list.

Visual Acuity (VA): Minimum Legible Using a LogMAR Chart

PURPOSE   To measure the clarity of vision or the ability of the visual system to resolve detail, the same as when taking VA with a Snellen chart. In a LogMAR chart, the incremental size of letters is determined according to the base ten logarithm of the critical detail in minutes of arc of the letters. The critical detail in minutes of arc of the smallest recognizable letters is considered to be the patient's minimum angle of resolution (MAR).

INDICATIONS

LogMAR charts should be used when a precise, quantitative assessment of visual acuity is needed. Visual acuity in LogMAR should be used in all research studies in which visual acuity is a dependent variable.

EQUIPMENT

- Visual acuity chart calibrated according to the LogMAR system. Visual acuity charts calibrated according to the LogMAR system have several special properties that render them more precise and accurate than Snellen charts. See Note 1 for a discussion of the rules for constructing a LogMAR visual acuity chart.
- Occluder.
- Lamp.
- Score sheet for the chart being used. (See note 2.)

SET-UP

- The patient wears his habitual correction for the distance being tested. When the examiner wants to measure the patient's VA both with (cc) and without (sc) correction, the acuity should be measured without correction first.
- The patient holds the occluder. The doctor holds the score sheet.
- A full LogMAR acuity chart is shown. (Lines or individual letters are not isolated.)

STEP-BY-STEP PROCEDURE

1. Instruct the patient to cover his left eye and not to squint.
2. To the extent possible, observe the patient, not the chart. Because you must make marks on the score sheet as the patient reads the chart, it will be necessary to look at the score sheet some of the time. Nevertheless, it is necessary to assure that the patient maintains occlusion of the non-tested eye and does not squint or in some other way modify his ability to read the chart.
3. Instruct the patient to read the letters on the chart (or identify the symbol in the case of charts using drawings), beginning at the top line. (See note 3.)
4. On the score sheet, circle each letter correctly identified and put a line or "X" through each letter incorrectly identified. Adjacent to the letters, in the space provided, record the number of stimuli correctly identified on each line.
5. Encourage the patient to continue reading smaller and smaller letters, even if he has to guess.
6. Proceed until he incorrectly identifies at least four of the five letters on a line.
7. Instruct the patient to unocclude his left eye and occlude his right eye, and repeat steps 2 to 6. (See note 4.)
8. When you have completed taking the VA on the patient's left eye, add up the number of letters or symbols correctly identified by each eye.
9. Apply the appropriate formula to calibrate LogMAR VA.

   The formula: In general, multiply the number of letters read correctly by 0.02 and subtract this product from 0.10 more than the LogMAR of the first line read, as illustrated in the following examples:

   (1) In the standard case in which the patient began reading at the top line of the chart (1.00 line), multiply the total number of letters read correctly by 0.02 and subtract this product from 1.10, or

   $$LogMAR\ VA = 1.10 - (0.02 \times \#\ letters\ correctly\ read)$$

   (2) If the patient began reading at the 0.80 line, the formula is

   $$LogMAR\ VA = 0.90 - (0.02 \times \#\ letters\ correctly\ read)$$

   (3) If he began reading at the 0.40 line, the formula is

   $$LogMAR\ VA = 0.50 - (0.02 \times \#\ letters\ correctly\ read).$$

   (See note 5.)

10. If the patient cannot read any of the letters on the largest line, initiate the following testing sequence, stopping at the level at which the patient can respond accurately:

    a. *Counting fingers* (CF): At a distance of approximately 1 foot, expose a selected number of fingers. Ask the patient to tell you how many fingers you are holding up. Increase the distance from the patient until his responses are no longer accurate. Move back toward the patient until he can reliably report the number of fingers presented.

    b. *Hand motion* (HM): Using a moving hand as the target, ask the patient if he can see the hand moving. Begin at approximately 1 foot and increase the distance until the patient reports he no longer detects the motion. Then move back toward the patient until he detects the motion once again.

    c. *Light projection* (LProj): Holding a penlight or transilluminator at a distance of approximately 20 in from the patient, position the light in different areas of the patient's visual field. Each time ask the patient to point at the light and note the areas of the field in which the patient has vision.

    d. *Light perception* (LP): Direct a penlight or transilluminator at the patient and ask if he can see the light.

11. Now test near visual acuity. Repeat steps 1 through 9 at near using the following set-up:

    a. Provide high illumination on a near point card calibrated according to the LogMAR system. The light source should be either above or slightly behind the patient. Care should be taken so that the light is not directed at the patient's eyes.

    b. Instruct the patient to hold the card at the appropriate distance, usually 40 cm.

RECORDING

- Write Vcc, or VAcc: cc, means "with correction." If the VA is taken without correction, use sc, instead of cc. If the patient's acuity is taken through contact lenses, record "cCL."

- Record each eye separately and then both eyes together. Use the abbreviation of OD for the right eye, OS for the left eye and OU for the two eyes together.

- Record the patient's distance acuity first, followed by the near acuity, followed by the distance at which the near acuity was measured.

- For each eye, record the result of the calculation of the formula (see Step 9, above) as a decimal carried to the second decimal place. Because both + and − VAs are possible, always record the sign of the VA.

- If the patient could not correctly identify any of the letters on the VA chart,

LogMAR VA cannot be obtained. Proceed with the VA as described in Step 10 above.

- If the patient's distance vision is so poor that a LogMAR acuity could not be obtained, record the acuity that applies, as follows:
  a. Counting fingers (CF) _____ (distance).
  b. Hand motion (HM) _____ (distance).
  c. Light projection (LProj). Record the areas of the visual field for which this was true.
  d. Light perception (LP). Record the areas of the visual field for which this was true.
  e. No light perception (NLP).

EXAMPLES

- VAcc   OD   +0.26, +0.20 @ 40 cm
           OS   +0.14, +0.02 @ 40 cm
- VAcc   OD   −0.02, 0.00 @ 40 cm
           OS   −0.12, +0.08 @ 40 cm (read very slowly)

EXPECTED FINDINGS

- A LogMAR visual acuity of 0.00 or better is considered normal. Young, healthy adult patients can be expected to have a best-corrected LogMAR VA of −0.1 to −0.20 (one to two lines better than 0.00) with a between-person standard deviation of approximately 0.10.
- LogMAR VA declines gradually as a function of age. Healthy seniors can be expected to have best-corrected VA of approximately 0.00 with a standard deviation of approximately 0.05.
- The difference between the two eyes should be no greater than 0.16.
- Like all measurements, LogMAR VA is subject to variability or measurement error. In general, measurement error (standard deviation) of LogMAR VA has been reported to be in the order of 0.08 to 0.10, which is equivalent to slightly less than one line on the chart. Therefore, interpreting these data very conservatively, consider that the patient's visual ability might have changed only if changes in their LogMAR VA exceed 0.10.
- Any abnormality in VA must be addressed in the course of the examination and explained in the problem and plan list.
- A LogMAR VA of +0.30 (Snellen equivalent 10/20) or better is considered normal for a healthy 3-year-old child. A LogMAR visual acuity of +0.20 (Snellen equivalent 10/16) or better is considered normal for a healthy 4-year-old child.
- Any abnormality in VA must be addressed in the course of the examination and explained in the problem and plan list. In the event of a failure on screening, the child must be referred for an eye examination by a licensed professional.

NOTES

1. "LogMAR" is a system for calibrating the size increments of targets on a visual acuity chart. Most such charts use block letters selected from the Roman alphabet. LogMAR charts are also available in Lea symbols. Theoretically, any type of stimulus can be used, provided it conforms to the rules of the system (see the following discussion and the section below, Special Properties of LogMAR Charts). LogMAR charts obey the rule that spacing between stimuli is proportional to letter size. Therefore, LogMAR charts are wide at the top, where the larger letters appear. As a result of the spacing requirement, it is very expensive to make a projected system calibrated according to LogMAR, and most LogMAR systems use printed charts. Both distance and near LogMAR charts are commercially available. The most commonly encountered examples for distance VA measurement are black Roman letters on a white, translucent background designed to be viewed via back illumination. Most near charts are black stimuli printed on white plastic and are intended to be illuminated by an overhead lamp. The requirement for proportionality limits the practical maximum letter size on LogMAR charts, because charts with stimuli with critical detail larger than LogMAR 1.0 would be very large, difficult to make, and expensive.

2. The score sheet (Table 2–2) contains the line-by-line identity of each letter or symbol on the chart, and has a space to the right of each line to record the number of stimuli correctly identified on each line. It is useful to preprint the formula for calibrating VA at the bottom of the score sheet (see Step 9).

3. To save time when taking the acuity, it is permissible to start at a line lower than the top line; this requires a modification of the formula for calibrating VA described in detail in Step 9. However, this is permissible only if the patient correctly identifies all five letters on the initial line read. If he fails to do so, then he must start reading the chart at a higher line with larger letters, such that he can correctly identify all five of the letters on the starting line. The only exception to this requirement is when the patient fails to read all of the letters on the top line of the chart. Because there is no larger line, he may begin on the top line (also, see Step 10).

4. It is desirable, but not necessary, to switch to a different LogMAR chart when switching from the right eye to the left eye to minimize the effects of stimulus memorization.

5. The formulas are to be applied literally. Thus, a patient can have a VA with a positive value, a VA with a negative value, or a VA of 0.00. A negative VA means that the critical detail, or MAR, is smaller than 1.0 minutes of arc, as is the case for any patient whose Snellen VA is better than 20/20.

TABLE 2–2. LOGMAR VISUAL ACUITY RECORDING FORM: PRECISION VISION SERIES ETDRS CHART 1

LogMAR	Snellen						Number Correct
1.00	200	N	C	K	Z	O	_____
0.90	160	R	H	S	D	K	_____
0.80	125	D	O	V	H	R	_____
0.70	100	C	Z	R	H	S	_____
0.60	80	O	N	H	R	C	_____
0.50	63	D	K	S	N	V	_____
0.40	50	Z	S	O	K	N	_____
0.30	40	C	K	D	N	R	_____
0.20	32	S	R	Z	K	D	_____
0.10	25	H	Z	O	V	C	_____
0.00	20	N	V	D	O	K	_____
−0.10	16	V	H	C	N	O	_____
−0.20	12.5	S	V	H	C	Z	_____
−0.30	10	C	Z	D	V	K	_____
					Total Number Correct		_____

Line A = 0.1 more than LogMAR of start line
Line B .02 × number correct
Subtract line B from line A = LogMAR VA.

SPECIAL PROPERTIES OF LOGMAR CHARTS

- The lines of letters on LogMAR charts are in steps of equal difficulty of recognition rather than in steps proportional to their physical size. This is the rationale for adjusting letter sizes according to the logarithm of the critical detail of adjacent lines, which differs by exactly 0.10.
- Every 0.10 LogMAR between the largest and the smallest targets is represented; no letter sizes are omitted. On most commercially available charts, the largest targets have a critical detail whose log is 1.0 (critical detail of 10 minarc, equivalent to 20/200 letters), and the smallest letters or symbols have a critical detail whose log is −0.30 (critical detail of 0.5 minarc, equivalent to 20/10).
- Letters are selected to be of a uniform difficulty of recognition.
- The spacing between letters on each line is proportional to letter size rather than being physically equal. Thus, the smaller the letter, the smaller is the between-letter gap. (See note 1.)
- Each line contains the same number of letters or visual stimuli (usually five).
- In general, distance LogMAR charts are calibrated for a 4.0 m viewing distance, and near LogMAR charts are calibrated for a viewing distance of 40 cm.

Visual Acuity (VA): Minimum Legible Using the Massachusetts Visual Acuity Test With Lea Symbols

 PURPOSE To measure the clarity of vision of 3- and 4-year-old children who do not know the alphabet. To screen for the presence of amblyopia and/or significant ametropia in 3- and 4-year-old children.

INDICATIONS

The Massachusetts Visual Acuity Test With Lea Symbols was designed specifically for vision screenings in young children who do not yet know the alphabet.

EQUIPMENT

- Massachusetts Visual Acuity Test With Lea Symbols (Fig. 2–2), manufactured and sold by Precision Vision, Lasalle, IL, 61301, catalog number 2590; designed by Luisa Mayer, PhD and Bruce Moore, OD; Lea Symbols developed by Lea Hyvarinen, MD.
- Occluder or eye patch
- Lamp

SET-UP

- The patient wears his habitual correction for the distance being tested. When the examiner wants to measure the patient's VA both with (cc) and without (sc) correction, the acuity should be measured without correction first. The habitual ophthalmic correction of most 3- and 4-year-olds is expected to be plano (no glasses).
- The child holds the occluder or one eye is patched during testing.
- The child also holds the square sheet containing large versions of the four Lea symbols.
- Establish accurate communication between yourself and the child, as follows:

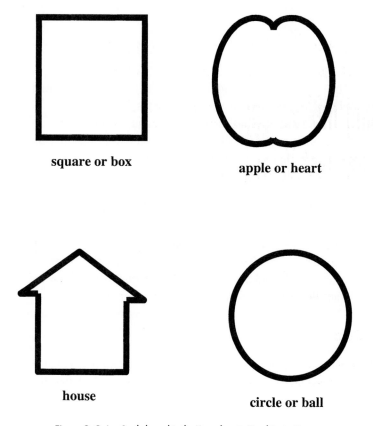

square or box

apple or heart

house

circle or ball

Figure 2–2. Lea Symbols used in the Massachusetts Visual Acuity Tests.

1. Standing 2 to 3 ft from the patient in good light, hold up one of the isolated Lea symbols.
2. Ask the child to name the picture he sees, noting what word he uses for each symbol. Note that there is no "right" or "wrong" name for a picture; for example, the child may call the square "square," "box," or something else. The purpose of this step is to ensure that the child uses a different word for each symbol and to identify the word the child will use when he correctly identifies the symbol.
3. Expose cards until you have gone through the full set of four symbols.
4. Repeat the exposure of each symbol, but now ask the child to point to the picture on the square sheet containing large versions of the four symbols that is the same as the one you are holding up.
5. Once the child is responding appropriately, proceed to screening or to VA measurement.
- As an alternative, use one of the cards marked "P" (for practice) in the upper corners instead of the small cards with isolated symbols.

STEP-BY-STEP PROCEDURE

A. Screening

1. Have the patient cover his left eye and tell him not to squint. If the patient is unable to hold the occuluder, patch his left eye.

2. To the extent possible, observe the patient, not the chart.

3. From a distance of 3 or 4 ft show the child one of the flip charts marked with a "P" in the upper left or right corner. As you point to each symbol ask the child either to name it or to point to the one just like it on the square sheet containing large versions of the four symbols.

4. If the child correctly identifies all symbols, move back to a distance of 3.0 m (10 ft) and show him the card with "R" in the upper corners and with his age (either 3 or 4) at the bottom center, and once again ask him to name the one you are pointing to or to point to the matching symbol on the square chart that he is holding. As you point to each symbol, do not break the contour interaction bar with your finger or other pointer (Fig. 2–3).

5. Correctly identifying four or five of the symbols is a pass. Identifying two or more symbols incorrectly is a fail.

6. Have the child cover his right eye to test his left eye, and show him the card with "L" in the upper corners and with his age (either 3 or 4) at the bottom center. Once again ask him to name the one you are pointing to or to point to the matching symbol on the square chart that he is holding.

7. Correctly identifying four or five of the symbols is a pass. Identifying two or more symbols incorrectly is a fail.

B. Visual acuity measurement

1. Have the patient cover his left eye and tell him not to squint.

2. To the extent possible, observe the patient, not the chart. Throughout the procedure, point to each symbol as you want the patient to identify it, making sure you unambiguously point to only one symbol at a time. As you point to each symbol, do not break the contour interaction bar with your finger or other pointer.

3. From a distance of 3 m (10 ft) with bright light illuminating the test card, show the child the +0.50 (equivalent to Snellen 10/32) card with "R" in the upper corners. If he correctly identifies the first two symbols, flip to the +0.40 card for the right eye (this may require flipping more than one card).

4. If the child correctly identifies the first two symbols on that card, proceed to the next smaller card of symbols for the right eye. (The symbols are incremented in steps of 0.10 LogMAR when viewed from 3 m.) Continue showing incrementally smaller targets until the child misses one of the first two symbols on a line.

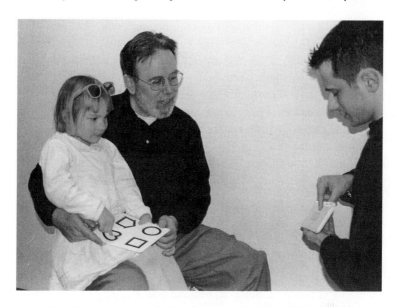

Figure 2–3. Patient viewing the Massachusetts Visual Acuity Test With Lea Symbols.

5. At that point go back to the card with the next larger set of symbols and ask the child to identify all of the symbols. If the child correctly identifies four or five of these symbols, go to the next smaller set of targets, and so on, until the child misidentifies more than one of the five symbols.
   a. The child's visual acuity is the card with the smallest targets on which he accurately identifies four or more symbols. If he misses one of the five targets, it is permissible to record a "−1" after the VA. Acuity can be recorded in Snellen equivalent, in LogMAR, or in one of the other notations at the bottom of each card.
6. Instruct the child to cover his right eye and tell him not to squint.
7. To the extent possible, observe the patient, not the chart.
8. From a distance of 3 m with bright light illuminating the test card, show the child the +0.50 (equivalent to Snellen 10/32) card with "L" in the upper corners. The "L" indicates that this card is for testing the left eye. If he correctly identifies the first two symbols, flip to the +0.40 card for the left eye (this may require flipping more than one card).
9. If the child correctly identifies the first two symbols on that card, proceed to the next smaller card of symbols for the left eye, and so on, until the child misses one of the first two symbols on a line.
10. At that point, go back to the next larger card of symbols for the left eye and ask the child to identify all of the symbols. If the child correctly identifies four or five of these symbols, go to the next smaller set of tar-

gets, and so on, until the child misidentifies more than one of the five symbols.

    a. The child's VA is the card with the smallest targets on which he accurately identifies four or more symbols. If he misses one of the five targets, it is permissible to record a "−1" after the VA. Acuity can be recorded in Snellen equivalent, in LogMAR, or in one of the other notations at the bottom of each card.

RECORDING

- Write Vcc, or Vacc; cc, means "with correction." If the VA is taken without correction, use sc instead of cc.
- Record each eye separately. Use the abbreviation of OD for the right eye, OS for the left eye.
- Record the child's distance acuity followed by the distance at which the acuity was measured (even if the standard distance of 3 m was used).
- If recording in LogMAR notation, because both + and − VAs are possible, always record the sign of the VA.
- If the child could not correctly identify any of the letters on the card with the largest symbols (the practice card has 0.60 targets), the actual visual acuity cannot be obtained with the Massachusetts Visual Acuity Test. Record "worse than +0.60" or "worse than 20/80."

EXAMPLES

For screening:

- OD pass/OS pass
- OD fail/OS pass

For VA measurement:

- VAsc   OD   10/32
              OS   10/8-1
- VAsc   OD   0.00
              OS −0.10
- VAsc   OD   +0.20
              OS   +0.30

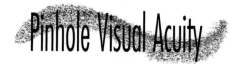

Pinhole Visual Acuity

PURPOSE To determine if a decrease in vision is correctable by lenses. Viewing the acuity chart through a pinhole will increase the patient's depth of focus and decrease the retinal blur. If the retina and visual pathway are free of abnormalities the patient's acuity will improve.

INDICATIONS

Pinhole acuities are taken when the VA is worse than 20/30 at distance and near through the habitual or induced correction.

EQUIPMENT

- Projector with VA slide or wall mounted acuity chart.
- Pinhole (PH) disc with 1.0- to 1.5-mm diameter pinhole(s).
- Occluder.

SET-UP

- The patient wears his distance correction while looking at the distance VA chart.
- Pinhole acuities are taken only at distance.

STEP-BY-STEP PROCEDURE

1. The patient is asked to occlude the eye not being tested. If both eyes are to be tested, test the right eye first.
2. Instruct the patient to position the PH disc until the chart is as clear as it will get and then read the smallest line of letters he can.
3. Encourage the patient to read the next smallest line, even if he has to guess. Continue until the patient has missed more than half the letters on a line.

RECORDING

- Write "PH" followed by the visual acuity. This notation is usually recorded next to the distance VA through correction.
- "PHNI" may be used to indicate no improvement in VA with the pinhole.

EXAMPLES

- VAcc   OD: $20/50^{+2}$ PH: $20/30^{+2}$
         OS: 20/40   PH: 20/25
- Vsc   OD: $20/40^{+1}$ PHNI
         OS: 20/100   PH: 20/50

EXPECTED FINDINGS

- If the cause of the patient's decreased acuity is due to an uncorrected refractive error, VA is expected to improve through the pinhole.
- If the cause of decreased acuity is not optically based, no improvement, and possibly a decrease, will occur through the pinhole.
- A refraction should improve the acuity level of the patient at least to the level obtained through the pinhole.

Amplitude of Accommodation: Push-Up Method

PURPOSE This procedure measures in diopters a patient's ability to change the focus of the eye's crystalline lens in response to a near stimulus.

EQUIPMENT

- Near point visual acuity card.
- Tape measure in centimeters.
- Occluder.

SET-UP

- The patient is tested wearing his habitual distance correction. This test may also be performed behind the phoropter as a part of the postrefraction phorometry sequence.
- Either the patient or the examiner may hold the near point card.
- The near point card should be well illuminated.

STEP-BY-STEP PROCEDURE

1. Instruct the patient to occlude his left eye to test his right eye.
2. Direct the patient's attention to a row of letters one or two lines larger than his near VA.
3. Instruct the patient to keep the letters clear.
4. Slowly move the chart closer to the patient and ask the patient to report when the letters become and remain blurry.
5. Measure the distance from the chart to the patient's spectacle plane in centimeters. The linear measurement is referred to as the *near point of accommodation.*
6. Convert the linear distance into diopters by dividing the near point of accommodation in centimeters into 100. The resulting dioptric value represents the patient's amplitude of accommodation.

7. Occlude the right eye and test the left eye using Steps 1 to 6.
8. An alternative method of measurement is to start with the letters close to the patient and move them away until the patient reports that the letters are clear. This method is helpful when testing young children who may not understand the concept of blur.

RECORDING

- Record the method of testing used.
- Record the amplitude of accommodation in diopters (round off to the nearest half diopter).
- Separately record the results for the right and left eyes.

EXAMPLES

- Amp (push up)   OD 7D   OS 7D
- Amp (push up)   OD 6D   OS 6D

EXPECTED FINDINGS

- The expected amplitude of accommodation decreases with age. The two most commonly used systems for obtaining the expected amplitude of accommodation are
  a. Hofstetter's formulas
     1. Minimum expected amplitude = 15-0.25 (age)
     2. Average expected amplitude = 18.5-0.30 (age)
     3. Maximum expected amplitude = 25-0.40 (age)
  b. Donders' table (see Table 2–3)
- The amplitude of accommodation of the two eyes should be within one diopter of each other.

TABLE 2–3. DONDER'S TABLE FOR AGE-REFERENCED AMPLITUDE OF ACCOMMODATION

Age	Amplitude	Age	Amplitude
10	14.00	45	3.50
15	12.00	50	2.50
20	10.00	55	1.75
25	8.50	60	1.00
30	7.00	65	0.50
35	5.50	70	0.25
40	4.50	75	0.00

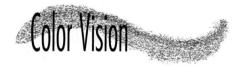

Color Vision

PURPOSE   To screen for acquired or hereditary color vision defects. These clinical
screening tests are particularly significant for the assessment of
macular cone and optic nerve function.

EQUIPMENT

- Occluder.
- Lamp of the correct color temperature for the particular test book used.
- Test book containing pseudoisochromatic plates (PIPs) or other material.

SET-UP

- The patient wears his habitual correction for near.
- The patient holds the occluder.
- The examiner holds the test book 50 cm from the patient.

STEP-BY-STEP PROCEDURE

1. Instruct the patient to occlude his left eye to test his right eye.
2. Observe the patient to make sure that only one eye can see the test plates.
3. Turn the pages one at a time, asking the patient to identify the number or figure on each page.
4. Instruct the patient to occlude his right eye.
5. Repeat Steps 2 and 3 to test the left eye.

RECORDING

- For each eye, write the number of correctly identified plates, a slash mark, and then the number of plates tested (ie, a fraction). Remember that the first plate in many PIP booklets is for demonstration purposes and does not actually test the patient's ability to see color. Therefore, it should not be counted when recording the number of plates tested.
- Record the type of test used.

EXAMPLES

- Color: OD   12/13   OS   11/13 Ishihara
- Color: OD   13/14   OS   8/14 AO

EXPECTED FINDINGS

Each PIP test booklet comes with instructions. These should be read to ascertain what is considered normal for that particular test. In some tests it is normal to make as many as 4 mistakes out of 13 PIPs tested.

Approximately 8% of the general population will have color vision anomalies; most of these patients are males.

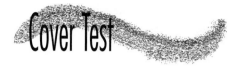

Cover Test

PURPOSE   To assess the presence and magnitude of a phoria or a strabismus (tropia). The cover test assesses the presence or absence of motor fusion. When motor fusion is present (ie, when there is no strabismus), the cover test determines the magnitude of the demand placed on a patient's fusional vergence system.

EQUIPMENT

- VA chart.
- Near cover test target.
- Occluder.
- Overhead lamp.
- Horizontal and vertical prism bars.

SET-UP

- The patient wears his habitual correction for the distance being tested.
- Set up the target.

    For distance: an isolated letter, one line larger than the VA in the patient's poorer seeing eye (with best correction).

    For near: an accommodative target held at 40 cm. Use a reduced Snellen letter one line larger than the visual acuity in the patient's poorer seeing eye or a picture target of comparable detail. The patient may hold the target.
- The examiner holds the occluder.
- The examiner or patient holds the prism bar or bars.
- The room illumination must be sufficient to allow the examiner to observe the patient's eye movements. The cover test may be done with full room illumination.
- The examiner must be positioned to see the patient's eyes easily without interfering with the patient's view of the target.

STEP-BY-STEP PROCEDURE

The cover test consists of two parts: the Cover–Uncover test, which differentiates between a phoria and a tropia, and the Alternating Cover Test, which determines the direction and the size of the deviation. Both parts of the cover test are done at distance and at near. Because occlusion can cause an intermittent tropia to become a constant tropia, the Cover–Uncover test is done first.

COVER–UNCOVER TEST

Differentiates between a phoria and a tropia and determines if a tropia is alternating or unilateral (Figure 2–4). The **cover** part of the cover–uncover test differentiates phorias from tropias by determining the position of the visual axis of each eye when both eyes are open to view the target. If the patient has a phoria, each visual axis will be aligned with the target when both eyes are open. If the patient has a tropia, one visual axis will be aligned with the target and the other visual axis will be misaligned with the target when both eyes are open. During the cover–uncover test, only the unoccluded eye is observed to determine the position of its visual axis.

The **uncover** part of the cover–uncover test differentiates alternating tropias from unilateral tropias (constant right or constant left tropias). A patient with an alternating tropia is able to keep either the right or left visual axis aligned with the target when both eyes are open. A patient with a unilateral tropia habitually fixates with one eye when both eyes are open, and only fixates with the troping eye when the fixating eye is occluded. The examiner observes the eye that is not covered by the occluder.

1. Instruct the patient to look at the target and to keep it clear. To test the left eye, start with both eyes open and cover the patient's right eye. Observe the left eye for movement as soon as the right eye is covered. If there is no movement, it indicates that the left eye was fixating on the target at the start of the test when both eyes were open. Remove the occluder and allow 2 to 3 seconds for the two eyes to resume their normal relationship to one another. Repeat a few times to be certain of the position of the left eye.

2. Instruct the patient to look at the target and to keep it clear. To test the right eye, start with both eyes open and cover the patient's left eye. Observe the right eye for movement as soon as the left eye is covered. If there is no movement, it indicates that the right eye was fixating on the target at the start of the test when both eyes were open. Remove the occluder and allow 2 to 3 seconds for the two eyes to resume their normal relationship to one another. Repeat a few times to be certain of the position of the right eye.

3. If there is no movement in either Step 1 or 2, the patient has a ***phoria.*** Under normal binocular conditions both visual axes are aligned with the target.

4. If there is movement in either Step 1 or 2, the patient has a ***tropia.*** To differentiate between an alternating tropia and a monocular (right or left)

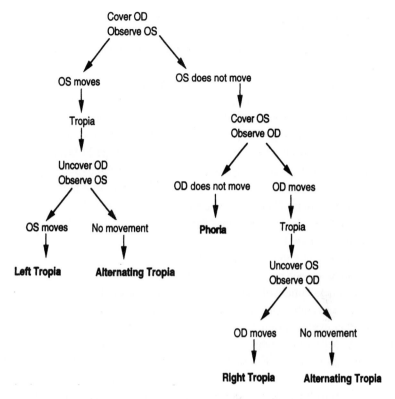

Figure 2–4. Flowchart showing the diagnosis of phorias and tropias on the cover–uncover test.

tropia, start with one eye covered and observe the uncovered eye for movement as soon as the occluder is removed.

a. If the left eye moved when the right eye was covered during Step 1, uncover the right eye and observe the left eye.

  (1) If the left eye does not move when the right eye is uncovered, the patient has an alternating tropia.

  (2) If the left eye does move when the right eye is uncovered, the patient has a constant left tropia (i.e., when both eyes are open, the right eye is aligned with the object and the left eye is not).

b. If the left eye did not move during Step 1 when the right eye was covered, but the right eye moved during Step 2 when the left eye was covered, then uncover the left eye and observe the right eye.

  (1) If the right eye does not move when the left eye is uncovered, the patient has an alternating tropia.

  (2) If the right eye moves when the left eye is uncovered, the patient has a constant right tropia, (i.e., when both eyes are open, the left eye is aligned with the object and the right eye is not).

ALTERNATING COVER TEST

Determines the direction and the magnitude of a phoria or tropia but does not differentiate a phoria from a tropia.

5. Instruct the patient to look at the target and to keep it clear.

6. Place the occluder in front of the patient's right eye for 2 to 3 seconds.

7. Quickly move the occluder from the patient's right eye to the left eye, observing the just-uncovered right eye for direction of movement.

8. Leave the occluder in front of the left eye for 2 to 3 seconds.

9. Quickly move the occluder from the patient's left eye to the right eye, observing the just-uncovered left eye for direction of movement.

10. Repeat steps 7 through 10 several times. It is important to keep one of the eyes covered at all times during the alternating cover test to keep fusion disrupted.

11. Identify the direction of the deviation based on the direction of movement of each eye as it was uncovered (see Table 2–4).

12. The magnitude of the deviation can be measured using a prism bar. To measure a phoria or an alternating tropia, place the prism bar over either eye as close to the eye as possible with the base in the appropriate direction (see Table 2–5). Repeat the alternating cover test while increasing the amount of prism held before one eye until no movement is observed on the alternating cover test. Experienced examiners frequently estimate the size of the deviation, particularly for patients with phorias.

13. The alternating cover test and the cover–uncover test are done at distance and at 40 cm with the patient or the examiner holding the near target at eye level in good illumination (Figure 2–5).

14. If a constant right or constant left tropia was found on the cover–uncover test, then both a primary and secondary deviation must be measured.

15. The primary deviation is measured with the normally fixating eye looking at the target and the occluder and prism placed over the deviating eye. The occluder is moved to the fixating eye while the examiner watches for movement of the deviating eye. The prism is increased until there is no movement of the deviating eye.

16. The secondary deviation is measured with the usually deviating eye looking at the target and the occluder and prism placed over the usually fixating eye. The occluder is moved to the deviating eye while the examiner watches for movement of the fixating eye. The prism is increased until there is no movement of the fixating eye.

17. If the size of the deviation in Steps 15 and 16 are the same, the patient has a comitant deviation. If the size of the deviation in Steps 15 and 16 vary by 5Δ or greater, the patient has a noncomitant deviation.

TABLE 2–4. RELATIONSHIP BETWEEN EYE MOVEMENT AND THE DIRECTION OF DEVIATION ON THE ALTERNATING COVER TEST

Direction of Eye Movement as Eye is Uncovered	Direction of Deviation
In	Exo
Out	Eso
Up	Hypo
Down	Hyper

TABLE 2–5. RELATIONSHIP BETWEEN THE DIRECTION OF DEVIATION AND THE PRISM NEEDED FOR NEUTRALIZATION ON THE ALTERNATING COVER TEST

Direction of Deviation	Direction of Prism Base for Neutralization
Exo	Base in
Eso	Base out
Hypo	Base up
Hyper	Base down

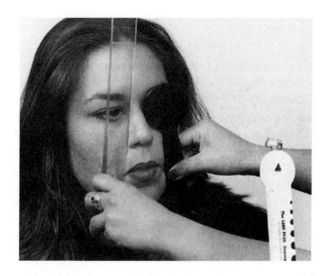

Figure 2–5. The examiner neutralizes an eso deviation on the alternating cover test with base out prism. The patient holds the target.

COVER TEST *at a glance*

PURPOSE	TECHNIQUE
Determine if the deviation is a phoria or tropia	"Cover" part of the cover–uncover test
Determine if a tropia is an alternating, constant right, or constant left tropia	"Uncover" part of the cover–uncover test
Determine the direction of deviation	Alternating cover test
Measure the deviation	Repeat the alternating cover test using prism to measure the deviation

RECORDING

- Write "cover test" or "CT."
- Write "sc" (without correction) or "cc" (with correction).
- Record separately for distance "D" and for near "N." The near results can also be indicated by adding a prime (') after the findings.
- Record the amount of prism that was required to neutralize the deviation.
- Record the direction of deviation, using the following abbreviations:
    E for eso, X for exo
    RH for right hyper, LH for left hyper
    ⏀ No horizontal deviation
    ⊖ No vertical deviation
    ⊕ Ortho: no deviation
- Record the type of deviation (phoria or tropia) using the following abbreviations:
    P for phoria
    T for tropia
- If the deviation is a tropia, record "R" or "L" or "alt" for right, left, or alternating tropia.
    Note: Lateral phorias reflect the relationship between the two eyes in the absence of fusion. Therefore, they do not need to be identified as right, left, or alternat-

ing. However, right or left must be recorded for all vertical phorias and right, left, or alternating must be recorded for all tropias. The term *hypo* is generally used only for downward-deviating unilateral tropias. The terms *right hyper* or *left hyper* are used for phorias or for alternating tropias.

- A T written in parentheses (T) indicates an intermittent tropia. If the tropia is intermittent, the percentage of time that the tropia is present should be estimated and recorded.
- If the patient has a noncomitant strabismus, both a primary and secondary deviation should be recorded.

EXAMPLES

- CT cc $\oplus$ at D and N
- CT sc 20Δ RXT; 10Δ XP'
- CT cc $\oplus$ at D; 25Δ alt E(T)' (75% T)
- CT sc 25Δ RET with 10Δ RHT at D and N
- CT sc RET OD fixating 30Δ; OS fixating 45Δ at D and N

EXPECTED FINDINGS

- 1Δ exophoria (±2Δ) at D; 3Δ exophoria (±3Δ) at N
  Note: Studies of phoria measurements by the Von Graefe method show that presbyopes have larger exophorias at near than the phorias of the nonpresbyopic population. This can also be expected on the cover test.

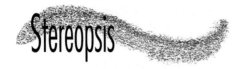

Stereopsis

PURPOSE To measure a patient's fine depth perception through his ability to fuse stereoscopic targets.

EQUIPMENT

- Polaroid glasses or red-green glasses depending on the test used.
- Stereo test booklet (eg, Randot, Titmus, Bernell, TNO Test).
  Note: There are stereo tests available that do not need Polaroid or red-green glasses (eg, the Frisby Stereotest, the Lang Stereotest). These are used chiefly in examining young children who will not tolerate wearing the test glasses. Stereo may also be tested at distance using the American Optical Vectographic Slide with the patient wearing Polaroid glasses.

SET-UP

- The patient wears Polaroid glasses or red-green glasses over his near correction.
- The patient holds the stereo target at 40 cm (Figure 2–6).
- The overhead lamp is directed toward the target.

STEP-BY-STEP PROCEDURE

1. Direct the patient's attention to the smallest set of targets. Frequently this is a set of three or four circles. Ask the patient to tell you what he sees. If the patient is unresponsive, ask him to identify which of the circles in set number one appears closest or seems to be floating above the page.
2. If the patient appreciates stereopsis on the first set of targets, instruct him to go on to the next set. If the patient does not appreciate stereopsis, go to Step 4.
3. Continue testing until the patient gives two consecutive incorrect answers.
4. If the patient is unable to correctly identify the floating object in the smallest set of targets, repeat Steps 1 and 2 using the medium-sized targets. Ask the patient again to identify the object that is floating above the page. If the patient identifies all of these correctly, go back and try the smallest set of targets again.
5. If the patient is unable to correctly identify any of the medium-sized tar-

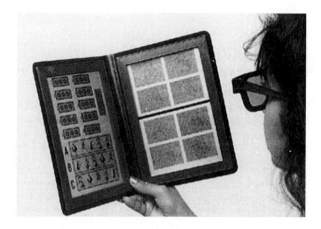

Figure 2–6. A patient viewing the Randot stereo test.

gets, show the patient the large targets and ask him to identify what he sees. To verify a correct response, ask the patient to show you in space where he sees the target. If the patient identifies all of the large targets correctly go back and try the medium and small sets of targets again.

RECORDING

- Write "Stereo at N" (near).
- If done without correction, record "sc"; if done with correction, record "cc."
- Record the amount of stereopsis in seconds of arc (taken from the instructions that come with the stereo test) for the last correct response the patient gave before two consecutive incorrect responses.
- If the patient is not able to correctly identify any of the small targets on the test, record the amount of stereopsis in seconds of arc for the smallest target the patient was able to correctly perceive.
- If the patient does not perceive any of the stereo targets, record "No stereo."
- Record the name of the test used.

EXAMPLES

- Stereo at N sc 40 sec, Titmus
- Stereo at N sc 20 sec, Randot
- Stereo at N sc 3000 sec, Stereo Fly
- Stereo at N cc none, Randot

EXPECTED FINDINGS

- Stereo at near: 20 seconds of arc.

Screening Stereopsis Using the Random Dot E

PURPOSE   To screen for the presence of third-degree fusion.

EQUIPMENT

- Polaroid glasses.
- Random Dot E cards: stereo E, blank card, and model E training card.

SET-UP

- The patient wears Polaroid glasses over his near correction. If the patient is reluctant to wear the Polaroid glasses, the examiner may wear a pair of the glasses to encourage the patient.
- The test should be done in good illumination with the light directed toward the cards.

STEP-BY-STEP PROCEDURE

1. Hold the model E card at a distance of 50 cm. Point to the E and say to the patient, "See the E."
2. Pick up the blank card and shuffle it and the Model E behind your back.
3. Show the blank card and the model E to the patient and ask the patient to point to the card with the "E" on it.
4. Repeat Step 3 until the patient correctly identifies the model E three out of four times. Randomly vary the position of the model E during each presentation (up, down, right, or left). If the patient is unable to identify the model E, stop the test and record that the patient is unable to do the test.
5. Replace the model E with the stereo E card. Shuffle the two cards (the blank card and the stereo E card) behind your back. Place the two cards side by side or one above the other and ask the patient to identify the card with the "E" on it.
6. Be careful to hold the cards with the upper edges tilted slightly toward the examiner so that light from above falls on the card without any glare (Figure 2–7).

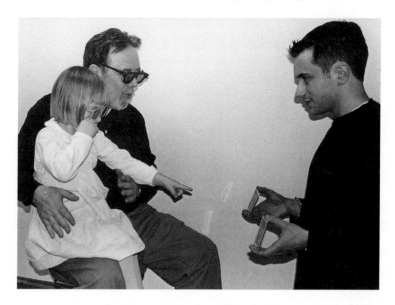

Figure 2–7. A patient viewing the Random Dot E.

7. Repeat Step 5 at 50 cm four times. If the patient is unable to identify the stereo E three out of the four times, stop the test and record "Unable to do Random Dot E at 50 cm."
8. If the patient correctly chooses the stereo E three out of four times at 50 cm, repeat the test (Step 5) at 150 cm.

RECORDING

- Write "Random Dot E at 150 cm," the number of correct responses, and the number of presentations.
- If done without correction, record "sc"; if done with correction, record "cc."
- If the patient is unable to identify the model E, record "Patient unable to identify model E."
- If the patient is able to identify the model E but unable to identify the stereo test E at 50 cm, record "No stereo."
- If the patient does not perceive any of the stereo targets, record "No stereo."
- Record the name of the test used.

EXAMPLES

- Random Dot E sc unable to identify model E
- Random Dot E cc [4/4] at 50 cm
- Random Dot E cc [3/4] at 150 cm

RANDOM DOT E *at a glance*

1. Teach the test to the patient	• Show the patient the model E and the blank E • Test the patient with the stereo E and the blank E at 50 cm
2. Screen for stereopsis	• Test the patient with the stereo E and the blank E at 150 cm

EXPECTED FINDINGS

The patient should be able to identify the stereo E three out of four times at 150 cm.

Note: The Random Dot E can also be used to measure the stereoacuity threshold by varying the distance of the target from the patient's eyes. At 50 cm the Random Dot E has a disparity of 504 seconds; at 150 cm, the Random Dot has a disparity of 168 seconds. Adults with normal stereopsis can appreciate stereopsis with the Random Dot E at distance up to about 2 m (126 seconds).

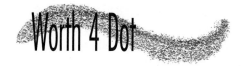

Worth 4 Dot

PURPOSE   To assess the patient's flat fusion ability at distance and at near. The hand-held Worth 4 Dot flashlight is also used to detect a small unilateral central scotoma.

INDICATIONS

The Worth 4 Dot test is indicated when stereopsis is below 40 seconds of arc. It is also used in the differential diagnosis of unilateral decreased VA.

EQUIPMENT

- Worth 4 Dot target.
- Red-green glasses.

SET-UP

- The patient wears his habitual correction for the distance being tested.
- The patient wears the red-green glasses over his correction, with the red lens over his right eye and the green lens over his left eye.
- The examiner turns on the Worth 4 Dot box mounted at the end of the examination room for distance testing. The Worth 4 Dot flashlight is used for near testing and for testing for a central suppression scotoma. The near target is initially held at 40 cm.

STEP-BY-STEP PROCEDURE

TO TEST THE PATIENT'S FLAT FUSION ABILITY AT DISTANCE OR AT NEAR

1. Show the patient the Worth 4 Dot target with the white dot at the bottom and the red dot at the top.
2. Ask the patient how many spots of light he sees.
   a. If the patient reports that he sees four dots, he has normal flat fusion.
   b. If the patient reports that he sees two red dots, he is using only his right eye and is suppressing his left eye.
   c. If the patient reports that he sees three green dots, he is using only his left eye and is suppressing his right eye.

d. If the patient reports that he sees five dots, ask the patient where the green ones (seen by the patient's left eye) are located: to the right, left, above, or below the red ones (seen by the patient's right eye). Based on the patient's response, determine the relationship of the visual axes of the two eyes. If the red dots are to the right of the green dots, the patient has an eso deviation. If the red dots are to the left of the green dots, the patient has an exo deviation. If the red dots are above the green dots, the patient has a left hyperdeviation. If the red dots are below the green dots, the patient has a right hyper deviation (Figure 2–8).

TO TEST FOR A CENTRAL SUPPRESSION SCOTOMA

This can be done only if the patient has normal flat fusion with the Worth 4 Dot at 16 in.

1. Hold the Worth 4 Dot flashlight 40 cm from the patient with the white dot at the bottom and the red dot at the top.
2. Instruct the patient to continue fixating on the flashlight and to report if the number of dots changes from four dots to either two or three dots at any time.
3. Slowly begin to move away from the patient. Ask the patient to report any changes in the number of dots he sees.
4. Stop when the patient reports a change in the number of dots. Estimate the distance at which this occurs. If the patient still reports seeing four dots at a distance of 3 m, stop the test and record "no suppression to 3 m."
5. Determine which eye is suppressing. Then ask the patient to cover the eye that is not suppressing and to report whether or not the suppressed dots reappear. If the dots reappear, the patient has a suppression scotoma that occurs only under binocular conditions. If the dots do not reappear, the patient has a unilateral scotoma.

RECORDING

For testing flat fusion:

- Record the distance at which the test was done.
- If the patient sees four dots, record "Fusion."
- If the patient sees two dots, record "Suppression OS."
- If the patient sees three dots, record "Suppression OD."
- If the patient sees five dots, record "Diplopia" and the type of deviation:
  a. Green dots to the left of red dots: "eso" (uncrossed diplopia).
  b. Green dots to the right of red dots: "Exo" (crossed diplopia).
  c. Green dots above red dots: "R hyper."
  d. Green dots below red dots: "L hyper."
  e. Combinations of vertical and horizontal deviations are possible.

WORTH 4 DOT

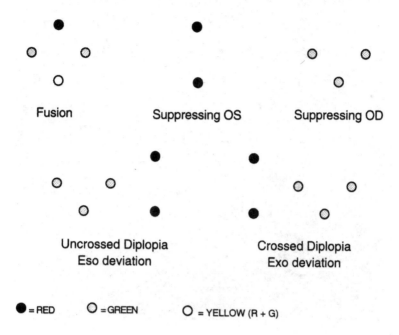

Fusion   Suppressing OS   Suppressing OD

Uncrossed Diplopia   Crossed Diplopia
Eso deviation   Exo deviation

● = RED   ○ = GREEN   ○ = YELLOW (R + G)

Figure 2–8. Examples of the appearance of the Worth 4 Dot as seen by the patient. The red lens is over the patient's right eye and the green lens is over the patient's left eye.

When using the Worth 4 Dot flashlight to detect a central suppression scotoma, record the distance at which suppression occurred, which eye is suppressing, and whether the dots reappeared or not when the seeing eye was occluded.

EXAMPLES

For flat fusion testing at distance or near:

- Worth 4 Dot—fusion at distance
- Worth 4 Dot—fusion at 40 cm
- Worth 4 Dot—fusion at distance; suppression OS at 40 cm
- Worth 4 Dot—diplopia, R hyper eso at 40 cm

For central suppression scotoma testing:

- Fusion at 40 cm and no suppression to 3 m.
- Fusion at 40 cm, suppresses OS at 2 m, dots reappear when OD occluded.

Near Point of Convergence (NPC)

PURPOSE To determine the patient's ability to converge the eyes while maintaining fusion.

EQUIPMENT

- Penlight or transilluminator.
- Red glass.
- Near accommodative target (reduced Snellen letter taped to a penlight or tongue depressor: four different sizes in the range of 20/25 to 20/200 are needed).
- Overhead lamp.

Note: The penlight or transilluminator is used as a target for initial screening. The penlight with red glass and the accommodative target are used when the near point of convergence is greater than 5 cm/7 cm or when a complete binocular workup is being done.

SET-UP

- The patient wears his habitual near correction.
- The overhead lamp is directed toward the target.
- The penlight (or other target) is held by the examiner at 40 cm.

STEP-BY-STEP PROCEDURE

1. Instruct the patient to look at the light (or other target) and to report how many targets he sees. If the target appears double, move it further from the patient until it appears single before proceeding with the test.
2. Move the target toward the patient, observing the patient's eyes until the patient reports that the target appears double or until you see one eye lose fixation on the target. Note the distance from the patient's eyes at which the patient reports that the target doubles or at which you note that the patient loses bifixation. This is the break point.
3. Move the target away from the patient's eyes and note the distance at which the patient's deviated eye regains fixation. The patient will report

single vision at this distance if he reported diplopia in Step 2. This is the recovery point.

4. If break and recovery are closer to the patient than 5 cm, record the results. If the NPC is greater than 5 cm record the results and then repeat the test using the penlight with a red glass placed over the patient's right eye or with the patient wearing red-green glasses. Then repeat the NPC a third time using an accommodative target.

RECORDING

- Record NPC and sc or cc.
- Record the target used:
  "Lite" for penlight
  "RG" for penlight with red glass
  "Accomm." for accommodative target
- Record the linear distance (in cm, mm, in, or ft) at which the eye deviated or at which the patient reported diplopia (break).
- Record the distance (in cm, mm, in, or ft) at which the eye regained fixation or at which the patient reported single vision (recovery).
- Record which eye deviated and in which direction, if you were able to make this observation.
- Record "diplopia" if the patient reported seeing two targets. Record "suppression" if the patient did not report seeing two targets but a break was observed.
- If the examiner was able to move the target to the bridge of the patient's nose without the patient's losing fixation, record TTN (for "to the nose").
- Repeat this recording for each target used.

EXAMPLES

- NPC cc lite—TTN
- NPC sc lite 10 cm/12 cm OS out, suppression
         RG 15 cm/20 cm OS out, suppression
         accomm. 8 cm/10 cm OS out, suppression

EXPECTED FINDINGS

Break: 5 cm
Recovery: 7 cm

A break point of greater than 5 cm is considered abnormal. The recovery point is expected to be within 7 cm. These figures reflect the mean finding for a normative adult population. It is normal for the patient to report diplopia at the break point. If there is a differece of >5 cm for the break or a difference of >8 cm for recovery between the accommodative target and the penlight with red glass, the patient may have convergence insufficiency.

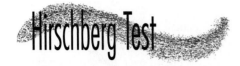

Hirschberg Test

PURPOSE To determine the approximate positions of the visual axes of the two eyes under binocular conditions at near. This test is used to identify a strabismus when other more precise methods cannot be used.

EQUIPMENT

- Penlight.
- Occluder.

SET-UP

- The patient removes his glasses.
- The examiner holds the penlight.

STEP-BY-STEP PROCEDURE

1. Direct the penlight toward the patient's eyes from a distance of 50 to 100 cm.
2. Instruct patient to look at the light.
3. Occlude the patient's left eye.
4. Place your eye directly behind the penlight and observe the location of the corneal light reflex in the right eye. There are three possible positions for the corneal reflex:
   a. the center of the pupil (zero angle lambda)
   b. slightly nasal to the center of the pupil (positive angle lambda)
   c. slightly temporal to the center of the pupil (negative angle lambda)
5. Occlude the patient's right eye. Repeat Step 4 observing the left eye.
6. Remove the occluder. Position your eye directly behind the penlight and observe the location of the corneal light reflexes in each of the patient's eyes with both eyes open.
7. Compare the locations of the corneal reflexes in each of the two eyes relative to where they were located with each eye fixating separately:
   a. If the reflexes are in the same relative positions in each of the two eyes, the patient does not have a strabismus (Figure 2–9).

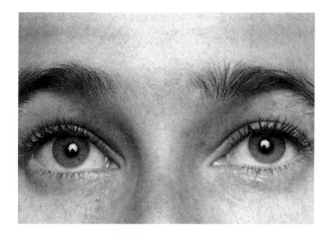

Figure 2–9. The appearance of Hirschberg reflexes in a patient with no manifest deviation.

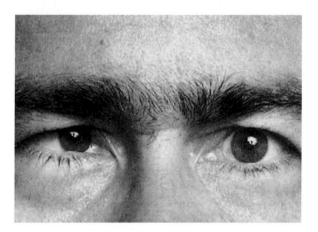

Figure 2–10. The appearance of the Hirschberg reflexes in patient with a right esotropia.

   b. If the reflexes are not in the same relative positions, the patient has a strabismus (Figure 2–10). Determine the direction of the deviation by observing the position of the two reflexes relative to the position of angle lambda in the fixating eye (Table 2–6).

   c. The size of the strabismus can be estimated by measuring (in mm) the distance from the position of the reflex in the deviated eye to the position where the reflex would be if the patient did not have a strabismus. One millimeter of deviation of the reflex is equal to 22Δ.

8. The angle of strabismus can be measured by placing a prism over the deviating eye (as it would be for measuring a deviation on the cover test;

TABLE 2–6. RELATIONSHIP BETWEEN THE POSITION OF THE CORNEAL REFLEX AND THE TYPE OF
DEVIATION ON THE HIRSCHBERG TEST

Position of Corneal Reflex Relative to Position of Angle Lambda in the Fixating Eye	Type of Deviation
Nasal	Exo
Temporal	Eso
Above	Hypo
Below	Hyper

see Table 2–6). The apex of the prism is placed in the direction that the reflex of the deviating eye needs to move to match the reflex in the fixating eye. The amount of prism is increased until the corneal reflex is in the same relative position in the deviating eye as it is in the fixating eye. This method of measurement is known as the Krimsky Test.

RECORDING

- Record the name of the test used.
- If there is no strabismus, record "symmetry" or "ortho."
- If there is a strabismus, record the eye that is deviated, the size of the deviation, and the direction of the deviation.

EXAMPLES

- Hirschberg: ortho
- Hirschberg: 22Δ LXT; Krimsky 25Δ LXT

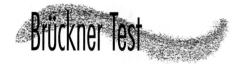

Brückner Test

PURPOSE   To assess the symmetry of binocular fixation by comparing the brightness of the red reflex in each of the two eyes. This test is used to screen for strabismus, anisometropia, media opacities, and posterior pole anomalies in infants and young preverbal children.

EQUIPMENT

- Direct ophthalmoscope.

SET-UP

- The patient removes his correction.
- Room illumination should be dim.
- The examiner holds the ophthalmoscope.
- Use the large spot beam and a +1D lens.
- The Brückner test should be done with nondilated pupils.

STEP-BY-STEP PROCEDURE

1. Direct the ophthalmoscope toward the patient's eyes from a distance of 80 to 100 cm with the beam of light illuminating both pupils.
2. Instruct patient to look at the light.
3. The examiner positions his eye directly behind the peephole of the ophthalmoscope and dials in the lens that gives a clear view of the patient's pupils (for a distance of 100 cm, this should be a +1D lens).
4. Observe the Hirschberg reflexes against the red reflex in the pupil (see Hirschberg procedure).
5. Compare the brightness of the red reflexes in each of the two eyes.
    a. If the two reflexes are equally bright, there is binocular fixation.
    b. If the two reflexes are not equally bright, the darker red reflex indicates the fixating eye and the brighter, lighter, or whiter reflex indicates the nonfixating eye. The difference in brightness may be caused by strabismus, anisometropia, anisocoria, media opacities, or posterior pole abnormalities (Figure 2–11).

Patient A

Patient B

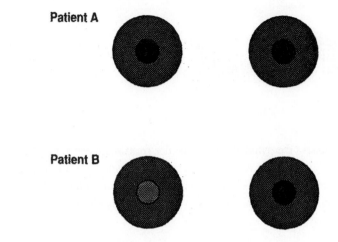

Figure 2–11. Appearance of the red fundus reflex in the Brückner test. Patient A has bifixation. Patient B is fixating with the left eye.

RECORDING

- Record which eye appears whiter and brighter, if applicable.
  or
- Record that the two eyes appear equally bright.

EXAMPLES

- Brückner test: OD=OS
- Brückner test: OD brighter than OS

Extraocular Motilities (EOM)

PURPOSE   To assess the patient's ability to perform conjugate eye movements.

EQUIPMENT

• Penlight.

SET-UP

• The patient removes his spectacles.
• The examiner holds the penlight.

STEP-BY-STEP PROCEDURE

1. Perform the Hirschberg procedure as described earlier in the chapter.
2. Instruct the patient to follow the light with his eyes without moving his head. Ask him to tell you if he ever sees the light double, or become two, or if he feels any pain, strain, or discomfort while moving his eyes.
3. Start with the penlight directly in front of the patient. This is called the "primary position."
4. Move the light to the eight additional positions shown in Figure 2–12. The order in which the positions are tested is not important. It is critical, however, to test gaze in all nine positions. In this Step you are tracing the pattern of a large letter H bisected by a vertical line as shown in Figure 2–12.
5. Throughout Step 4, point the light at the patient's eyes as they follow the penlight. Look for changes in the relative positions of the corneal reflections, as in the Hirschberg test. Do not move the penlight too far. At a test distance of 30 to 40 cm, a movement of the light 30 to 40 cm from the primary position will detect ocular deviations of about 40°. This is sufficient to uncover weak extraocular muscles.
6. Throughout the procedure observe
   a. the smoothness of movement.
   b. the accuracy of following the penlight.
   c. the extent of movement.
7. If the patient reports diplopia in any position of gaze, perform the Mus-

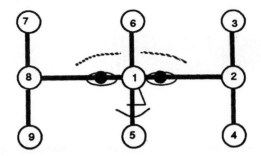

Figure 2–12. Schematic diagram showing the sequential order of positions of gaze for EOM testing seen from the perspective of the examiner looking at the patient.

cle Field with Red Lens, Ductions, and Saccades procedures described in Chapter 8.

RECORDING

- If the patient follows the light smoothly to all positions of gaze with both eyes and never reports diplopia (double vision) or discomfort, write SAFE or FESA. These letters stand for: S: Smooth, A: Accurate, F: Full, E: Extensive.
- If the patient shows any problem, record only the letters that apply and describe the problem, for example:
  jerky, unsteady, nystagmoid
  failure to follow into (give the location)
  restricted, lagging, noncomitant
- Identify the direction(s) of gaze that result in diplopia and/or discomfort.
- If only one eye is the abnormal one, be sure to identify it.

EXAMPLES

- EOM: SAFE
- EOM: diplopia on up-right gaze, OD lagging
- EOM: FESA, OD pain on left gaze

EXPECTED FINDINGS

- FESA.
- No pain or diplopia.
- At the extreme limits of a healthy patient's gaze it is normal to observe a low-amplitude nystagmus, a so-called endpoint nystagmus.

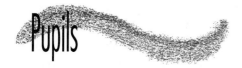

Pupils

PURPOSE   To assess the afferent and efferent neurological pathways responsible for pupillary function.

EQUIPMENT

- Penlight or transilluminator.
- Distant fixation target (e.g., 20/400 E).

SET-UP

- Use ambient illumination that is as dim as possible, but permits a clear view of both of the patient's pupils.
- Position yourself within 25 cm of the patient, but not in his line of sight (i.e., off to one side, sitting or standing).
- Instruct the patient to remove his spectacles.

STEP-BY-STEP PROCEDURE

1. Instruct the patient to look at the distant target.
2. Shine the light into his right eye and observe the size and the speed of the pupillary constriction in this eye (This is the direct response).
3. Repeat Step 2 twice.
4. Shine the light into the right eye and observe the size and the speed of the pupillary constriction in the left eye (This is the consensual response).
5. Repeat Step 4 twice.
6. Repeat Steps 2 through 5 shining the light into the left eye, again observing the direct and consensual responses of the appropriate pupils.
7. *Swinging Flashlight Test:* Move the light between the eyes rapidly, leaving it on each eye for 3 to 5 seconds. Observe the response (dilation or constriction) and the size of each pupil at the moment when the light first arrives there and during the 3- to 5-second observation period. Be sure to shine an equal intensity of light into each eye on the same relative part of the retina.
8. The swinging flashlight test should be repeated for two or three complete cycles.

9. Throughout the test, judge the roundness of each pupil.
10. If the pupils are unequal in size, perform the dim-bright pupillary test (see Chapter 8).
11. If either or both pupils fail to respond directly or consensually, or if their responses are sluggish, test the accommodative response of the pupil (see Chapter 8).

RECORDING

- If all the pupillary responses are normal, write PERRL no APD (pupils equal round responsive to light; no afferent pupillary defect). Record only those that apply, omitting the others.
- Separately describe abnormalities, such as inequality of size, shape, or rate of response (see also, Recording, under dim-bright pupillary test).
- If pupillary escape is observed on the swinging flashlight test, record +RAPD (positive relative afferent pupillary defect), or +MG (positive Marcus Gunn) followed by the affected eye.
- "D" is for direct and "C" is for consensual.

EXAMPLES

- PERRL, +RAPD OS
- PRRL, no RAPD, OD>OS by 1 mm in dim and bright
- OD: RRL D no MG
  OS: irregular, sluggish D and C

EXPECTED FINDINGS

- PERRL, no RAPD

Screening Visual Fields

PURPOSE   To screen for previously unnoted visual field defects. This technique is generally effective only for substantial field losses.

EQUIPMENT

- Overhead lamp.
- Target (white sphere, 3 mm or less in diameter, mounted on matte black wand).
- Occluder.

SET-UP

- Instruct the patient to remove his glasses.
- The examiner faces the patient at eye level, about 50 cm away.
- The space between the patient and the examiner should be brightly illuminated, but light should not shine directly into either the patient's or the examiner's eyes.
- The rest of the testing room should be dimly illuminated.
- The patient holds the occluder.

STEP-BY-STEP PROCEDURE

1. Hold a finger in front of the eye being tested at a distance of 40 to 60 cm. Instruct the patient to maintain fixation on the tip of your finger throughout the test.
2. Show the target to the patient.
3. Tell him that you are going to bring the target into his side vision. Instruct the patient to tell you as soon as he sees it. Repeat the instruction to keep looking at the tip of your finger.
4. Instruct the patient to cover his left eye with the occluder.
5. Throughout the test, the target should remain 1 to 2 inches from the patient's facial structures (Figure 2–13).
6. Place the target where the patient cannot see it; then slowly move it toward his line of sight, noting the location at which he first reports seeing it. Note that because the target is close to the patient's face, even small movements cover large angles and rapid movements will cover large angles quickly.

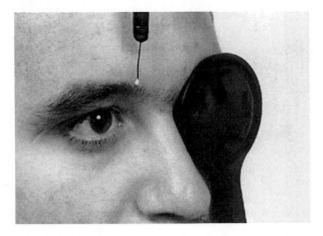

Figure 2–13. An example of the position of the test target relative to the patient's eye during screening visual fields. The superior nasal field of the patient's right eye is being tested.

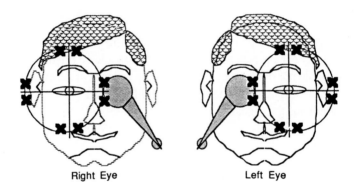

Right Eye   Left Eye

Figure 2–14. Schematic diagram of the eight locations to be tested within the visual field of each eye during screening visual fields.

> *Note*: As you perform this test, try to visualize where the limits of the patient's field ought to be. In this test you are comparing where the patient sees the target to where, in your judgment, he ought to be able to see it.

7. Test the appropriate eight locations in the field, on each side of the four visual field meridia (see Figure 2–14).
8. When you have mapped the field for the right eye, instruct the patient to occlude his right eye and repeat Steps 6 and 7 on the left eye.
9. Throughout the test, monitor the patient's fixation and keep reminding him to maintain fixation on your fingertip.

RECORDING

- Record the results for each eye separately.
- If the field is normal, write "full."
- If the field is abnormal, write "restricted" followed by the location of the restriction.

EXAMPLES

- VF: OD full
         OS full
- VF: full OD, restricted temporally OS
- VF: restricted upper right quadrant OD and OS

EXPECTED FINDINGS

- Right eye full and left eye full.

Finger Counting Visual Fields

PURPOSE   To screen for previously unnoted visual field defects. This technique is generally effective only for substantial field losses.

EQUIPMENT

- Overhead lamp.
- Occluder.

SET-UP

- Instruct the patient to remove his glasses.
- The examiner faces the patient at eye level at a distance of 60 to 80 cm from the patient.
- The space between the patient and the examiner should be brightly illuminated, but the light should not shine directly into either the patient's or the examiner's eyes.
- The rest of the testing room should be dimly illuminated.

STEP-BY-STEP PROCEDURE

1. Instruct the patient to occlude his left eye.
2. Tell him that you are going to show him your fingers in his side vision and that you will hold up one, two, or four fingers. Instruct the patient to tell you how many you are holding up. Tell him to keep looking at your left eye at all times. Avoid holding up three fingers because this stimulus is too easily confused with two or four fingers.
3. Close your right eye.
4. Place your closed fist in the peripheral visual field. Your hand should be in the far periphery, but at a location where you will be able to distinguish the number of fingers exposed. Finger counting fields are actually a form of visual acuity of the peripheral visual field, so the fingers should not be moved or wiggled. In finger counting fields, the patient's visual field is compared to the examiner's field, which is presumed to be full.

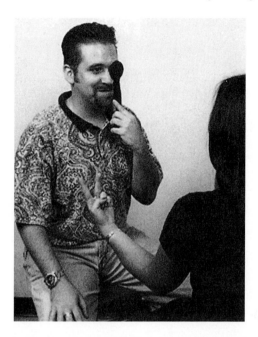

Figure 2–15. An example of finger counting visual fields. The examiner is exposing two fingers in the inferior temporal field of the patient's right eye.

5. Expose one, two, or four fingers, taking care that they are brightly illuminated, that the darkened exam room (not your hand or arm) provides the background, that they are not pointing toward the patient, and that the fingers are in a plane midway between you and the patient (Figure 2–15).
6. Repeat Step 5 in the appropriate eight locations in the field, on each side of the four visual field meridia.
7. When you have mapped the field for the right eye, have the patient occlude his right eye and repeat Steps 4 through 6 on the left eye.
8. Throughout the test, monitor the patient's fixation and keep reminding him to maintain fixation on your open eye.

RECORDING

- Record the results for each eye separately.
- Use FCF (Finger Counting Fields) to identify the procedure.
- If the field is normal, write "full."
- If the field is abnormal, write "restricted" followed by the location of the restriction.

EXAMPLES

- FCF: OD full, OS full
- FCF: full OD, restricted temporally OS
- FCF: restricted upper right quadrant OD and OS

EXPECTED FINDINGS

- Right eye full and left eye full.

Interpupillary Distance (PD)

PURPOSE To determine the distance in millimeters between the entrance pupils of the two eyes for a given viewing distance.

EQUIPMENT

- An easy-to-hold ruler marked in mm.

SET-UP

- The examiner sits directly in front of the patient at eye level.
- The examiner's face should be located at the patient's customary near working distance (usually 40 cm).

STEP-BY-STEP PROCEDURE

FOR NEAR PD

1. Close your right eye and instruct the patient to look at your open left eye, the tip of your nose, or some other near target. Align the zero-point of the ruler on a landmark of the patient's right eye. Stabilize the ruler by resting two or three fingers on the patient's face and by lightly resting the ruler on the bridge of the patient's nose.
2. Still using your left eye, measure to the corresponding landmark on patient's left eye. For example, if you set the zero on the nasal pupillary edge of the patient's right eye, measure to the temporal pupillary edge of his left eye (Figure 2–16).

FOR DISTANCE PD

3. Instruct the patient to look at your open left eye. Close your right eye.
4. Align the zero-point of the ruler on a landmark of the patient's right eye (eg, nasal pupillary edge). Stabilize the ruler by resting two or three fingers on the patient's face and by lightly resting the ruler on the bridge of the patient's nose.
5. Close your left eye. Instruct the patient to look at your now open right eye.

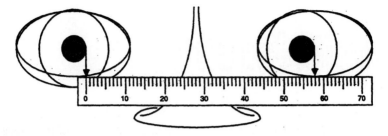

Figure 2–16. Schematic diagram of the near PD measurement showing the zero set to the nasal pupillary border of the patient's right eye and the measurement taken at the corresponding point, the temporal pupillary border of the patient's left eye.

6. Measure to the corresponding landmark on the patient's left eye, as described in Step 2.
7. Recheck the entire procedure.
   Note: By following Steps 3 through 7, although the patient never looks at distance, you measure his distance PD, with each eye pointing straight ahead, as if the patient had been looking at distance (Figure 2–17).

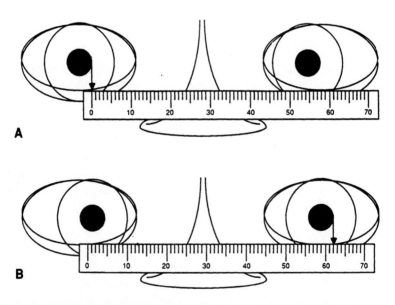

Figure 2–17. Schematic diagram of the distance PD measurement. **A.** The zero is set to the nasal pupillary border of the patient's right eye with the patient's right eye looking straight ahead at the examiner's open left eye and the patient's left eye converged to look at the examiner's open left eye. **B.** The measurement is taken at the corresponding point, the temporal pupillary border of the patient's left eye, with the patient's left eye looking straight ahead at the examiner's open right eye and the patient's right eye converged to look at the examiner's open right eye.

RECORDING

- Write the distance PD in mm, a slash, then the near PD in mm.

Note: Although you measure the near PD before the distance PD, record the distance PD followed by the near (see Examples).

- Sometimes the eyes are not centered with respect to the nose, and separate, monocular PDs are recorded for each eye relative to the center of the bridge of the patient's nose.

EXAMPLES

- 64/61
- 62/58
- OD 30/28   OS 32/30

EXPECTED FINDINGS

- The average measurement for adults is 64/60.

Summary of Expected Findings

TABLE 2–7. EXPECTED FINDINGS FOR ENTRANCE TESTS

Visual Acuity (VA or V)	20/20 or better No more than 1 line difference between eyes
LogMAR VA	0.00 or better
Mass VA With Lea Symbols	Appropriate for child's age
Amplitude of Accommodation (Amp) Hoffstetter's formulas:	Minimum $= 15 - 0.25$ (age) Average $= 18.5 - 0.30$ (age) Maximum $= 25 - 0.40$ (age)

<table>
<tr><th colspan="2" align="center">Donders' Table</th><th colspan="2" align="center">Donders' Table</th></tr>
<tr><td>Age</td><td>Amplitude</td><td>Age</td><td>Amplitude</td></tr>
<tr><td>10</td><td>14.00</td><td>45</td><td>3.50</td></tr>
<tr><td>15</td><td>12.00</td><td>50</td><td>2.50</td></tr>
<tr><td>20</td><td>10.00</td><td>55</td><td>1.75</td></tr>
<tr><td>25</td><td>8.50</td><td>60</td><td>1.00</td></tr>
<tr><td>30</td><td>7.00</td><td>65</td><td>0.50</td></tr>
<tr><td>35</td><td>5.50</td><td>70</td><td>0.25</td></tr>
<tr><td>40</td><td>4.50</td><td>75</td><td>0.00</td></tr>
</table>

Color Vision (CV): Ishihara, 16 plate (Number of errors allowed varies by test)	No more than 3 errors No difference between eyes
Cover Text (CT)	1 Δ XP at distance (mean, SD= 2Δ) 3 Δ XP at near (mean, SD = 3Δ)
Stereopsis	20 seconds of arc
Random Dot E	[3/4] at 150 cm (168 seconds of arc)
Near Point of Convergence (NPC) (Penlight)	Break: 5 cm Recovery: 7 cm
Hirschberg Test	Symmetry of reflexes
Extraocular Motilites (EOM)	FESA (Full, Extensive, Smooth, Accurate)
Pupils	PERRL,-RAPD
Screening Visual Fields (VF)	OD full OS full
Interpupillary Distance (PD)	Average adult: 64/60

REFRACTION

Daniel Kurtz, OD, PhD

CHAPTER AT A GLANCE

INTRODUCTION TO REFRACTION

Refraction is a multistep process that involves a combination of psychomotor skill and intellectual problem solving. The process allows the examiner to arrive at one individualized prescription, from a universe of approximately 200,000 possible prescriptions.

The goal of refraction is to render the retina conjugate with optical infinity through the application of lenses in front of the eye. However, refraction is done for people, not eyeballs, and the goal is restated here in functional terms: to identify the lenses that will allow the patient to achieve clear and comfortable vision, to which he will adapt rapidly, and that will do no harm to the patient. That is, to see everything he needs and wants to see and to use his eyes for as long as he desires without strain or discomfort. The process of the routine refraction can be divided into three parts.

In the first part, made up of the *starting points,* the examiner collects preliminary information about the refractive status of the patient. Based on the information, the examiner makes predictions about the outcome of the refraction, and, in rare instances, can actually write a prescription.

The second part of the routine refraction is the *refinement.* In this phase, predictions from the starting points are tested and refined. The principal tool of the refinement is the *phoropter.* The examiner makes changes in the targets or the phoropter lenses. The patient makes a response to indicate how each change affects what he sees. Because it relies heavily on patient response the refinement includes most of what is generally termed the *routine subjective refraction.*

The third part of the routine refraction is made up of the *endpoint techniques.* These include the *binocular balance* and the *demonstration* or *trial frame technique.* The endpoint is not only technical, but is intellectual as this is when the patient's refractive problems must be solved. To arrive at a single prescription that will provide the patient with clarity and comfort of visual function, the examiner must weigh all the available information, including the starting points, the results of the refinement, and the endpoint tests. The examiner must also factor in his knowledge of geometric and ophthalmic optics, his assessment of the patient's ability to adapt to changes in the correction, and the patient's lifestyle and attendant visual needs. Finally, exercising his professional judgment, the examiner chooses a prescription for the patient. But the intellectual process does not stop there.

Both health and visual function problems can manifest themselves as the apparent need for glasses or changes in the eyeglass prescription. Decisions about spectacles and contact lenses can have important implications for the patient's safety, health, and visual function. Refractive problems must always be addressed within the context of both a health and a visual function analysis. The authors of this text subscribe to and agree completely with the resolution passed at the 1995 American Optometric Association Congress: "A refraction for the purposes of determining the need for corrective lenses is but one component of an eye health and vision evaluation. A refraction without a corresponding eye health evaluation can result in the failure to diagnose vision and life threatening diseases to the irreparable harm of the individual." Although it is treated in the text as an isolated set of procedures, refraction should not be thought of as separate from the other processes that make up the comprehensive ocular examination.

This chapter includes a group of problem-specific refractive tests. These side trips from the routine refraction allow the examiner to obtain additional refractive data about the patient and to refract the unusual or difficult patient.

Finally, readers should remember that refraction is a problem-solving, not merely a technical, exercise. The goal is not to perform certain steps and procedures, but to ascertain what lenses to prescribe to serve the best interests of the patient. By using all of the information available, the examiner can often determine an appropriate prescription without performing every one of the steps in the routine refraction. The process of refraction is summarized in the following flow chart (Figure 3–1).

FLOW of the ROUTINE DISTANCE REFRACTION

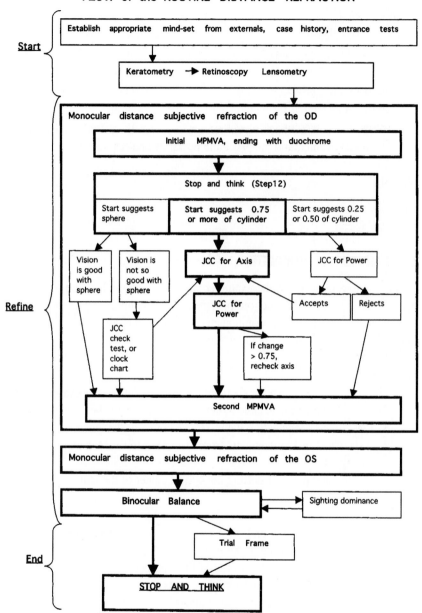

Figure 3–1. Flowchart of routine distance refraction. The main route or standard sequence of tests is shown on the left. Recommended side trips, or secondary tests, are presented on the right.

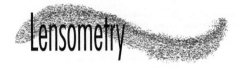

PURPOSE   To measure the back vertex refractive power, the cylinder axis, the optical center, and the prismatic power of prescription lenses.

EQUIPMENT

- Lensometer.
- Loose lenses.

BASIC COMPONENTS OF A LENSOMETER

Because lensometers differ, the examiner should review the location of the components and the specific instructions provided by the manufacturer for the lensometer he is using. The following components are common to all lensometers and are important to the examiner in reading a lens prescription.

External Parts

1. Adjustable eyepiece for focusing the instrument for the examiner's eye.
2. Lens holder and lens table to support the lens that is being measured.
3. Power wheel for reading the refractive power of the lens.
4. Axis wheel in 1° increments from 1° to 180° to read the axis of cylindrical lenses.
5. Inkwell and pens for dotting the optical center of the lens.

Internal Parts

1. Reticle for focusing and for determining prism power. The reticle is focused by the eyepiece of the instrument.
2. A target consisting of two sets of lines perpendicular to one another for reading the power of the lens. These lines are focused by the power wheel.
3. To distinguish the sphere and cylinder lines for your particular lensometer, with no lenses in place set the axis wheel to 180 and focus the mires. The vertically oriented mires are the sphere lines and the horizontally oriented mires are the cylinder lines. At this time it is also useful to see what the power wheel actually reads; because there is only air in place, the reading should be zero diopters, but often a small offset may be detected. Findings should be adjusted for any offset observed at this time.

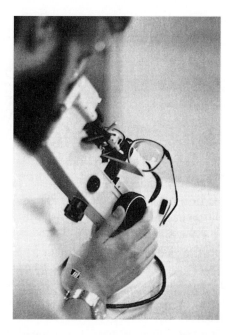

Figure 3–2. A clinician reads the prescription of the right lens in a pair of glasses.

SET-UP

- With the power wheel set on zero, the examiner focuses the eyepiece by turning the eyepiece as far counterclockwise as possible, and then slowly turning it clockwise until the reticle first comes into sharp focus.
- If testing a pair of glasses, always check the right lens first.
- Place the lens or pair of glasses in the lensometer with the ocular surface away from you. The lens is held in place by the lens holder and is held level on the lens table (see Figure 3–2).
- Center the lens by moving it so that the image of the lensometer target is aligned in the center of the eyepiece reticle. *Note:* If the lens has been made with prism ground into it, it may be impossible to center the target in the reticle. See the section in this chapter for methods to deal with prism.

STEP-BY-STEP PROCEDURE

SINGLE-VISION LENSES

1. Determine which part of the target is used for determining the spherical power of the lens and which part is used for determining the cylindrical

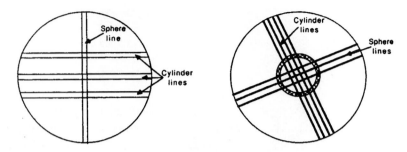

Figure 3–3. Two types of lensometer targets are shown, with the sphere and cylinder components identified.

power of the lens. This varies depending on the manufacturer of the lensometer, as shown in Figure 3–3.

2. Rotate the power wheel until the target comes into sharp focus. If the spherical and cylindrical lines of the target come into focus at the same time, the lens is spherical. Read the power of the lens from the power wheel and record.

3. If the spherical and cylindrical lines do not come into focus at the same time, the lens has a cylindrical component. To read the power of a spherocylindrical lens, start with enough plus power to blur the lensometer target, then rotate the power wheel toward less plus until the spherical line comes into focus. At the same time, orient the axis wheel of the lensometer so that the spherical line is perfectly continuous. Read the power from the power wheel and record it as the spherical portion of the prescription.

4. Focus the cylindrical line by rotating the power wheel toward more minus power. The difference between the power when the spherical portion of the target is in focus and the cylindrical portion of the target is in focus is the amount of minus cylinder power in the lens. The axis of the cylinder is read directly from the lensometer's protractor.

5. Before moving the glasses, dot the optical center (OC) of the lens with the lensometer's marking device. The lensometer target should be in the exact center of the reticle lines when dotting the OC.

6. Repeat steps 2 to 5 for the left lens.

7. When both lenses have been measured and dotted, measure the distance between the optical centers of the lenses and compare it to the patient's interpupillary distance. If the patient's PD and the PD of the spectacles are not the same, or if there is a vertical discrepancy in the heights of the optical centers of the two lenses, calculate the amount of induced prism using Prentice's rule (see step 4 under Prism).

8. The power of rigid and soft contact lenses can also be read in the lensometer. The procedures are described in Chapter 6.

Multifocal Lenses

1. Read and record the power of the distance portion of each of the two lenses (the carrier) as described in steps 1 to 7 above.
2. Turn the glasses around so that the ocular surface faces you.
3. Recheck one meridian in the carrier and compare the power in this meridian to the power in the *same meridian* through the near portion (the segment) of the lens (i.e., compare the spherical power to the spherical power or the cylindrical power to the cylindrical power). The difference between these powers is the add. It is often necessary to reset the axis orientation during this step.
4. Although the adds in the right and left lenses are usually the same, the add should be determined separately for each lens.
5. Progressive addition lenses are read in the same manner as other multifocal lenses, but the examiner must use the guidelines of the manufacturer for locating the near portion of the lens.

Prism

1. Locate the center of the target in the center of the eyepiece reticle.
2. Dot this location on the lens. This is the optical center of the lens.
3. Subsequently dot the location of the patient's line of sight on the lens.
4. When the optical center of the lens and the location of the patient's line of sight do not coincide, compute the induced prism using Prentice's rule:

$$\Delta = DC/10$$

where D is the power of the lens in diopters and C is the linear distance between the patient's line of sight and the optical center of the lens in millimeters. Vertical and horizontal prism are calculated separately.
5. If the lens has been made with prism ground into it, it may be impossible to center the target in the reticle. In this case, dot the lens at the location of the patient's line of sight and position the lens so the dot is in the center of the reticle. Read the amount of prism using the prism scale in the lensometer.
   Note: With high amounts of prism, it is difficult or impossible to locate the center of the target. In this case, hand held prisms are added to center the target and to determine the amount of prism in the lens.
6. Record the amount and direction of prism in the glasses.
   Note: First calculate the prism induced by each lens separately. The prism induced by the spectacles is the net discrepancy between the prism induced by each of the two lenses.

RECORDING

- Record the Rx for each lens separately in standard Rx form.
- Record the amount of induced prism in the glasses, if applicable.

EXAMPLES

- OD   −2.75sph
  OS   −2.25 = −1.00 × 10
- OD   +2.75 = −1.50 × 90, Add +2.00
  OS   +3.25 = −1.25 × 110, Add +2.00
- OD   −2.00 = −1.00 × 180, Add +1.50
  OS   +2.75 = −1.50 × 160, Add +2.00
- OD   +2.00 = −1.00 × 165 = 2 Δ BI, Add +1.00
  OS   +2.00 = −1.00 × 10 = 2 Δ BI, Add +1.00

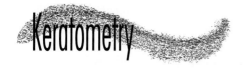

PURPOSE To assess the curvature, power, and toricity of the cornea. Keratometry may also be used to assess the integrity of the corneal/tear surface.

EQUIPMENT

• Keratometer or ophthalmometer.

BASIC COMPONENTS OF THE KERATOMETER

Because keratometers differ, the examiner should review the specific instructions provided by the manufacturer for the keratometer or ophthalmometer he is using. The following components are common to all keratometers.

• Adjustable eyepiece for focusing the instrument for the examiner's eye.
• Adjustable chin rest and forehead rest to support the patient's head during testing.
• A knob to raise and lower the instrument to align it with the patient's eye.
• Two power wheels to measure the corneal power in each of the two principal meridians.
• An axis scale to indicate the location of the two principal meridians. The barrel of the instrument can be rotated to align the keratometer appropriately.
• Target (known as *mires*), which is reflected onto the patient's cornea.
• Focus control knob or joystick to focus the mires on the patient's cornea.

SET-UP

• Disinfect the chin rest and forehead rest of the keratometer.
• The patient removes his glasses or contact lenses.
• Focus the eyepiece of the keratometer.
    a. Turn on the power.
    b. Set the adjustable eyepiece as far counterclockwise as possible.
    c. Place a white paper in front of the instrument objective to retroilluminate the reticle.
    d. Turn the eyepiece clockwise until the reticle is first seen in sharp focus.
• Adjust the height of the patient's chair and the instrument to a comfortable position for both the patient and the examiner.

- Unlock the instrument controls. This is necessary on some keratometers.
- Instruct the patient to place his chin in the chin rest and his forehead against the headrest.
- Raise or lower the chin rest until the patient's outer canthus is aligned with the hash mark on the upright support of the instrument or with the pointer on the side of the instrument.

STEP-BY-STEP PROCEDURE

1. From outside the instrument, roughly align the barrel with the patient's right eye by raising or lowering the instrument and by moving it to the left or right until a reflection of the mires is seen on the patient's cornea (see Figure 3–4).
2. Instruct the patient to look at the reflection of his own eye in the keratometer barrel.
3. Look into the keratometer and refine the alignment of the image of the mires (3 circles) on the patient's cornea (see Figure 3–5A).
4. Focus the mires and adjust the instrument so that the reticle is centered in the lower right hand circle (see Figure 3–5B).
5. Lock the instrument in place. This is necessary on some but not all types of keratometers.
6. Adjust the horizontal and the vertical power wheels until the mires are in close apposition.
7. To locate the two principal meridians of the patient's cornea, rotate the telescope until the two horizontal spurs on the mires are perfectly continuous with one another (see Figure 3–5C).
8. Adjust the horizontal power wheel until the horizontal mires are coincident (see Figure 3–5D).
9. Adjust the vertical power wheel until the vertical mires are coincident (see Figure 3–5D).
   Note: If the corneal astigmatism is irregular, the two principal meridians will not be 90° apart. In this case, after the power reading for the horizontal meridian is made, the examiner must readjust the barrel of the instrument to align the vertical components of the mires before adjusting the power wheel.
10. Throughout the procedure, adjust the focus and recenter the reticle as needed.
11. Observe the integrity of the cornea by observing the condition of the mires.
12. Roughly align the telescope with the patient's left eye as described in step 1.
13. Repeat steps 2 to 11 on the patient's left eye.

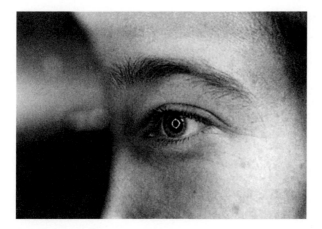

Figure 3–4. Aligning the keratometry mires on the patient's cornea from outside the instrument.

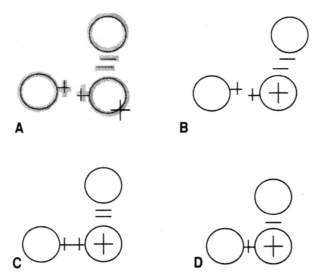

Figure 3–5. The appearance of the keratometric mires on the patient's cornea from inside the instrument. **A.** The appearance of the blurry mires when the telescope has first been aligned with the patient's cornea. **B.** The appearance of the mires when they have been focused and the reticle has been placed in the lower right hand circle. **C.** The appearance of the mires when the two principal meridians have been properly located. **D.** The appearance of the mires when the horizontal and vertical power wheels have been properly adjusted.

TABLE 3–1. CORRECTION FACTORS FOR EXTENDING THE RANGE OF THE KERATOMETER WITH AUXILIARY LENSES.

	Extender Lens Used		
	+1.25	**+2.25**	**−1.00**
Correction factor*	1.166	1.3126	0.8576

*Actual correction factors vary with the specific brand of keratometer. However, the above multipliers are close to those of keratometers in common use and their use will probably not result in significant errors.

EXTENDING THE RANGE

Sometimes the power in a meridian falls outside the power range of the ker-atometer. In such cases extend the range of the keratometer in the following man-ner: Tape or hold a +1.25 sph, +2.25 sph (for corneal powers above the range of the keratometer), or –1.00 sph (for corneal powers below the range of the ker-atometer) lens over the opening of the keratometer barrel and perform the mea-surement as described in steps 1 to 11. To calculate the actual power of the merid-ian, multiply the keratometer reading by the *correction factor* that corresponds to the extender lens used (see Table 3–1).

RECORDING

- Record for each eye separately.
- Record the power and the meridian for the horizontal meridian first (the primary meridian).
- Write a slash mark after the primary meridian and record the power and merid-ian for the vertical meridian (the secondary meridian).
- Record the amount of corneal astigmatism in diopters.
- Record the type of astigmatism:
  WR—with the rule (more power in the vertical meridian)
  AR—against the rule (more power in the horizontal meridian)
  OBL—oblique (major meridians within 15° of 45 and 135)
  Irregular—the two principal meridians are not 90° apart
- Record the conditions of the mires: mires clear and regular (MCAR) or mires ir-regular and distorted.

EXAMPLES

- OD   42.50 at 180/ 43.50 at 90; 1.00 D WR, MCAR
  OS   47.37 at 180/ 41.37 at 90; 6.00 D AR, mires distorted
- OD   41.75 at 180/ 43.75 at 70; 2.00 D irregular astig; mires distorted
  OS   43.12 at 135/ 41.87 at 45; 1.25 D OBL; MCAR

KERATOMETRY *at a glance*

PURPOSE	TECHNIQUE
Prepare the instrument for the examiner	Focus the eyepiece
Prepare the instrument for the patient	Wipe the chinrest and forehead rest with alcohol. Set the chinrest so that the patient's outer canthus is aligned with the marker.
Align the instrument	From outside the instrument align the keratometer so the image of the mires can be seen on the patient's cornea. Look into the keratometer and refine the alignment by placing the reticle in the lower right hand circle.
Locate the principal meridians	Rotate the telescope so that the spurs of horizontal mires are continuous with one another.
Measure the power in each of the principal meridians	Adjust the horizontal and the vertical power wheels so the mires are coincident.
Examine the integrity of the cornea	Observe the quality of the image.
Record the data	Record the power and location of each of the two principal meridians, the amount and type of astigmatism, and the condition of the mires.

If only the secondary meridian is recorded, the position of the primary meridian is assumed to be 90° away.

OD   42.00/ 43.00 at 90; 1.00 WR MCAR
OS   42.00/ 42.00 at 90; sphere MCAR

If both meridians have exactly the same power, it is permissible to record that power a single time followed by the abbreviation "sph" rather than to record each meridian's power separately. (e.g., 42.12 sph)

EXPECTED FINDINGS

- Average K readings are 43.00 D to 44.00 D.
- The two principal meridians are expected to be 90° apart.

Introduction to the Phoropter

Introduction to the Phoropter

PURPOSE The phoropter is a complex lens holder designed to allow the examiner to change lenses efficiently and easily. It consists of four groups of controls. Controls that are labeled in Figure 3–6 are *italicized* in the text.

I. Lens controls

The heart of the phoropter is its two sets of lens controls, one for spherical and one for minus-plano-cylindrical lenses.

A. Spherical lens control

The control for the spherical lenses is a large wheel at each side of the phoropter called the *weak sphere dial*. There is a *strong sphere control* that allows ±3.0 or 4.0 diopter changes in sphere. Inside the housing of the machine there are two sets of lenses mounted on large wheels. One wheel carries a set of lenses in 0.25 diopter steps. The other carries lenses in 3.0 or 4.0 diopter steps. The two wheels work together to provide total lens powers in the range of +20 D to −20 D in 0.25-D steps.

The net spherical power is shown on the *sphere power scale*.

B. Minus-plano-cylinder control

Minus-plano-cylindrical lenses are mounted in a wheel that rotates to bring different powers of lenses before the patient's eye. The lenses in the cylinder wheel can also be rotated to vary the axis.

The cylinder is controlled by two knobs, the *cylinder power knob* and the *cylinder axis knob*. The cylinder power is shown on the *cylinder power scale*. The *cylinder axis indicators* display the axis of the minus cylinder by the position of an arrow on a standard ophthalmic protractor, the *cylinder axis reference scale*.

II. Auxiliary Lens Knob/Aperture Control

The *auxiliary lens knob/aperture control* determines what the patient looks through when behind the phoropter. The most frequent positions are **O**pen, in which the aperture contains the lenses, and **BL**ank or **OC**cluded, in which the eye is completely occluded.

Most phoropters also contain a **R**etinoscopy **L**ens aperture, a +1.50 or +2.00 diopter spherical lens placed in the aperture in addition to the lenses indicated by the power scales. Additional apertures that are available on

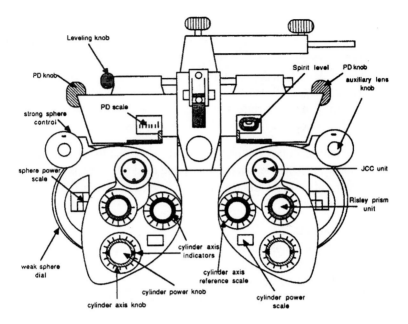

Figure 3–6. Schematic diagram of a generic phoropter in common use today.

some phoropters include ±0.50 diopter Jackson Cross Cylinders (JCCs), pinholes (PH), red lens (RL), Maddox rod (RMH/RMV), Polaroid (P), +.12 D, and horizontal (10ΔI) or vertical (6ΔU) prisms.

III. Ancillary Units

The phoropter has two or three ancillary lenses, that can rotate in front of the aperture when desired.

A. Jackson Cross Cylinders Unit (JCCs)

The JCCs are marked with red dots or lines to indicate their minus-cylinder axis and with white marks to indicate their plus-cylinder axis. The handles are positioned 45° away from the cylinder axes.

B. Rotary Prism Unit

The rotary (or Risley) prisms have an indicator for the direction of the prism base and a scale to indicate their net prism power. With the zero in the horizontal meridian, the indicator is placed above the zero for base up prism and below zero for base down prism. With the zero in the vertical meridian, the indicator is placed toward the nose for base in prism and away from the nose for base out prism.

C. Maddox rod

In some phoropters the Maddox rod is included as an ancillary lens rather than in the aperture.

IV. Adjustments

The phoropter contains controls for adjusting the phoropter to fit the patient.

A. *PD knob*

B. *Leveling knob with spirit level*

C. Vertex distance control

D. Pantoscopic tilt control

Static Retinoscopy

PURPOSE To objectively determine the distance refractive status of the patient's eyes. The results of this technique serve as a starting point for the subjective refraction or as the patient's final prescription if the patient is unable to respond to subjective testing.

EQUIPMENT

- Streak retinoscope.
- Phoropter, lens rack, or loose trial lenses. The technique described here refers to lenses in the phoropter, because that is the usual clinical method of retinoscopy. The same principles can be applied to retinoscopy using loose lenses or a retinoscopy rack instead of the phoropter.
- Fixation target: 20/400 E projected through a red/green filter.

SET-UP

- The patient removes his corrective lenses.
- Adjust the height of the examination chair so that the patient's eyes are at the same level as yours.
- Disinfect patient contact surfaces of the phoropter.
- Place the phoropter in front of the patient with the interpupillary distance (PD) set to match the patient's distance PD. Level the phoropter so the patient's eyes are centered in the apertures.
- Instruct the patient to keep both eyes open during retinoscopy. Ask the patient to inform you if your head blocks his view of the fixation target. It may be necessary to rotate the phoropter slightly or to move the target off the screen and onto the wall to allow the patient to see the target while you maintain alignment along the patient's visual axis.
- During retinoscopy, the examiner keeps both of his eyes open and examines the patient's right eye with his right eye and examines the patient's left eye with his left eye.
- The examiner holds the retinoscope 20 in (50 cm) or 26 in (67 cm) from the patient's eye. The retinoscope is held in the examiner's right hand to examine the patient's right eye and in the examiner's left hand to examine the patient's left eye.

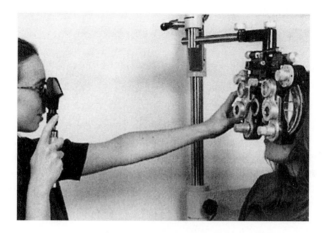

Figure 3–7. Static retinoscopy technique is demonstrated.

- Retinoscopy is most easily done in dim illumination. An illustration of the performance of static retinoscopy is provided in Figure 3–7.

STEP-BY-STEP PROCEDURE

1. Instruct the patient to look at the fixation target. Examine the patient's right eye.
2. Determine if the refractive error is spherical or astigmatic by changing the position of the sleeve of the streak retinoscope and the distance between the examiner and the patient until the reflex is enhanced. Then rotate the streak of the retinoscope through 360°, looking for the break phenomenon, the thickness phenomenon, the skew phenomenon, or changes in the brightness of the reflex within the pupil.
   a. If the error is spherical, the reflex within the pupil will be continuous with the intercept of the streak on the patient's face (i.e., there will be no break phenomenon). If the error is astigmatic, the reflex within the pupil may not be continuous with the intercept on the patient's face (i.e., there will be a break phenomenon) (see Figure 3–8).
   b. As the streak is rotated through 360°, the thickness of the reflex within the pupil will be constant in a spherical error and vary in an astigmatic error (thickness phenomenon) (see Figure 3–9). Moreover, as the streak is rotated, the brightness of the pupillary reflex will remain constant in a spherical error and may vary in an astigmatic error. The principal meridians correspond to the orientations of the streak that provide the thickest and thinnest reflexes and/or the brightest and dimmest reflexes.

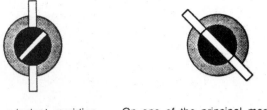

Not on principal meridian   On one of the principal meridians

Figure 3–8. Diagram of the appearance of the retinoscopic reflex when using the break phenomenon to locate the principal meridians of an astigmatic eye.

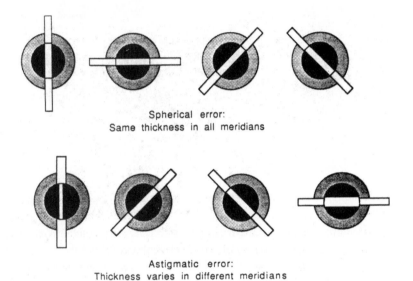

Spherical error:
Same thickness in all meridians

Astigmatic error:
Thickness varies in different meridians

Figure 3–9. Diagram of the appearance of the retinoscopic reflex when using the thickness phenomenon to locate the principal meridians of an astigmatic eye.

    c. In an astigmatic error, as the streak is swept across the patient's pupil, the reflex within the pupil will move parallel to the movement of the streak on the patient's face when the streak is aligned with one of the two principal meridians. The reflex will move in a different direction than the streak when the streak is not aligned with one of the principal meridians (skew phenomenon). There will be no skew phenomenon in a spherical error (see Figure 3–10).

3. If the error is spherical, observe the reflex for *with* or *against* motion and add plus or minus lenses until there is no motion of the reflex. The type of lens needed for neutralization depends on the patient's refractive error,

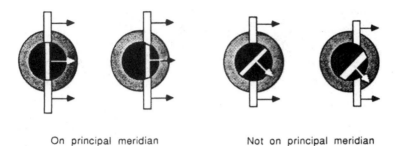

On principal meridian   Not on principal meridian

Figure 3–10. Diagram of the appearance of the retinoscopic reflex when using the skew phenomenon to locate the principal meridians of an astigmatic eye.

the position of the sleeve of the retinoscope (plane mirror position or short concave mirror position), and the type of motion seen (with motion or against motion) (see Table 3–1).

Note: With motion is easier to observe and to neutralize than against motion. However, if with motion is present, the patient may accommodate, particularly if minus lenses were added. When against motion is initially seen, it can be changed to with motion, without affecting the patient's accommodation, by changing the sleeve of the retinoscope from the plane mirror position to the short concave mirror position.

4. To neutralize an astigmatic error, first identify the two principal meridians (see step 2). Then neutralize each meridian separately. When using a phoropter with minus cylinders, one meridian is neutralized with sphere only. The other meridian is neutralized with a combination of sphere and minus-cylinder. The least myopic or most hyperopic meridian is neutralized with sphere. The most myopic or least hyperopic meridian is neutralized with cylinder in addition to the sphere.

Because it may be difficult for a novice retinoscopist to determine which meridian is the least myopic, either meridian can be neutralized first. The other meridian can then be checked and adjustments can be made in the sphere power if necessary. If using a plane mirror retinoscope, when one meridian is neutralized the other meridian must show against motion to be neutralized with minus-cylinder power. If the retinoscopist neutralizes the most myopic meridian first, one meridian will show neutrality while the other shows with motion. To correct this, the retinoscopist can add more plus to the sphere power to neutralize the second meridian. This will leave the first meridian showing against motion. The newly created against motion can now be neutralized by adding minus-cylinder power with the cylinder axis aligned with the orientation of the streak.

It is often observed, particularly when the pupils are large, that the motion of the reflex in the periphery of the pupil differs from that observed near the center of the pupil. For purposes of refraction, it is necessary to achieve neutrality only at the center of the pupil, ignoring peripheral reflex movements.

5. When both principal meridians are neutralized, recheck the meridian neutralized with sphere and adjust the spherical power if necessary.

6. When neutrality is reached, recheck all meridians with the sleeve of the retinoscope in both the plane mirror position and the short concave mirror position. If true neutrality is achieved, all meridians will look neutral regardless of the position of the sleeve of the retinoscope. If neutrality is not reached in all meridians, make necessary adjustments.

7. The lens (or combination of lenses) that produces neutrality is called the *gross retinoscopy finding.* The gross finding makes the patient's fundus conjugate with the examiner's entrance pupil. Leave the gross static finding in front of the patient's right eye and neutralize the patient's left eye by following steps 2 to 6. When the patient's left eye is neutralized, recheck the right eye and adjust the sphere or cylinder if necessary.

8. To convert the gross retinoscopy finding to a net finding, algebraically add a spherical minus lens equal to your working distance in diopters to the spherical lens that produced neutrality. For example, -2.00 D for a working distance of 20 in; -1.50 D for a working distance of 26 in. This is the *net static retinoscopy finding,* or the *net static,* that makes the patient's retina conjugate with infinity.

9. Measure the patient's visual acuity in each eye through the net static retinoscopy finding.

RECORDING

- Record the net static for each eye separately.
- Record the patient's visual acuity for each eye through the net static retinoscopy finding.

EXAMPLES

- OD   +4.75 sphere   20/60
  OS   +1.50 = -0.50×175 20/20
- OD   +1.00 = -1.25×10 20/15
  OS   +1.00 = -0.75×165 20/15

Routine Distance Subjective Refraction With the Phoropter

PURPOSE   To determine the refractive status of the eye using the patient's subjective responses. When the distance subjective refraction is completed, a distant point stimulus should form a point image on the retina with accommodation fully relaxed.

EQUIPMENT

- Projector, VA slide, screen.
- Standard phoropter.

SET-UP

- The patient should be seated comfortably.
- Disinfect patient contact surfaces of the phoropter.
- Set the phoropter PD to match patient's distance PD.
- Position the phoropter in front of the patient.
- Level the phoropter.
- Project the full-screen VA chart with the 20/15 line at the bottom.

SUBJECTIVE REFRACTION *at a glance*

PURPOSE	TECHNIQUE
Component: Monocular Subjective (OD first, then OS)	
Finding a working sphere	Fog to 20/40 to 20/60
	MPMVA
	Initial duochrome
Refine the cylinder	JCC axis check
	JCC power check
	Recheck axis, if needed
Refine the sphere	Fog to 20/40 to 20/60
	MPMVA endpoint
Component: Binocular Balance	
Balance the two eyes	Fog by +0.75 D to 20/25
	or worse
	Dissociate with prism
	Equalize blur
Refine the sphere	Binocular MPMVA Endpoint

Step-by-Step Procedure for the Routine Distance Subjective Refraction With the Phoropter

The pages that follow describe the step-by-step procedure for the entire routine distance refraction, which consists of several individual procedures. These individual procedures often have names and are labeled within the step-by-step procedure. The numbering of the steps is continuous for the entire routine distance refraction. Side trips are described at the end of the step-by-step procedure of the routine refraction. The Flow of Refraction chart (Figure 3–1) shows how the individual procedures, including the side trips, are organized to make up the entire distance subjective refraction.

I. MONOCULAR DISTANCE SUBJECTIVE REFRACTION

Initial MPMVA (Maximum Plus to Maximum Visual Acuity)

PURPOSE   To determine the maximum plus (minimum minus) spherical power that provides the patient with his maximum visual acuity. The initial MPMVA begins with the net static retinoscopy findings in the phoropter.

1. Open the right eye and occlude the left eye.
2. Fog the eye to a visual acuity of 20/40 to 20/60. This will usually require the addition of about +1.00 sphere to (or the removal of -1.00 diopter sphere from) the net static retinoscopy finding or the clock chart finding. Check the patient's VA through the fogging lenses to be sure he is fogged to the correct level.
3. Predict the final sphere by comparing the patient's VA under fog to Egger's chart. Remember that the patient should obtain approximately one additional line of VA for each 0.25 D of minus-sphere added (or each 0.25 diopter of plus-sphere that is removed) during the MPMVA.
4. Reduce the plus (add minus) 0.25 D at a time, checking VA and encouraging the patient to read the next smaller line each time.
5. Keep in mind that each 0.25 D should allow the patient to read smaller letters. Having the chart look "better" to the patient is not sufficient justification to give him more minus.

Initial Duochrome (Bichrome, Red-Green Test)

PURPOSE   To determine the correcting spherical lens power. The duochrome should be used as the endpoint procedure for the initial MPMVA.

6. Put the projector's red-green filter over the chart of letters.
7. Direct the patient's attention to the 20/25 line or to the letters one line above his best VA so far. For some patients it may be necessary to isolate this line of letters.
8. Tell the patient to look from the green side to the red side and back to the green side. Have him state which side has the sharper and clearer (not "better," "darker," or "brighter") letters or to state if the two sides are equally clear. Because this test works on the principle of chromatic aberration, it will work for color anomalous patients. For such individuals, it may be necessary to tell them to look at the left or right sides of the chart rather than at the green or red sides.
9. If the letters on the red side are clearer or if the letters on both sides are equally clear, introduce an additional 0.25 D of minus-spherical power. If the letters on the green side are clearer, take away 0.25 D of minus (or add another 0.25 D of plus-sphere).
10. Repeat steps 8 and 9 until you find the minimum amount of minus power (or maximum plus) at which the patient reports that the green side has the clearer letters. Then the patient is "one into the green."
11. Remove the red-green filter and recheck the VA.
    Note: Some patients are unresponsive to this test and seem to choose one side or the other, regardless of the lens powers in place. Be alert to this possibility and abandon the duochrome test in favor of some other endpoint to the MPMVA (see step 31).
12. Consider the following:
    a. Does the amount of minus added correlate with the amount of improvement in VA over the starting point with the patient fogged? The correct refraction will yield a close match between the actual and the predicted changes in lens power.

b. If the phoropter contains a tentative cylinder of –0.75 diopter or greater from static retinoscopy or some other test, proceed with the Jackson Cross Cylinder test (step 13). Remember that a visual acuity of 20/20, or sharp, clear vision may not be possible at this point in the refraction, because the cylindrical part of the prescription has not yet been refined.

c. If the patient has clear VA of 20/20 or better with spherical lenses and if you are refracting the right eye, proceed to the monocular refraction of the left eye. If the patient has clear VA of 20/20 or better with spherical lenses and if you are refracting the left eye, proceed to the binocular balance.

d. If the phoropter contains a tentative cylinder of –0.25 diopter or –0.50 diopter from static retinoscopy or some other test, perform the Jackson Cross Cylinder test for power before going further, starting with step 22. If the patient *rejects* the cylinder power, proceed with the second MPMVA (step 27). If the patient *accepts* the cylinder power, do not continue with the power check at this time, but resume the Jackson Cross Cylinder test at step 13.

e. If the static retinoscopy and other starting data do *not* indicate an astigmatism *and* the patient does *not* have clear 20/20 VA or better with a spherical correction, perform one or both of the side trips for astigmatism, the JCC Check Test or the Clock Chart, described later in this chapter, to search for a small, uncorrected astigmatism. These side trips may be called for if the static retinoscopy is unreliable for reasons such as opacities in the media or poor patient cooperation.

f. If the starting data and the side trips do not detect any astigmatism and the patient does not achieve 20/20 VA with spherical lenses, consider the possibility that the eye suffers from pathology or amblyopia.

The Jackson Cross Cylinder (JCC) Test

PURPOSE To refine the axis and power of the cylindrical component of the correction after the initial monocular MPMVA has determined the tentative spherical correction.

Ordinarily one should refine cylinder axis prior to refining cylinder power. However, if the tentative cylinder power is only –0.50 or –0.25, it is permissible to perform a power check, following steps 22 through 26, prior to refining the axis. If the patient accepts the cylinder power at this time, return to step 13, the axis check, followed by refinement of the cylinder power. If the patient rejects the cylinder power at this time, proceed to step 27, the second MPMVA.

PERFORM THE JCC AXIS CHECK

13. Isolate a line of letters one line above the best VA obtained so far in the monocular subjective refraction.
14. As shown in Figure 3–11, place the JCC lens before the eye such that its axes straddle at 45° angles the axis of the correcting cylinder in the phoropter. This is achieved by lining up the handle of the JCC with the axis of the cylinder in the phoropter.
15. Instruct the patient that you will show him two views of the line of letters and will identify each view with a number. Tell him that both views may be blurry, but to tell you which view is sharper or less blurry. Further instruct him to try to ignore differences in the shapes of the letters when comparing the views.
16. Have the patient look at the letters and tell him, "This is view number one."
17. After 2 to 5 seconds, flip the JCC and say, "This is view number two. Which view has the clearer letters?" If the views are equally blurry, the axis is set in the appropriate position. Go to step 21 to refine the cylinder power by the JCC.
18. If the views are not equally blurry or equally clear, move the axis of the phoropter cylinder by 15° toward the minus-cylinder axis (indicated by the red marks) that gave the clearer view. In Figure 3–11, if view num-

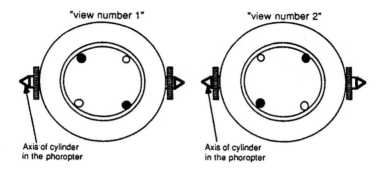

Figure 3–11. Schematic diagram of the JCC for axis refinement, showing the JCC in its two positions.

ber 1 provided the patient with clearer vision, the axis in the phoropter should be moved in a clockwise direction. If view number 2 provided the patient with clearer vision, the axis in the phoropter should be moved in a counterclockwise direction.

19. Shift the orientation of the JCC lens so that the handle remains aligned with the axis of the phoropter cylinder. In many phoropters, the JCC will rotate automatically along with the phoropter cylinder, so this step is unnecessary.

20. Repeat steps 14 through 19 as long as you have to keep adjusting the cylinder axis in the same direction (i.e., clockwise or counterclockwise). When the axis has to be moved in the opposite direction, repeat steps 14 through 19, but move the axis in 5° or 10° steps. Hone in on the correct axis by successively decreasing the step size.

    Note: The greater the cylinder power, the greater the need for precision in the axis. For cylinder powers greater than 5.0 diopters, the axis should be specified to the single degree. For cylinder powers less than 2.0 diopters, the axis should be specified to the nearest 5°. For cylinder powers between 2.0 and 5.0 D, exercise professional judgment.

21. End the JCC axis check when either of the following two conditions are met:

    a. Both views look the same to the patient.

    b. The patient's responses move the axis back and forth within a narrow range. In this event, select an axis in the middle of the range.

PERFORM THE JCC POWER CHECK

22. Place the JCC lens so that one axis is aligned with and the other axis is perpendicular to the axis of the correcting cylinder in the phoropter, as shown in Figure 3–12.

23. The instructions are the same as in steps 15, 16, and 17. It is often necessary to repeat them, however.

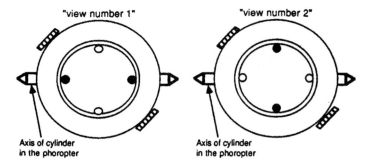

Figure 3–12. Schematic diagram of the JCC for power refinement, showing the JCC in its two positions.

24. Present the two views to the patient by flipping the JCC lens. If the patient prefers the view with the RED dots (minus-cylinder axis) aligned with the cylinder axis in the phoropter, view number one in Figure 3–12, increase the power of the minus-cylinder in the phoropter by −0.25 D. If the patient prefers the view with the WHITE dots (plus-cylinder axis) aligned with the cylinder axis in the phoropter, view number 2 in Figure 3–12, reduce the power of the minus-cylinder in the phoropter by −0.25 D.
25. Throughout the JCC power check, maintain the spherical equivalent of the MPMVA starting point. For each increase in minus-cylinder of −0.50 D that the patient accepts, add +0.25 D to the sphere or take away −0.25 D. For each decrease in minus-cylinder of −0.50 D, add −0.25 D to the sphere.
26. End the JCC power check when either of the following two conditions are met:
   a. Both views look the same to the patient.
   b. The patient's responses call for changes within a narrow range of powers. In this event, select the power that is closer to that found in his habitual prescription. If a habitual prescription is not available, select the less minus cylinder power.

   Note: If the results of the JCC power check call for a change in power of greater than 0.75 diopters, compared to the starting cylinder power, recheck the cylinder axis at this point.

   Note: For some patients, making the choice of which view is clearer is very difficult. Borish describes a variation on the JCC technique in which the whole VA chart, from the 20/50 to the 20/15 letters, rather than an isolated line of letters, is displayed. The patient is asked to report which view allows him to read farther down the chart. By having the patient try to read the chart, the examiner can exercise his professional judgment as to the view that provides the sharper retinal image.

   Upon reaching the conclusion of the JCC test for both axis and power, perform the second monocular MPMVA.

Second Monocular MPMVA

PURPOSE To determine the maximum plus-spherical power that provides the patient with his maximum visual acuity.

Note: During the second monocular MPMVA and the remainder of the distance refraction, the cylinder in the phoropter at the end of step 26 is not changed.

27. Fog the patient to a visual acuity of 20/40 to 20/60. This will usually require the addition of about +1.00 to, or the removal of −1.00 from, the spherical lens in the phoropter. Check the patient's VA through the fogging lenses to be sure he is fogged to the correct level.

28. Predict the final sphere by comparing the patient's VA under fog to Egger's chart. Remember that the patient should obtain approximately one additional line of VA for each 0.25 D of minus-sphere added or each 0.25 diopter of plus-sphere removed.

29. Reduce the plus (add minus) 0.25 D at a time, checking VA and encouraging the patient to read the next smaller line each time.

30. Keep in mind that each 0.25 D should allow the patient to read smaller letters. The patient reporting that the chart looks "better" is not sufficient justification to give him more minus.

31. Reach an appropriate stopping point. To decide when to stop the second monocular MPMVA, choose one of the following endpoints. The order of presentation here does not imply order of preference.

    a. **The DUOCHROME endpoint**
       (1) Put the projector's red-green filter over the chart of letters.
       (2) Direct the patient's attention to the line of letters one line above his best VA so far. For some patients it may be necessary to isolate this line.
       (3) Tell the patient to look from the green side to the red side and back to the green side. Have him state which side has the sharper, clearer (not "better," "darker," or "brighter") letters or to state if the two sides are equally clear.
       (4) If the letters on the red side are clearer or if the letters on the two sides appear equal, introduce an additional 0.25 D of minus-spherical power over the eye being tested. If the letters on the

green side are clearer, take away 0.25 D of minus (or add another 0.25 D of plus-sphere).

(5) Repeat steps 3 and 4 above until the patient is one into the green, the minimum amount of minus power at which the patient reports that the green side has the clearer letters. As an alternative, use a red-green balance, the point at which both sides appear equally clear, rather than one into the green, as the endpoint.

(6) Remove the red-green filter and recheck the VA.

Note: Some patients always seem to choose one side or the other, regardless of the lens powers in place. Be alert to the possibility that your patient is unresponsive to this test and abandon the duochrome test in favor of one of the other endpoints described here.

b. **The smaller/darker endpoint**

(1) Introduce one more 0.25 D of minus (or remove 0.25 D of plus).

(2) Ask the patient whether the change makes the letters clearer or just "smaller," "darker," or "better."

(3) If the change makes the letters subjectively clearer to the patient, accept the change and repeat steps (1) and (2) above. If the change makes the letters "smaller, darker, or better, do not accept the change and take away the 0.25 D added in step (1).

c. **The 20/20 endpoint**

If the patient has subjectively clear 20/20 vision, and if the lenses in the phoropter at step 28 match the prescription that was predicted from the starting information, the second monocular MPMVA may be stopped. The amount of minus added (plus taken away) should correlate with the amount of improvement in VA over the starting point with the patient fogged (step 27). The correct refraction must yield a close match between the actual and the predicted changes in lens power.

32. Record the sphere power, cylinder power, cylinder axis in the phoropter, and the VA achieved through these lenses.

33. Repeat steps 2 to 32 with the right eye occluded and the left eye open.

II. BINOCULAR BALANCE

PURPOSE   To equalize the stimulus to accommodation for the two eyes. The primary purpose of binocular balance is to match the accommodative stimulus for the two eyes. It serves a secondary purpose of relaxing the accommodation. With both eyes open, the accommodative responses of the two eyes should be maximally relaxed and equal. For many patients, binocular balance serves the additional function of matching the visual acuity in the two eyes through the new prescription.

INDICATIONS

Because this binocular balance procedure calls upon the patient to match the VA under fog in the two eyes, perform it only if the two eyes achieved the same VA during their monocular refractions. If the best corrected VAs of the two eyes differ after the distance monocular subjective refractions, the binocular balance procedure should be skipped. If the best corrected VAs of the two eyes differ and there is reason to believe that the accommodation differs in the eyes following their distance monocular subjective refractions, perform the prism dissociated duochrome test.

34. Make sure that neither eye is occluded and that both eyes can see the projector screen.
35. Fog each eye by +0.75 D sphere relative to the endpoint of its respective monocular refraction. Measure the patient's binocular VA and continue adding +0.25 sphere in front of both eyes until the binocular VA is 20/25 or worse, if necessary.
36. Isolate a line of letters one line above the VA found at the end of step 35.
37. Place 3 to 4Δ base up over the right eye and 3 to 4Δ base down over the left eye using the phoropter's rotary (Risley) prisms, as shown in Figure 3–13.
38. Inform the patient that he should see two lines of letters, both of which should be blurry, as in Figure 3–14. Make certain that this is the case.
39. Have the patient look back and forth between the two lines of letters and have him tell you which line, the upper or the lower, is clearer.

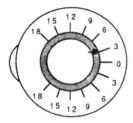 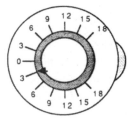

Figure 3–13. Schematic diagram of the phoropter's Risley (rotary) prisms set to 3∆ base up over the right eye and 3∆ base down over the left eye for performing binocular balance. With the prisms set in this way, the right eye will see the lower image, except in the rare case of a left hyper deviation greater than or equal to 6∆.

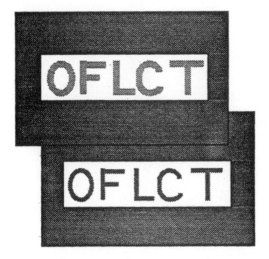

Figure 3–14. Schematic representation of the 20/30 line fogged for both eyes during prism-dissociated binocular balance. In this example, there is more blur for the left eye, which sees the upper image, than for the right eye, which sees the lower image.

40. Add +0.25 (take away −0.25) sphere to the eye that sees the clearer line (i.e., make it blurrier). For example, if the patient reports that the lower line is clearer, as in Figure 3–14, add +0.25 sphere (take away −0.25 from) to the clearer seeing right eye.

41. Repeat steps 39 and 40 until the patient reports equal blurriness of the two lines or until the patient is simply switching back and forth between the two. If it is not possible to achieve a close match between the blurriness of the two eyes, perform the sighting-dominance check. Then leave the sighting-dominant eye with the subjectively clearer vision.

   Note: As long as both lines remain legible, continue to add fog to the better-seeing eye in +0.25 diopter steps. However, because the letters must remain legible at all times, after the first or second repetition of steps 39 and 40, it may be necessary to make the blurrier eye clearer. Do this by adding −0.25 D sphere to it (taking away +0.25 D) rather than continuing to blur the clearer eye. Take care to ensure that both eyes remain fogged and target letters remain legible until the end of the binocular balance procedure.

42. When equality of the vision of the two eyes is reached, or the sighting-dominant eye is left with the slightly clearer vision, remove the Risley prisms to allow fusion.

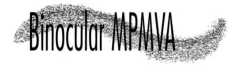

Binocular MPMVA

To determine the maximum plus spherical power that provides the patient with his maximum visual acuity through both eyes simultaneously.

43. The patient's eyes should still be equally fogged or the sighting-dominant eye should be slightly clearer from step 42. Check the patient's binocular VA through the fog.
44. Predict the final sphere by comparing the patient's VA under fog to Egger's chart. Remember that the patient should obtain approximately one additional line of VA for each 0.25 D of minus-sphere added (or each 0.25 diopter of plus-sphere removed) during the MPMVA.
45. Reduce the plus (or add minus) 0.25 D at a time over both eyes simultaneously, checking VA and encouraging the patient to read the next smaller line each time.
46. Keep in mind that each 0.25 D should allow the patient to read smaller letters. The patient reporting that the chart looks "better" is not sufficient justification to give him more minus.
47. Reach an appropriate stopping point. To stop the binocular MPMVA, choose one of the following endpoints. The order of presentation here does not imply order of preference.
   a. **The smaller/darker endpoint**
      (1) Introduce one more 0.25 D of minus (less plus).
      (2) Ask the patient whether the change makes the letters clearer or smaller, darker, or "better."
      (3) If the change makes the letters subjectively clearer to the patient, accept the change and repeat steps (1) and (2). If the change makes the letters smaller, darker, or "better," do not accept the change and take away the 0.25 D added in step (1).
   Note: When this technique is used, patients often accept 0.25 D more minus than the lens power that provided them with maximum visual acuity. Although this outcome is acceptable, never give a patient more than 0.25 D beyond the lenses that gave him maximum VA.
   b. **The DUOCHROME endpoint**
      (1) Put the projector's red-green filter over the chart of letters.

(2) Direct the patient's attention to the 20/25 line or to the letters one line above his best VA so far. For some patients it may be necessary to isolate this line of letters.

(3) Tell the patient to look from the green side to the red side and back to the green side. Have him state which side has the sharper, clearer (not "better," darker, or brighter) letters or to state if the two sides are equally clear.

(4) If the letters on the red side are clearer or if the letters on the two sides appear equal, introduce an additional 0.25 D of minus (take away 0.25 D of plus) spherical power over both eyes. If the letters on the green side are clearer, take away 0.25 D of minus (or add 0.25 D of plus sphere) from both eyes.

(5) Repeat steps (3) and (4) until the patient is one into the green, the minimum amount of minus power at which the patient reports that the green side has the clearer letters. As an alternative, use a red-green balance, the point at which both sides appear equally clear, rather than one into the green, as the endpoint.

(6) Remove the red-green filter and recheck the VA.

Note: Some patients always seem to choose one side or the other, regardless of the lens powers in place. Be alert to the possibility that your patient is unresponsive to this test and abandon the duochrome test in favor of one of the other endpoints.

c. **The 20/20 endpoint**

If the patient has subjectively clear 20/20 vision, and if the lenses in the phoropter at step 46 match the prescriptions that were predicted from the starting information for both eyes, the binocular MPMVA may be stopped. The correct refraction must yield a close match between the actual and the predicted changes in lens power.

Note: The results of subjective refraction are susceptible to measurement error and may vary in sphere and/or cylinder power by ±0.25 diopter in the absence of any change in the patient's actual refraction.

RECORDING

- Record the sphere power, cylinder power, and cylinder axis in the phoropter for each eye.
- Measure and record the VA for the right eye, the left eye, and for both eyes together.

Note: The patient's final eyeglass prescription may differ from the results of the distance subjective refraction with the phoropter. Some examples will illustrate this point. If the prescription is greater than ±4.0 D, it is necessary to adjust it for the vertex distances of the phoropter versus the patient's spectacles. Be conservative about changing the cylindrical components (particularly the axis) of a prescription that is comfortable for the patient. For high amounts of cylinder, it may be necessary to prescribe a different axis and power in glasses that will be used for reading as opposed to distance viewing.

EXAMPLE

Monocular Subj.

OD	$+1.75 = -1.00 \times 165$	20/15
OS	$+1.75 = -1.00 \times 10$	20/15

Binocular Bal.

OD	$+2.00 = -1.00 \times 165$	20/15
OS	$+2.00 = -1.00 \times 10$	20/15
OU		20/15

Use of the Trial Frame to Modify a Prescription

PURPOSE To demonstrate a new prescription for the patient and to modify the subjective refraction findings for maximum patient comfort.

EQUIPMENT

- Trial lens set.
- Trial frame.
- Distance visual acuity chart.
- Near visual acuity chart.
- Reading material—newspaper, magazine, phone book, music.

SET-UP

- Place the trial frame on the patient. Adjust the trial frame so that it sits comfortably on the patient's face and the patient's eyes are centered relative to the lens wells of the frame. See the section on trial frame refraction in this chapter.
- If the patient has a previous pair of glasses and the change is spherical, the trial lenses can be held directly over the patient's current glasses to demonstrate the change in prescription, as shown in Figure 3–15.

STEP-BY-STEP PROCEDURE

1. Instruct the patient to look at the distance acuity chart if the new prescription is for distance or at the near point card if the new prescription is for near. Alternatively, the patient may look out a window rather than at the distance acuity chart or at reading material rather than at the near acuity chart.
2. Ask the patient if things look clear and if he feels comfortable looking through the new prescription.
3. If the patient reports that things are not clear or are not comfortable through the new prescription, adjust the prescription in one of the following ways until the patient reports clear and comfortable vision:

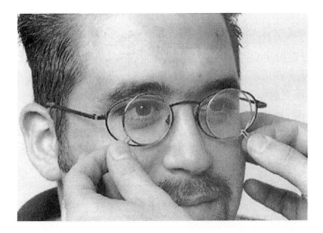

Figure 3–15. The clinician holds trial lenses over the patient's old glasses to demonstrate a change in prescription.

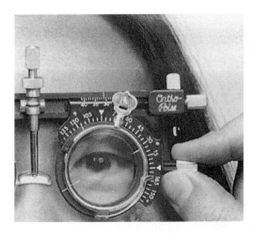

Figure 3–16. The clinician adjusts the axis of a proposed prescription in the trial frame.

    a. increase the minus-sphere in 0.25 D steps.
    b. increase the plus-sphere in 0.25 D steps.
    c. move the axis of the cylinder toward the axis in the patient's previous prescription or toward 90° or 180° (see Figure 3–16).
    d. decrease the cylinder power in 0.25 D steps, making concurrent changes in the sphere to maintain the spherical equivalent of the prescription.
  4. For prescriptions that are for near only, instruct the patient to move the reading material in until it blurs and out until it blurs to ensure that there is an adequate range for the patient's needs.

5. For prescriptions that are for near only, instruct the patient to look through the prescription at distance and explain that it is normal for distance objects to look blurry through a near prescription.

RECORDING

- Record all of the prescriptions that were tested.
- Record the patient's response to each of the trial framed prescriptions.

EXAMPLES

- TF

OD   −4.75 sphere 20/20
OS   −3.50 = −0.50 × 175   20/20
patient comfortable at D and N.

- TF for near

1. OD   +1.00 = −1.00 × 10
   OS   +1.00 = −1.00 × 165

2. OD   +1.00 sph
   OS   +1.00 sph

3. OD   +0.50 sph
   OS   +0.50 sph

Patient was 20/20 with each—most comfortable with +1.00 sph OU. Range adequate for patient's near needs.

- TF +2.00 OU for near; patient reports clear, comfortable vision for reading, but blurry at the computer screen. TF +1.75 OU and +1.50 OU for computer; patient most comfortable with +1.50 OU at CRT.
- TF +0.25 OU and +0.50 OU over patient's current near glasses; patient prefers +0.50 OU.

III. SIDE TRIPS FROM THE ROUTINE DISTANCE SUBJECTIVE REFRACTION

Clock Chart (Sunburst Dial)

PURPOSE   To determine the cylindrical component of the refractive error by a subjective technique.

INDICATIONS

The clock chart is performed if 20/20 VA cannot be achieved with spherical lenses and the starting points of the refraction do not indicate a need for cylinder. It is also indicated if there is reason to believe that the tentative cylindrical correction from the static retinoscopy is inaccurate. The clock chart is done one eye at a time.

STEP-BY-STEP PROCEDURE

1. Remove any cylinder that may have been in the phoropter and fog the eye to a VA of 20/40 with spherical lenses.
2. Show the patient the clock chart (see Figure 3–17).
3. Ask the patient to identify the darkest, sharpest set of lines in the clock chart according to their position on the face of a clock e.g., 2 and 8 o'clock, 3 and 9 o'clock. If all the lines appear equally blurry, the test is terminated. Return to step 12 of the routine distance subjective refraction.
4. If one set of lines appears clearer or darker than the others, set the AXIS of the minus cylinder in the phoropter to *30* times the smaller o'clock from the patient's report e.g., if the patient reports the 2 and 8 o'clock lines are darkest, set the cylinder axis to 30 × 2 = 60° on the phoropter. This is known as the *rule of thirty.*
5. If two sets of lines seem about equally dark or sharp, select an axis value midway between e.g., if 1 and 7 and 2 and 8 are equally sharp, set the cylinder axis to 30 × 1.5 = 45° on the phoropter.

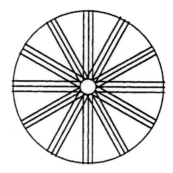

Figure 3–17. Diagram of a typical clock dial, clock chart, or sunburst dial target.

6. Add −0.25 D cylinder power. Again ask the patient if one set of lines is clearer or darker than the others.
7. If the patient still reports that one set of lines is clearer or darker than the others, repeat step 6. If the patient reports that all of the lines are about equally sharp and dark or if a different set of lines becomes sharper and/or darker, return to step 12 of the monocular distance subjective refraction. *Note*: In the clock chart test it is not necessary to maintain the spherical equivalent of the starting point.

Jackson Cross Cylinder (JCC) Check Test for Uncorrected Astigmatism

PURPOSE   To test for the presence of a small amount of uncorrected astigmatism.

INDICATIONS

The JCC check test is indicated if the starting techniques of the refraction show no need for cylinder in the correction but the patient does not achieve sharp vision with a spherical correction.

SET-UP

• The phoropter contains the sphere from the end of the initial MPMVA.

STEP-BY-STEP PROCEDURE

1. Place −0.50 D of cylinder in the phoropter and remove −0.25 D from (add +0.25 to) the sphere in the phoropter.
2. Using the JCC lens, do a power check on the cylinder at axis 180, 45, 90, and 135. If the letters appear clearer to the patient with the minus-cylinder axis of the JCC aligned with the axis of cylinder in the phoropter, do not test the other axes. Leave the cylinder power in the phoropter and return to step 13 of the distance subjective refraction.
3. If the letters appear clearer to the patient when the plus-cylinder axis of the JCC is aligned with each of the four axes of cylinder in the phoropter, the patient probably has no significant uncorrected astigmatism. Continue with step 12 of the distance subjective refraction.

Prism-Dissociated Duochrome Test

PURPOSE To equalize the stimulus to accommodation for the two eyes.

INDICATIONS

Perform the prism-dissociated duochrome test at the conclusion of the monocular subjective refraction of the left eye only if the two eyes did not reach equal VAs during their monocular refractions *and* there is reason to believe that the accommodation differs in the two eyes.

STEP-BY-STEP PROCEDURE

1. Make sure neither eye is occluded and that both eyes can see the visual acuity chart on the screen.
2. Isolate a line of letters one line above the VA of the poorer seeing eye at the end of the monocular subjective refractions. Fogging lenses are not added.
3. Place the red-green filter over the isolated line of letters.
4. Using the phoropter's Risley prisms, place 3 to 4Δ BU over the right eye and 3 to 4Δ BD over the left eye.
5. Inform the patient that he should see two lines of red-green letters. Make certain that this is the case.
6. Direct the patient's attention to the lower line of letters.
7. Tell the patient to look from the green side to the red side and back to the green side. Have him state which side has the sharper, clearer (not "better," darker, or brighter) letters or to state if the two sides are equally clear.
8. If the letters on the red side are clearer or if the letters on both sides are equally clear, introduce an additional 0.25 D of minus spherical power. If the letters on the green side are clearer, take away 0.25 D of minus (or add another 0.25 D of plus-sphere).
9. Direct the patient's attention to the upper line of letters and repeat step 7 and 8.
10. Repeat steps 6 through 9 until the patient is one into the green, the min-

imum amount of minus power at which the patient reports the green side has the clearer letters, for both the upper and the lower line letters. As an alternative endpoint use a red-green balance, the point at which both sides appear equally clear, rather than one into the green.

11. Remove the red-green filter and recheck the VA in each eye separately and in both together.

    Note: Some patients always seem to choose either the red or the green side regardless of the lens powers in place. Be alert to the possibility that your patient is unresponsive to the duochrome test and abandon it in favor of the smaller/darker endpoint for each eye separately (see step 31b). If this side trip was taken, the subjective distance refraction is completed. Record the results.

Sighting-Dominance Check

PURPOSE   To identify the patient's sighting-dominant eye.

INDICATIONS

A sighting-dominance check is performed when a subjective match in the clarity of the two lines of letters is not achieved during the binocular balance, even though the two eyes are correctable to the same VA under monocular conditions.

EQUIPMENT

- No special equipment is needed, although sighting-dominance typically will be performed with the patient looking through the phoropter.

SET-UP

- Have the patient form a triangular "window," 5 cm or 2 in on a side, with his hands.

STEP-BY-STEP PROCEDURE

1. Instruct the patient to extend his arms fully in front of him, and, with both eyes open, to look at your dominant eye through the window he has made with his hands.
2. Note which eye the patient uses to look at your eye. This is his sighting-dominant eye. Leave this eye with the slightly clearer vision during the binocular balance when the patient is unable to match the clarity of his two eyes.
3. Return to step 41 of the binocular balance.

Trial Frame Refraction

PURPOSE   To determine the refractive state of the eye when a phoropter is un-
available or contraindicated. The trial frame is also used to confirm
and modify phoropter-based refraction results.

INDICATIONS

This method of refraction is particularly useful with patients having high refractive errors (including aphakes), low vision, accommodative instability, or ambulatory restrictions.

Note: The technique described here is a modification of a phoropter-based refraction. It is critical to point out that substeps of the procedure may be applied or eliminated depending on the patient and the refractive error. The substep sequence may
also be modified to enhance the efficiency of the trial frame refraction. Prior to
reading this section, the examiner should be thoroughly familiar with routine distance subjective refraction with the phoropter.

EQUIPMENT

- Trial frame.
- Retinoscopy rack.
- Trial lens kit.
- Hand held Jackson Cross Cylinder (JCC): Hand held JCCs come in a variety of
  powers. The power used will depend on the patient's acuity level. For patients
  with normal acuity, a ± 0.25 D JCC is recommended.

SET-UP

- Have the patient remove any corrective lenses.
- Place the trial frame on the patient. Be certain to adjust the trial frame so that it
  sits comfortably on the patient's face and the patient's eyes are centered relative
  to the lens wells of the frame. This requires adjustment of the following (see Figure 3–18):
  a. the temple length to minimize vertex distance.
  b. the frame height via the nose pad adjustment.
  c. the pantoscopic tilt and leveling of the frame.
  d. the interpupillary distance.

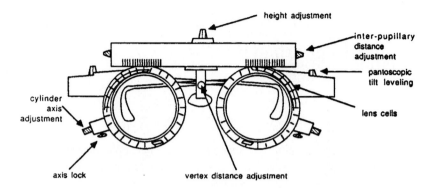

Figure 3–18. Schematic diagram of a typical trial frame with the adjustment mechanisms labeled.

- Fixation target: 20/400 E projected through a red-green filter. An illustration of the trial frame on the patient is shown in Figure 3–19.

STEP-BY-STEP PROCEDURE

Retinoscopy

1. Tell the patient to look at the large E, or another large, nonaccommodative target.
2. The retinoscope should be held at the examiner's customary working distance.
3. Using the retinoscopy rack neutralize the patient's right eye:
   a. locate the two major meridians.
   b. determine the power required to obtain neutrality in each meridian.
4. Calculate and place the gross retinoscopy finding for the right eye into the trial frame. The lenses should be placed in the trial frame with the sphere in the lens cell closest to the patient (behind the facade of the trial frame), and the cylinder in the next closest cell (located in the front of the trial frame) (see Figure 3–20). Adjust the cylinder to the appropriate axis. The lens cell closest to the patient approximates the vertex distance of a spectacle correction.
5. Perform retinoscopy on the left eye repeating steps 3 and 4.
6. With your gross retinoscopy finding for the left eye in the trial frame, recheck the right eye for neutrality.
7. Change the lenses in the trial frame so your net retinoscopy findings are in place.
8. Take and record monocular VAs and record the net retinoscopy findings in minus cylinder form.

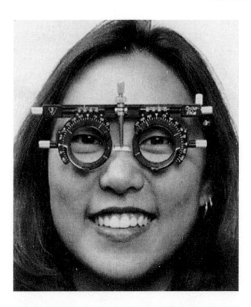

Figure 3–19. Patient wearing a trial frame. The patient's eyes should be centered in the lens apertures and the temples adjusted to provide a snug fit.

Monocular Subjective Refraction

9. Occlude the patient's left eye.
10. Perform an initial MPMVA on the right eye leaving the patient over-minused by 0.25 D or one into the green. This may be done by using hand held lenses (several in one hand, eg, +0.25, +0.50, +0.75), or a lens rack. Modify the sphere in the trial frame to reflect the results of the MPMVA.
11. Perform the JCC test using a hand held JCC. To increase manual control, a long handled JCC is recommended.
12. Refine the cylinder axis by flipping the JCC in front of the trial frame with the axis of the cross cylinders 45° away from the correcting cylinder axis. This is generally the case when the handle of the JCC is aligned with the correcting cylinder axis. Rotate the lens cell of the trial frame to change the cylinder axis.
13. Refine the cylinder power using the JCC. Adjust the power of the cylinder in the trial frame. Unnecessary lens changes may be avoided by changing the cylinder power in the trial frame by an amount equal to twice the power of the JCC. For example, if a ±0.25 D JCC is being used, and the patient prefers minus, add −0.50 D to the correcting cylinder and maintain the spherical equivalent by adding +0.25 D (or removing −0.25D) to the sphere. If on the next comparison the patient prefers minus you will have saved a step. Similarly, if the patient prefers plus, you can extrapolate that the endpoint is 0.25 D less minus.

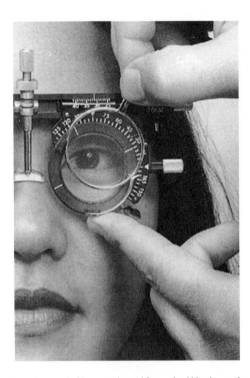

Figure 3–20. The insertion and removal of lenses in the trial frame should be done with care. The sphere is placed in the lens cell behind the facade of the frame and the cylinder in the cell before the facade.

14. Perform an MPMVA using loose lenses or a lens rack and make the final adjustment to the spherical component of the patient's correction.
15. Record your monocular subjective results and the VA for the right eye.
16. Occlude the right eye and repeat steps 10 through 15 for the left eye.

Binocular Balance

Perform this step only if each eye achieved the same VA following the monocular subjective refraction. As with a phoropter-based refraction, the binocular balance may be done via prism dissociation using the loose prisms included in the trial lens kit. The technique described here, the alternate occlusion method, is preferred for a trial frame refraction. Although it is not quite as precise as the prism-dissociation method, it is less cumbersome.

17. Make sure neither eye is occluded and both eyes can see the VA chart. Fog with +0.75 D OU and take the VA.
18. Direct the patient's attention to a single line of letters, one line above the patient's best VA. If you are using a projector and VA slide, isolate the line.

19. Cover the patient's left eye and then move the occluder to the right eye.
20. Ask the patient through which eye the target appears clearer.
21. Add +0.25 D to the better seeing eye.
22. Repeat steps 19 through 21 until the two eyes are equally clear or a reversal occurs. If a reversal occurs, select the dioptral values for which the clarity of the images in the two eyes is closest.
23. Perform a binocular MPMVA using loose lenses in each hand.
24. Measure and record the VA for the right eye, the left eye, and both eyes.

RECORDING

• Record the technique used.
• Record the final correction for the left eye and the right eye.
• Record the VA for the left eye, the right eye, and both eyes.

EXAMPLE

• Trial Frame Refraction:

Static:	OD	$-3.00 = -0.50 \times 135$	$20/20^{-1}$
	OS	$-2.75 = -0.50 \times 45$	20/20
Subj:	OD	$-2.75 = -0.50 \times 130$	20/20
	OS	$-2.25 = -0.50 \times 50$	20/20
	OU		20/20

Note: Recommendations for performing efficient trial frame refractions:
• Avoid changing the lenses in the cells of the trial frame. This may be accomplished by holding lenses in front of the trial frame, rather than placing lenses in the lens cells. Learn to insert and remove lenses smoothly to promote patient comfort.
• If the patient has reduced acuity, be sure to use lens increments and JCC powers that allow the patient to make comparative judgments. For example, if a patient can only see 20/40 try using a ±0.50 D JCC instead of a ±0.25 D or ±0.37 D JCC.

Stenopaic Slit Refraction

PURPOSE   To subjectively determine the power required to correct the refractive error of each major meridian individually.

INDICATIONS

The stenopaic slit refraction is useful for confirming the results of other refraction techniques for patients with irregular astigmatism or reduced visual acuity. It is helpful for patients who have difficulty understanding the complex instructions associated with other subjective techniques.

It is important to note that, like the pinhole, the stenopaic slit may be used diagnostically to determine a patient's potential visual acuity.

EQUIPMENT

- Trial frame.
- 1-mm stenopaic slit (2 to 3 slits of various widths are usually included in trial lens kits).
- Trial lens kit or lens rack.
- Distance visual acuity chart.

SET-UP

- Place the trial frame on the patient's face so the patient is comfortable and his eyes are centered relative to the lens wells (see the section on trial frame refraction).
- Project the visual acuity chart. Expose a range of letters in which the patient's best known acuity corresponds to the lowest line. For example, if the patient's VA is 20/40, expose lines ranging from 20/70 down to 20/40.

STEP-BY-STEP PROCEDURE

1. Occlude the patient's left eye.
2. Using a lens rack, perform an MPMVA on the right eye.
3. Add +1.00 to +1.50 diopters to the result found in step 2 and place a lens of this power in the rear cell of the trial frame.
4. Place a 1-mm wide stenopaic slit in the trial frame in front of the fog-

ging lens. If the patient's acuity is significantly reduced, it may be necessary to use a wider slit.

5. Rotate the slit until the position of best acuity is found. At this time, the slit will run parallel to the axis of the correcting minus cylinder.

6. Decrease the fog, using a lens rack, until MPMVA is achieved.

7. The combined power of the lens in the lens rack and the fogging lens is the correction for the meridian that runs parallel to the stenopaic slit. Record the power and the meridian on an optical cross.

8. Remove the lens rack from in front of the eye and rotate the stenopaic slit until the position of worst acuity is found. If this is not 90° away from the meridian found in step 5, an irregular astigmatism is present.

9. Again, reduce the fog using an MPMVA.

10. Record the resulting power and meridian as in step 7.

11. Calculate the resulting spherocylindrical correction and place the correction in the trial frame. Remember to remove the stenopaic slit and the fogging lens. If an irregular astigmatism is present, the resulting spherocylindrical correction may be determined by placing two cylinders in a trial frame and measuring the total power through the lensometer or by calculating the result using a formula for obliquely crossed cylinders.

12. Measure the patient's VA for the right eye.

13. Occlude the patient's right eye and repeat steps 2 through 12 for the left eye.

RECORDING

- Record the refraction technique used.
- If the patient has a regular astigmatism, record the spherocylindrical correction in minus cylinder form for each eye.
- If the patient has an irregular astigmatism record the correction for the major meridians separately.
- Record the visual acuity for each eye.

EXAMPLE

- Refraction (Stenopaic Slit)

OD	+1.00 = −1.00 × 90	20/20+2
OS	+0.75 = −1.25 × 90	20/20+1

- Refraction (Stenopaic Slit)

OD	−3.50 at 170, −5.75 at 105	20/70
OS	−4.00 at 160, −5.00 at 80	20/40

Note: "at" indicates the meridian of power, not the axis.

Cycloplegic Refraction

PURPOSE   To measure a patient's refractive error in the absence of accommodation. This is accomplished through the use of cycloplegic drugs that paralyze the ciliary body.

INDICATIONS

This procedure is useful when it is suspected that the patient has latent hyperopia, a strabismus of accommodative etiology, any strabismus in a child, an accommodative spasm, or when visual symptoms or visual acuity do not match objective assessment of the condition of the tissues of the eye or refractive measures. Cycloplegic refractions are most frequently used for examining children, and some authors recommend that the procedure be performed on all children under the age of 3. The examiner who elects to perform cycloplegic refractions must be aware of the contraindications and side effects of the drug selected for this purpose.
Note: Parental consent should be obtained prior to performing this technique on a child.

EQUIPMENT

- Retinoscope.
- Phoropter.
- Distance visual acuity chart.
- Topical anesthetic.
- Cycloplegic agent: Agents that may be used include cyclopentolate 1.0%, cyclopentolate 0.5% (particularly with infants), atropine 0.5% or 1.0%, scopolamine 0.25%, or homatropine 2% or 5%. Cyclopentolate 1.0% is recommended for routine cycloplegic refractions on patients above the age of 2 years. Atropine 0.5% or 1.0% should be used when absolute cycloplegia is called for, for example, in cases of preschool children with accommodative esotropia. Tropicamide 1.0% has been shown to be an effective cycloplegic agent in myopic children.

SET-UP

- A complete eye exam, including a "dry" (i.e., done without cycloplegic) refraction, should be conducted prior to cycloplegia. A postcycloplegic refraction is often done at a second visit.

STEP-BY-STEP PROCEDURE

1. Check the intraocular pressure and the anterior chamber angles of both eyes prior to instilling drops. These tests serve to rule out the risk of angle closure due to the mydriatic effect of cycloplegic agents. If the anterior chamber angle is estimated at less than 1\4 using the van Herick angle estimation technique, gonioscopy must be performed prior to inducing cycloplegia.
2. Instill one drop of topical anesthetic into the inferior cul-de-sac of each eye.
3. Instill two drops (gtts) of 1.0% cyclopentolate. Allow 5 minutes between drops. Maximum cycloplegia with cyclopentolate occurs 10 to 40 minutes after the instillation of drops.
4. Check each eye for cycloplegia after 30 minutes. There are several ways this may be done. Two are described here.
   a. Ask the patient to focus on an accommodative target set at a distance of 1 meter. Determine the accommodative near point using a push-up amplitude of accommodation technique. If there is adequate cycloplegia there should be less than two diopters of accommodation remaining prior to beginning the refraction.
   b. If the patient is too young to respond to the above procedure, the examiner can screen for accommodative activity with a retinoscope.
5. Perform retinoscopy or a monocular subjective refraction on both eyes using routine techniques.
6. Following the cycloplegic refraction recheck the intraocular pressure in both eyes.

RECORDING

- When using pharmacological agents always record the agent, concentration, number of drops, and time administered.
- Record the refraction technique, the correction found, and the resulting VA.

EXAMPLE

- Cycloplegic refraction:

1 gtt Ophthaine 0.5%, 2 gtts Cyclogel 1% @ 10:00 AM

Static:	OD	$+8.50 = -1.50 \times 95$	20/30+
	OS	$+7.00 = -1.00 \times 90$	20/20+
Subj:	OD	$+8.00 = -1.00 \times 90$	20/20
	OS	$+7.00 = -1.00 \times 90$	20/20
	OU		20/20

EXPECTED FINDINGS

- If routine refractive techniques were unable to relax the accommodative system, additional plus will be found in the spherical component of the patient's refraction under cycloplegia.
- Because of the high level of accommodative activity found in many children, the cylinder power measured during retinoscopy without cycloplegia is frequently inaccurate. The amount of cylinder found using cycloplegic drugs is likely to be more accurate.

Delayed Subjective Refraction

PURPOSE   To maximally relax a patient's accommodation and subsequently stimulate the acceptance of plus when determining the correction of a refractive error.

INDICATIONS

This technique is particularly useful for patients with suspected latent hyperopia or an accommodative spasm.

EQUIPMENT

- A phoropter with near point rod.
- Near point cards.
- Distance acuity chart.

SET-UP

- This technique is performed following a complete routine refraction.
- Perform the phorometry tests with the NRA test last (see Chapter 4).
- Leave the plus from the NRA test in the phoropter.

STEP-BY-STEP PROCEDURE

1. Isolate a line of letters equal to the patient's best distance acuity (but no smaller than 20/20).
2. Remove the near point rod and direct the patient to view the distance target. The patient should report that it is blurry.
3. Reduce the plus binocularly, in 0.25 D steps, until the letters are again clear.
4. Confirm the endpoint using the duochrome test (optional).

RECORDING

- Write "Delayed Subjective."
- Record the correction and the patient's visual acuities.

EXAMPLE

• Delayed Subjective:

OD	+1.50 = −0.75 × 175	20/15
OS	+1.25 = −0.25 × 010	20/15

EXPECTED FINDINGS

• If latent hyperopia or an accommodative spasm exists, this technique may produce a greater plus acceptance than was indicated by routine refractive procedures.

Convergence Controlled Refraction

PURPOSE To control the accommodative response by eliminating the convergence demand present in cases of high exophoria. Base in prism is used to neutralize the influence of the exo deviation. This technique may be performed alone or done in conjunction with the delayed refraction (Pierce-Borish test). The Pierce-Borish test is described here.

INDICATIONS

This technique is useful for patients with suspected accommodative dysfunction secondary to a high exophoria.

EQUIPMENT

- Phoropter with near point rod.
- Near point cards.
- Distance acuity chart.

SET-UP

- This technique is performed following a complete routine refraction.
- Perform the phorometry tests with the NRA test last (see Chapter 4).
- Leave the plus from the NRA test in the phoropter.

STEP-BY-STEP PROCEDURE

1. Reduce the plus in the phoropter by −0.25 D to allow the patient to clear the near target.
2. Using the Risley prisms, gradually introduce base in prism binocularly until the patient again reports a blur.
3. Remove the near point rod, leaving the plus and the base in prism in place.
4. Present a distance target consisting of an isolated line of letters equal to the patient's best distance acuity level.
5. Direct the patient to view the target, letting him know it may be quite blurry.

6. Leaving the prism in place, reduce the fog in both eyes simultaneously using 0.25 D steps until the letters are clear.
7. Confirm your endpoint with the duochrome test (optional).

RECORDING

- Record the technique used:
  a. Pierce-Borish Test
  b. Delayed Ref. with BI Prism
- Record the correction obtained and the patient's visual acuities.

EXAMPLE

- Refraction (Delayed with BI prism)

OD	+2.50 sphere	20/20
OS	$+2.00 = -0.50 \times 90$	20/20

EXPECTED FINDINGS

- The presence of an accommodative spasm may be confirmed if this technique yields a greater plus acceptance than that obtained using routine refraction techniques.

Binocular Refraction With the Vectographic Slide

PURPOSE To permit monocular refraction under binocular viewing conditions. Through the use of polarization, separate targets are shown simultaneously to the left and right eyes. The active involvement of the convergence system helps to stabilize accommodation.

INDICATIONS

Binocular refraction techniques are used as an alternative to the monocular subjective refraction with accompanying binocular balance. Due to the presence of binocularity during the refraction, this approach offers greater control of accommodation and a more accurate endpoint for the cylinder axis than a monocular subjective procedure. This method requires that a patient have binocular vision.

EQUIPMENT

- Phoropter with polarized filters.
- AO vectographic projector slide (see Figure 3–21).

SET-UP

- The patient should be comfortably positioned behind the phoropter. Take care to ensure that the phoropter and the patient are level. If there is misalignment, the effectiveness of the polarizing filters will decrease.
- Do not put the polarizing filters in place.
- Place the vectographic slide in the projector with the first line (20/200) projected. Without the polarizers, this will be seen by both eyes and is an appropriate fixation target for retinoscopy.

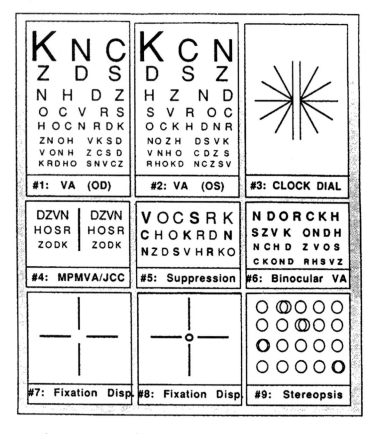

Figure 3–21. Schematic representation of the AO vectographic slide for adults. Each subchart has been numbered and labeled to coincide with the text.

STEP-BY-STEP PROCEDURES

Retinoscopy

1. Perform retinoscopy using the routine technique.
2. Remove your working distance so your net retinoscopy finding is in the phoropter.
3. Put the polarizing filters in place.
4. Check the patient's VAs in each eye. (The subchart numbers in the text refer to those illustrated in Figure 3–21.) Through the polarizers, the patient will see the first chart (#1) with his right eye and the second chart (#2) with his left eye.
5. Record your net retinoscopy and the patient's visual acuities.

Subjective Refraction

Clock Dial

This step in the refraction is optional. If the cylinder found with retinoscopy appears reasonably accurate or the acuity obtained with a spherical result is good (20/20 or better), the clock dial may be skipped. Proceed to step 13.

6. Remove the cylinder found with retinoscopy and fog the patient to 20/40 in each eye.
7. Expose the clock dial target (#3). The right eye will see the right side of the target and the left eye will see the left.
8. Direct the patient's attention to the right side of the clock dial.
9. Perform the clock dial test on the right eye.
10. Direct the patient's attention to the left side of the clock dial.
11. Perform the clock dial test on the left eye.

Bi-ocular MPMVA

12. Change the target to chart #4. The letters on the right side are seen only by the right eye. The letters on the left are seen only by the left eye.
13. Direct the patient's attention to the three lines on the right.
14. Perform an MPMVA test on the right eye.
15. Add one extra 0.25 D of minus in preparation for the Jackson Cross Cylinder test.
16. Direct the patient's attention to the three lines on the left.
17. Repeat steps 14 and 15 for the left eye.

Jackson Cross Cylinder

18. Isolate the line one line above the patient's best VA. If one of the three lines on chart #4 is not large enough, use the larger acuity charts (#1 and #2), although this is likely to decrease the patient's stimulus to fusion and accommodative stability.
19. Direct the patient's attention to the letters on the right and modify the correcting cylinder axis and power for the right eye using the JCC test.
20. Redirect the patient's attention to the letters on the left and modify the correcting cylinder axis and power for the left eye using the JCC test.

Bi-ocular MPMVA

21. Expose all three lines of chart #4.
22. Fog the patient binocularly with +0.75 D.
23. Perform an MPMVA on the right eye.
24. Perform an MPMVA on the left eye.

Binocular MPMVA

25. Go to chart #6 (four lines, 20/30 to 20/15, seen binocularly).
26. Fog the patient with +0.75 D spheres over both eyes and perform a binocular MPMVA to obtain the final sphere value.

RECORDING

- Specify the technique used for refraction.
- Record the patient's final correction.
- Record the visual acuities for the right eye, the left eye, and both eyes.

EXAMPLE

- Binocular Refraction (Vectographic)

OD	+4.00 sph	20/20
OS	+3.50 = −0.50 × 180	20/20
OU		20/15

EXPECTED FINDINGS

The refraction results for this technique are very similar to those obtained using a monocular subjective technique with a binocular balance. The spherical value may contain an additional +0.25 D. In patients with a cyclophoria, the cylinder axis may shift by as much as 5°.

Note: The vectographic slide comes with several other targets. These allow the examiner to evaluate a patient's binocular function at distance. Included are checks for suppression, the associated phoria with and without a central fusion stimulus, and stereopsis charts. It is also possible to screen for aniseikonia by comparing the two sides of chart #4.

Humphriss Immediate Contrast Method

PURPOSE   To allow for a subjective refraction under conditions that maintain peripheral fusion while testing foveal vision monocularly. This is accomplished by placing a fogging lens over the nontested eye to induce suppression of its central retina. Nonfoveal zones remain binocularly active and stabilize accommodation.

Note: This is generally considered a method of refinement, with retinoscopy or monocular subjective findings used as a starting point. The method described below uses retinoscopy as the starting point and assumes the visual acuity in each eye through the net static to be 20/20.

EQUIPMENT

- Distance acuity chart.
- Phoropter or trial frame.

SET-UP

- Perform retinoscopy. For the Humphriss technique to be successful, the retinoscopy findings must be reasonably accurate, within 0.50 D of neutrality.
- Place your net retinoscopy findings in the phoropter. Neither eye should be occluded.
- Display the distance visual acuity chart with the 20/15 to 20/50 lines exposed.

STEP-BY-STEP PROCEDURE

1. Place a +0.75 D fogging lens over the net retinoscopy finding of the left eye. The patient's visual acuity in the fogged eye should be either 20/30 or 20/40. This is checked quickly by briefly occluding the right eye and asking the patient to read the lowest line of letters he can.
2. Take the patient's acuity for the right eye through the net retinoscopy finding. Both eyes are open from this point on.

3. Fog the patient's right eye by adding +0.75 D of sphere and perform an MPMVA.
4. Isolate the 20/30 line.
5. Place an additional +0.25 D sphere over the right eye, then quickly replace this with a −0.25 D sphere. Ask the patient which lens makes the line of letters appear clearer. This is done most effectively by using loose lenses.
   a. If the patient reports that the −0.25 D sphere is clearer, add −0.25 D to the correction and continue step 5 until the two views appear equal.
   b. If the +0.25 is preferred, add a +0.25 to the correction and continue step 5. If on the next comparison the patient prefers the −0.25, add the −0.25 and proceed to step 6.
   c. If the two views appear equal, leave the correction as is and proceed to step 6.
6. Perform a cylinder axis check and power check using the JCC test.
7. Place +0.75 D fog in front of the right eye and proceed to refract the left eye.
8. Place an additional +0.25 D sphere over the left eye, quickly replace this with a −0.25 D sphere and ask the patient which lens makes the line of letters appear clearer. This is done most effectively by using loose lenses.
   a. If the patient reports that the −0.25 D sphere is clearer, add −0.25 D to the correction and continue step 8 until the two views appear equal.
   b. If the +0.25 is preferred, add a +0.25 to the correction and continue step 8. If on the next comparison the patient prefers the −0.25, add −0.25 and proceed to step 9.
   c. If the two views appear equal, leave the correction as is and proceed to step 9.
9. Perform a cylinder axis check and power check using the JCC test.
10. Remove the +0.75 D fogging lenses from both the patient's right and left eye.
11. Take the patient's VA for the right eye, the left eye, and both eyes.

RECORDING

• Specify the type of refraction performed.
• Record the patient's final correction and visual acuities.

EXAMPLE

• Binocular Refraction /Humphriss Immediate Contrast Method

OD	$-3.50 = -1.00 \times 45$	20/20+
OS	$-2.75 = -1.25 \times 135$	20/20+
OU		20/15+

EXPECTED FINDINGS

- Due to the binocular conditions under which the refraction occurs, there may be some additional plus acceptance and a small change in the cylinder axis to compensate for a cyclophoria.

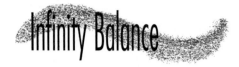

Infinity Balance

Based on "Turville Infinity Balance" as modified by Morgan, using a septum and a projected chart (rather than mirrors).

 To refine the refraction (sphere power and/or cylinder axis and power) at distance under binocular conditions when there is reason to believe that any of these parameters may differ from the results obtained during monocular refraction.

EQUIPMENT

- Phoropter.
- Septum of the proper width (preferably of the same color as the screen)—see calculations below.
- Rod or stand to hold the septum.

SET-UP

- In the phoropter, both eyes start with the results of the routine distance refraction, or, alternatively, with the retinoscopy results.
- Set the phoropter to the patient's far PD.
- Mount the septum on the rod or stand so that half of the distance VA chart is visible to each eye and the other half is occluded for each eye. The formulas necessary to calculate the distance of the stand from the patient and the width of the septum follow the examples of recording.

STEP-BY-STEP PROCEDURE

1. By alternately occluding each eye, determine that the septum is properly positioned such that half of the distance VA chart is visible to each eye and the other half is occluded for each eye. Note that if the patient has a lateral phoria at distance, the two halves of the chart will either appear separated in space or overlapping; if the patient has a vertical phoria, the halves of the chart may not appear at the same height. These variations

may be ignored provided at least two letters of each line are visible to each eye but to one eye only.

2. Adjust the projector slide so that the highest 20/20 line of letters is at the bottom of the chart.
3. If acuity is equal in both eyes, alternately add +0.25 of fog to each eye until the patient reports that both eyes are blurred (i.e., that each half of the chart is blurred).
4. Check for binocular balance.
    a. If the two halves of the chart are equal, alternately unfog (MPMVA) to best visual acuity in each eye, checking balance as you go.
    b. If the two halves of the chart are not equally blurry, adjust the sphere until they are balanced and slightly blurry; then alternately unfog (MPMVA) to best visual acuity in each eye, checking balance as you go.

RECORDING

- Indicate that the Infinity Balance (IB) technique was used.
- For each eye record the final Rx for sphere, cyl power, and cyl axis and monocular VAs.

EXAMPLE

- IB refraction

OD −2.50=−0.50 ×95	20/20
OS −1.75 sph	20/15

To Calculate Septum Distance and Width

1. Determine in centimeters for all measurements:
    D = the distance of the chart from the patient
    S = half the width of the visual acuity chart
    PD = the patient's PD
2. Calculate the necessary distance of the septum from the patient in centimeters by the following formula:

    Y (the distance) = (PD times D) divided by (S + PD) or
    $Y = (PD \times D) \neq (S + PD)$

3. Calculate the necessary septum width in centimeters by the following formula:

    X (septum width) = S times Y divided by D or
    $X = S \times Y/D$

Mohindra's Near Retinoscopy

PURPOSE   To determine the patient's distance refractive error while using the light of the retinoscope as the fixation target.

INDICATIONS

Although this method may be used with adults, it is particularly useful for determining the refractive error of infants and toddlers.

EQUIPMENT

* Retinoscope.
* Lens rack.

SET-UP

* The examiner should be 50 cm from the patient. During this procedure the examiner may use the same eye to examine both eyes of the patient.
* The room should be completely darkened.
* Set the intensity of the retinoscope to a level that allows for observation of the reflex without being aversive to the patient.

STEP-BY-STEP PROCEDURE

1. Occlude the left eye and test the right eye.
2. If you are examining an infant, the child will tend to fixate the light. If this does not occur, stimulate the child's attention by making sounds. If you are using this method on an older child or adult, instruct the patient to look at the light.
3. Scan and identify the major meridians.
4. Using a lens rack identify the power that neutralizes each meridian.
5. Calculate your gross retinoscopy finding in minus cylinder form.
6. Add a -1.25 D sphere to the spherical component of your findings. The resultant spherocylinder represents the patient's *distance* correction.
   Note: The -1.25 D sphere represents an empirically defined constant.

Consider adjusting the gross findings by -1.00 for children and -0.75 or -1.00 for infants, rather than using -1.25 for all patients.
7. Occlude the patient's right eye.
8. Repeat steps 2 through 6 for the left eye.
9. Take the patient's distance visual acuity through the resultant correction if it is possible to do so.

RECORDING

- Write "Mohindra's Near Retinoscopy."
- Record the correction and VA (if obtainable) for the right eye and for the left eye.

EXAMPLE

Mohindra's Near Retinoscopy

OD	$+1.00 = -0.50 \times 80$	VA unobtainable
OS	$+1.50$ sph	

Determining the Add for the Presbyope

PURPOSE To determine the near prescription for the presbyopic patient.
Note: Near corrections are generally prescribed based on the final distance refraction. The add is the difference between the distance correction and the near correction.

EQUIPMENT

- Phoropter with a near point rod.
- Trial frame.
- Trial lens set.
- Near point card with small block of 20/30 letters.
- Near VA card.

SET-UP

- Complete the distance refraction and leave these lenses in the phoropter for subsequent testing. This provides the distance portion on which to base the final near prescription.
- Seat the patient behind the phoropter, which is set to his near PD.
- Place the near point card with a block of 20/30 letters on the near point rod at 40 cm from the patient.
- Brightly illuminate the near point card.

STEP-BY-STEP PROCEDURE

1. Select the tentative add. Choose the tentative add by one of the following techniques. The order of presentation here is not meant to imply order of preference.
   a. Age and refractive status (see Table 3–2).
   b. Fused cross cylinder (see procedure in Chapter 4). The endpoint of the fused cross cylinder technique can be used as the tentative add.

TABLE 3–2. TYPE OF LENSES USED FOR NEUTRALIZATIONS DURING STATIC RETINOSCOPY BASED ON THE MOTION OBSERVED, THE POSITION OF THE SLEEVE OF THE RETINOSCOPE, AND THE PATIENT'S REFRACTIVE ERROR

Refractive Error	Motion Seen With Plane Mirror Retinoscope (sleeve down)	Motion Seen With Short Concave Mirror Retinoscope (sleeve up)	Lens Power Needed for Neutralization
Emmetrope	Wiith	Against	+
Hyperope			
Low myope			
Myope> working distance	Against	With	−

c. *Half the amp in reserve* rule: Convert the patient's customary near working distance into its dioptric equivalent. From this quantity subtract 50% of the patient's amplitude of accommodation, as determined by the push-up method (see procedure in Chapter 2). The remainder can be used as the tentative add (see Figure 3–22).

d. Entering prescription and VA: Add +0.25 D to the patient's entering net near prescription, as determined by lensometry, for each line of reduction in the near VA below 20/20. If the distance prescription is to be changed, this change must be taken into account in calculating the tentative add (see Figure 3–23).

2. Refine the add: Algebraically add the NRA and PRA findings (see Chapter 4) and divide the sum by 2. Algebraically add the resulting quantity to the tentative add from step 1.

3. Finalize the add.

a. To this point, testing has been done at 40 cm. However, large individuals tend to hold reading material at distances greater than 40 cm and small individuals tend to hold reading material at distances closer than 40 cm. Assess the stature of the patient and adjust the add by decreasing it by +0.25 D for the large patient and increasing it by +0.25 D for the small patient.

b. Compare the adjusted, refined near prescription to the patient's entering near prescription. If you plan to increase the near prescription, the amount of the increase should be as small as possible and should correspond to the increase in near VA.

c. Trial frame the adjusted, refined near prescription.

d. Through this correction, take the near VA monocularly and binocularly. The best corrected VA at near should be equivalent to the best corrected distance VA. If it is not, consider increasing the add.

e. Measure the linear range of clear vision: Instruct the patient to bring some printed material in toward himself until it just blurs. Measure the distance from the trial frame to the printed material. Then, instruct the

Example #1

Tentative add (based on "half the amp in reserve" rule)

+ 2.50 D	Patient's customary working distance (16"), converted to diopters
- 1.50 D	50% of patient's amplitude of accommodation of 3.0 D, determined by push-up method
+ 1.00 D	Tentative add

Refining the add (by the NRA/PRA)

Example : NRA/PRA = +1.25 / -0.75 (test done through tentative add of +1.00)

+ 0.25 D	Algebraic sum of the NRA and PRA findings divided by 2
+ 1.00 D	Tentative add, from step 1
+ 1.25 D	Refined add

Finalizing the add

+ 1.25 D	Refined add from step 2
+ 0.25 D	Increase add by 0.25 D to compensate for patient's small stature
+ 1.50 D	Adjusted add, to be trial framed

Trial frame : +1.50 Add OD 20/20 @ 16"   range 10" - 28"
+1.50 Add OS 20/20 @ 16"

Near VA and range of clear vision are satisfactory to patient, so final add of +1.50 would be prescribed.

Figure 3–22. Example #1 illustrates how to determine a tentative add by leaving half the amplitude of accommodation in reserve.

patient to move the material away from himself until it just blurs. Measure this distance. Record the blur in point and the blur out point in inches or centimeters.

f. The patient's customary near working distance should be at the dioptric midpoint of the linear range of clear vision. Increase the add if the midpoint of the range is too far removed from the patient. Decrease the add if the midpoint of the range is too close to the patient.

g. Recheck the near VA through the final add. The VA at near should be equivalent to the distance VA. If it is not, consider increasing the add and repeat step 3.

Example #2

1. Tentative add (based on patient's near VA through old near Rx)

    +1.75 D   Patient's old net near Rx (from old distance Rx of +0.75, with + 1.00 add

    +0.50 D   Increase in net near Rx based on near VA of J2 through old Rx
    _____

    +2.25 D   Total near Rx needed

  - +1.00 D   New distance refraction
    _____

    +1.25 D   Tentative add

2. Refining the add (by the NRA/PRA)

    Example : NRA/PRA = +0.75 / -1.25 (test done through tentative add of +1.25)

      - 0.25 D   Algebraic sum of the NRA and PRA findings divided by 2

      + 1.25 D   Tentative add, from step 1
      _____

      + 1.00 D   Refined add

3. Finalizing the add

      + 1.00 D   Refined add from step 2

      Trial frame :   +1.00 Add   OD 20/20 @ 16"   range 12" - 24"
                      +1.00 Add   OS 20/20 @ 16"

      Near VA and range of clear vision are satisfactory to patient,
      so final add of +1.00 would be prescribed.

Figure 3–23. Example #2 illustrates how to determine a tentative add based on the patient's near visual acuity from his old near prescription.

  h. The add should be responsive to the patient's visual needs. The final considerations are patient comfort and satisfaction with the add.

RECORDING

- For each eye write the word "add" followed by the dioptric power of the final add (not the net near Rx).
- Record the near VA for each eye through the final add.
- Write "range OU."
- Record the distance from the patient at which print first began to blur when the patient, with both eyes unoccluded, brought the material toward himself. This is his near point through the add.

DETERMINING THE ADD FOR THE PRESBYOPE
at a glance

PURPOSE	TECHNIQUE
Select a tentative add (see Table 3-3)	• Age and refractive status • FCC • 1/2 amp in reserve • Rx + VA
Refine the add	Balance the NRA/PRA
Finalize the add	• Trial frame • Measure VA and range • Adjust Rx as needed

TABLE 3–3. TENTATIVE ADD AS A FUNCTION OF THE PATIENT'S AGE AND REFRACTIVE STATUS

Age	Myopia Emmetropia	Low Hyperopia	High Hyperopia
33–37	pl	pl	+0.75
38–43	pl	+0.75	+1.25
44–49	+0.75	+1.25	+1.75
50–56	+1.25	+1.75	+2.25
57–62	+1.75	+2.25	+2.50
63 and over	+2.25	+2.50	+2.50

- Write a dash.
- Record the distance from the patient at which the print first began to blur when the patient, with both eyes unoccluded, pushed the material away from himself. This is his far point through the add.

EXAMPLE

OD   add +1.25 VA 20/20 @16=
OS   add +1.25 VA 20/20 @16=
Range OU 10" − 21"

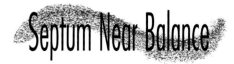

PURPOSE   To refine the cylinder axis and power at near when there is reason to believe that either may differ from the results of the distance refraction and/or refine the add when there is reason to believe the adds may differ between the two eyes.

EQUIPMENT

- Phoropter with near point rod.
- Near target for Septum Near Balance (SNB) (Figure 3–24).
- Septum for SNB (Figure 3–25)

SET-UP

- In the phoropter, both eyes start with the results of the distance refinements of the cylinder axis and power and the spheres either from binocular balance or from the refinement of the add.
- Set the phoropter to the patient's near PD.
- Mount the septum for SNB on the near point rod at about 20 cm from the phoropter.
- Mount the near target for SNB on the near point rod at 40 cm from the phoropter; make sure it is well illuminated.

STEP-BY-STEP PROCEDURE

Cylinder Refinement

1. With both eyes open, slowly slide the Septum toward the patient until the conditions as described on the card are satisfied; namely, that the right eye sees the words on the right, the left eye sees the words on the left, and both eyes see the words in the middle and at the bottom. For most PDs and a near target at 40 cm, this should occur when the septum is 15 to 25 cm from the phoropter.
2. Directing the patient's attention to the words on the right side of the near target for SNB, perform a Jackson Cross Cylinder axis refinement fol-

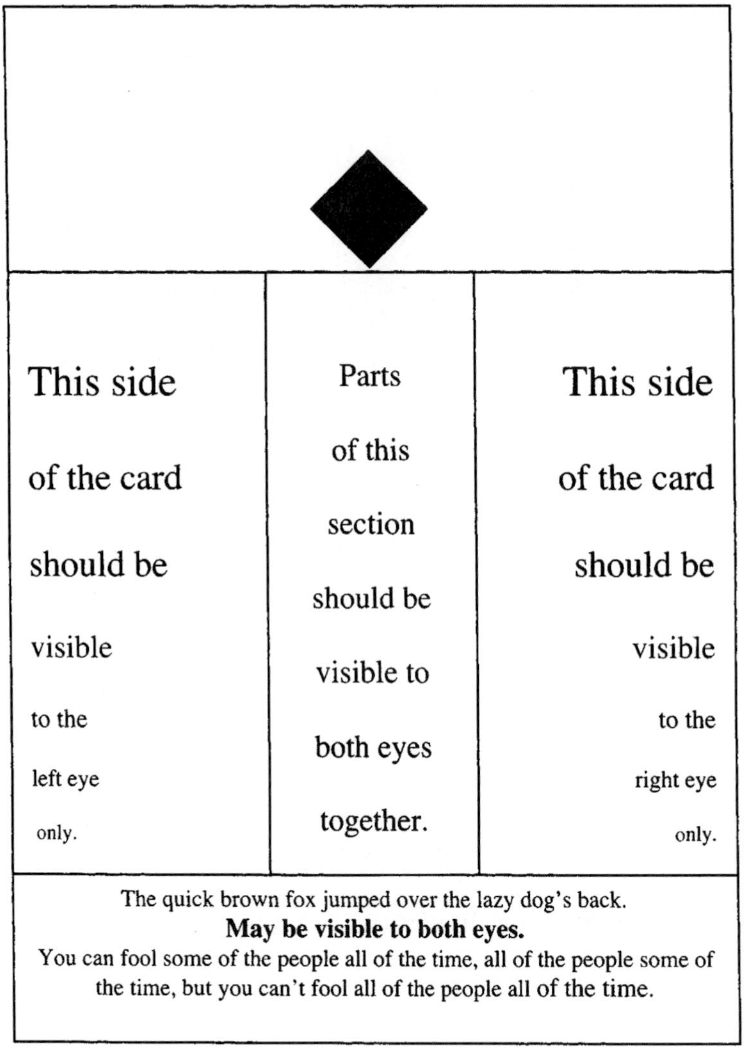

This side	Parts	This side
of the card	of this	of the card
should be	section	should be
visible	should be	visible
to the	visible to	to the
left eye	both eyes	right eye
only.	together.	only.

The quick brown fox jumped over the lazy dog's back.
May be visible to both eyes.
You can fool some of the people all of the time, all of the people some of the time, but you can't fool all of the people all of the time.

Figure 3–24. Near point card that may be used when performing the Septum Near Balance procedure.

lowed by a JCC for power refinement on the right eye according to the standard procedure.

3. Directing the patient's attention to the words on the left side of the near target for SNB, perform a Jackson Cross Cylinder axis refinement followed by a JCC for power refinement on the left eye according to the standard procedure.

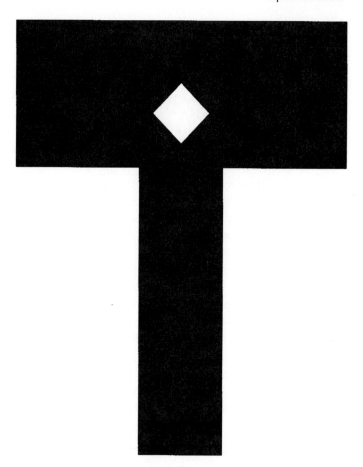

Figure 3–25. Septum for performing the Septum Near Balance procedure.

STEP-BY-STEP PROCEDURE

Monocular Add Determination

1. With both eyes open, slowly slide the Septum toward the patient until the conditions as described on the card are satisfied; namely, that the right eye sees the words on the right, the left eye sees the words on the left, and both eyes see the words in the middle and at the bottom. For most PDs and a near target at 40 cm, this should occur when the septum is 15 to 25 cm from the phoropter.
2. Directing the patient's attention to the words on the right side of the near target for SNB:

a. Add plus lenses over the right eye until the patient reports first sustained blur; note the amount of plus added relative to the starting point (distance refraction or tentative add).

b. Next add minus lenses over the right eye until the patient again reports sustained blur; note the amount of minus required relative to the starting point (distance refraction or tentative add).

c. Modify the tentative add so that the final add achieves a balance between the monocular plus to sustained blur and the monocular minus to sustained blur.

3. Directing the patient's attention to the words on the left side of the near target for SNB:

a. Add plus lenses over the left eye until the patient reports first sustained blur; note the amount of plus added relative to the starting point (distance refraction or tentative add).

b. Next add minus lenses over the left eye until the patient again reports sustained blur; note the amount of minus required relative to the starting point (distance refraction or tentative add).

c. Modify the tentative add so that the final add achieves a balance between the monocular plus to sustained blur and the monocular minus to sustained blur.

4. Have the patient compare the clarity of the letters on the right and left sides of the near target for SNB. If they are equally clear, stop. If they are unequal, add 0.25 of plus to the eye with the blurrier vision and recheck for equality.

RECORDING

- For each eye record the final near Rx for sphere, cylinder power, cylinder axis, and/or record the add.
- Measure and record the near VA for the OD, the OS, and for both eyes together.

EXAMPLE

- SNB: $OD-2.00 = -4.50 \times 87 + 1.50$ add VA: 20/20
          $OS +2.00 = -5.50 \times 103 + 2.00$ add VA: 20/20
                                              OU: 20/20

TO CALCULATE SEPTUM DISTANCE AND WIDTH (SAME FORMULAS AS FOR INFINITY BALANCE)

1. Determine in centimeters for all measurements:
   D = the distance of the chart from the patient
   S = half the width of the visual acuity chart
   PD = the patient's PD (*note:* in centimeters not in millimeters)

2. Calculate the necessary distance of the septum from the patient in centimeters by the following formula:

Y (the distance) = (PD times D) divided by (S + PD) or
$Y = (PD \times D)/(S + PD)$

3. Calculate the necessary septum width in centimeters by the following formula:

X (septum width) = S times Y divided by D or
$X = S \times Y/D$

TARGET AND SEPTUM

To create a target and septum, photocopy Figure 3–24 and Figure 3–25. Cut out the septum and target and mount them on thin cardboard or stiff paper, cutting out the diamond-shaped portion to allow them to slip over the near point rod. The septum length and/or width may need to be adjusted for particular phoropters.

Near Refinement of Cylinder Axis and Power Using the Borish Binocular Near Point Card

PURPOSE   To refine the cylinder axis and power under binocular conditions at near when there is reason to believe that either may differ from the results of the distance refraction and/or that the near cylinder axis or power may differ from the results of the distance refraction.

EQUIPMENT

- Phoropter with near point rod and Polaroid filters.
- Borish Binocular Near Point Card.

SET-UP

- In the phoropter, both eyes start with the results of the distance refinements of the cylinder axis and power and the spheres either from binocular balance or from the refinement of the add.
- Set the phoropter to the patient's near PD and insert the Polaroid filters over both apertures.
- Mount the Borish Binocular Near Point Card on the near point rod 40 cm from the phoropter with the three reduced Snellen charts facing the patient; make sure it is well illuminated.

STEP-BY-STEP PROCEDURE

1. Make sure that the patient sees all three reduced Snellen charts.
2. Direct the patient's attention to the right-hand chart and recheck his near acuity.
3. Direct the patient's attention to the line of letters one or two lines above his threshold acuity in his right eye.

4. Perform a standard Jackson Cross Cylinder refinement of cylinder axis followed by refinement of cylinder power of the right eye.
5. Upon completion of cylinder refinement of the right eye, direct the patient's attention to the left-hand chart and recheck his near acuity.
6. Direct the patient's attention to the line of letters one or two lines above his threshold acuity in his left eye.
7. Perform a standard Jackson Cross Cylinder refinement of cylinder axis followed by refinement of cylinder power of the left eye.

RECORDING

- For each eye record the final near Rx for sphere, cyl power, and cyl axis.
- Measure and record the near VA for the OD, the OS, and for both eyes together.

EXAMPLE

- Borish card: OD +4.00 =−1.00 × 85 = +2.00 add 20/20 @ 16″
  OS +3.50 =−1.25 × 100 = +2.00 add 20/20 @ 16″ NVO
  OU 20/20

Modified Humphriss for Near Refinement of Cylinder Axis and Power

PURPOSE
To refine the cylinder axis and power at near when there is reason to believe that either may differ from the results of the distance refraction.

EQUIPMENT

- Phoropter with near point rod.
- Reduced Snellen near point card.

SET-UP

- In the phoropter, both eyes start with the results of the distance refinements of the cylinder axis and power and the spheres either from binocular balance or from the refinement of the add.
- Set the phoropter to the patient's near PD.
- Mount the reduced Snellen near point card on the near point rod 40 cm from the phoropter; make sure it is well illuminated.

STEP-BY-STEP PROCEDURE

1. Occlude the OD.
2. At near, add plus over the OS until the patient is blurred to 20/40; this will typically take about 3.50 more plus than the distance subjective.
3. Unocclude the OD, leaving the OS open.
4. Make sure that the patient can read at least 20/30 with the OD on the near point card.
5. Directing the patient's attention to the 20/30 line on the card, perform a JCC for axis refinement followed by a JCC for power refinement on the OD.

6. Occlude the OS.
7. At near, add plus over the OD until the patient is blurred to 20/40; this will typically take about 3.50 more plus than the distance subjective.
8. Unocclude the OS, leaving the OD open.
9. Return the sphere power over the OS to the starting point (the results of the sphere either from binocular balance or from the refinement of the add).
10. Make sure that the patient can read at least 20/30 with the OS on the near point card.
11. Directing the patient's attention to the 20/30 line on the card, perform a JCC for axis refinement followed by a JCC for power refinement on the OS.

RECORDING

- For each eye record the final near Rx for sphere, cyl power, and cyl axis.
- Measure and record the near VA for the OD, the OS, and for both eyes together.

EXAMPLE

- OD +4.50 =−2.00 × 165 = +2.25 add 20/25 @ 16"
  OS +1.50 =−1.50 × 15 = +2.00 add 20/20 @ 16"NVO
  OU 20/20

FUNCTIONAL TESTS

Nancy B. Carlson, OD

CHAPTER AT A GLANCE

INTRODUCTION TO FUNCTIONAL TESTS

The evaluation of the patient's functional status consists of testing the accommodative system and the vergence system. To maintain clear, comfortable, binocular vision for all his visual tasks, a patient needs a number of well-functioning visual skills. The patient must be able to align his two eyes and maintain alignment for a sustained period of time. The patient must have sufficient accommodation to focus on the task and to sustain accommodation comfortably. The patient's accommodation must be accurate and efficient. Accommodation and convergence must interact appropriately. The techniques in this section allow the examiner to screen each of these visual skills and determine if the patient has a functional problem. These procedures allow the examiner to determine if the patient's functional problem can be corrected with a lens prescription, or if a more comprehensive binocular work-up or vision therapy is required.

Each examiner must decide which of these techniques to include in his core examination. The decision is based on the patient's age, symptoms, the results of the functional entrance tests, and the examiner's professional judgment. Because the functional test sequence is individualized, a flowchart with a main route and side trips is not included in this chapter (Table 4–1 provides a list of all functional tests and expected findings discussed in the chapter). This does not, however, imply that efficiency is not an important consideration. Once the examiner has selected the appropriate techniques to include, the following points are considered in determining the efficient flow of the functional testing. Tests done in the phoropter are done at the same time. Tests done out of the phoropter, or in free space, are done at the same time. Distance tests are grouped together and near tests are grouped together. Tests done through the same prescription are grouped together.

It is important to realize that the patient's prescription will influence the status of the accommodative and vergence systems. The examiner must take this into consideration and decide whether to do the tests through the patient's old correction (known as *habitual findings*), the correction found in the most recent subjective refraction (known as *induced findings*), or both.

TABLE 4–1. EXPECTED FINDINGS FOR FUNCTIONAL TESTS

Cover Test	1Δ XP (SD = 2Δ) at D; 3Δ XP (SD = 3Δ) at N
Near point of convergence	5 cm/7 cm
Stereopsis	20 seconds of arc
DLP (von Graefe)	1Δ exo
DVP (von Graefe)	Ortho
Horizontal vergences at D	Morgan's Expecteds
	BI X/7/4; BO 9/19/10
	Saladin and Sheedy
	BI X/8/5; BO 15/28/20
Vertical vergences at D	$3-4\Delta/1.5-2\Delta$
NLP (von Graefe)	3Δ exo
NVP (von Graefe)	Ortho
Horizontal vergences at N	Morgan's Expecteds
	BI 13/21/13; BO 17/21/12
	Saladin and Sheedy
	BI 14/19/13; BO 22/30/23
Vertical vergences at N	$3-4\Delta/1.5-2\Delta$
Vergence facility at N	12Δ BO/3Δ BI: 15 cycles/minute
Fused cross cylinder	+0.50 ($\pm$0.50 for nonpresbyopes)
NRA/PRA	+2.00 ($\pm$0.50)/-2.37 ($\pm$1.00)
Accommodative facility	Monocular
	Children 8–12 years: 7 cpm
	Adults: 11 cpm
	Binocular
	Children 8–12 years: 5 cpm
	Adults 13–30: 10 cpm
Dynamic retinoscopy (MEM)	+0.25 to +0.50
Dynamic retinoscopy (Bell)	17–14" to against/15–18" to with
Amp by minus lens method	2 D less Donders' Table

Distance Lateral Phoria by von Graefe Technique

PURPOSE   To determine the relative horizontal position of the visual axes of the eyes at distance when fusion has been broken.

EQUIPMENT

* Phoropter.
* A distance acuity chart that can isolate letters.

SET-UP

* The phoropter should contain the patient's distance correction and be set for the patient's distance PD.
* A single letter on the distance chart, one line larger than the patient's best corrected visual acuity in the poorer eye, should be displayed.
* Place the Risley prisms before both eyes. Instruct the patient to close his eyes while you are adjusting the prisms. Set the prism before the right eye at 12Δ base in and the prism before the left eye at 6Δ base up. The 12Δ base in prism serves as a measuring prism and the 6Δ base up prism serves as a dissociating prism for the lateral phoria test (see Figure 4–1).

STEP-BY-STEP PROCEDURE

1. Instruct the patient to open both eyes. Ask the patient how many targets he sees and where they are in relation to one another. The patient should see two targets: one up and to the right, one down and to the left.
   a. If the patient sees only one target, check to see if one eye is occluded or alternately occlude each eye to help the patient locate each of the images in space. An alternative method is to change the dissociating prism to 6Δ base down on the left eye or change the amount of base in prism in front of the right eye.
   b. If the patient sees two targets, but one is up and to the left and the other

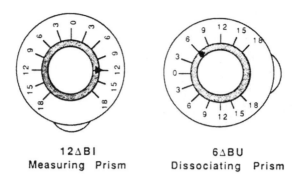

12△BI
Measuring Prism

6△BU
Dissociating Prism

Figure 4–1. To measure the distance lateral phoria by the von Graefe technique, the Risley prisms are placed in front of the phoropter lens apertures and oriented as shown.

is down and to the right, increase the amount of base in prism on the right eye. Do this until the targets are seen in the appropriate relationship, one up and to the right, one down and to the left.

2. Instruct the patient to look at the lower target, and to keep it clear.

3. Instruct the patient to look at the lower target, but think about the other, or upper one. Tell him that you will make the upper target move. Ask him to tell you when the two images or targets are vertically lined up in a straight line, one directly above the other. Inform him that he should always see double, to keep the images clear, and to continue to look at the lower target.

4. At about 2△ per second, reduce the base in prism until the patient reports vertical alignment of the two targets. Note the amount of prism and the direction of the base of the prism when the patient reports that the two targets are aligned.

5. Continue changing the measuring prism in the same direction (i.e., overshoot the point of alignment), until the patient sees the two targets as one up and to the left, one down and to the right.

6. Bring the measuring prism back in the other direction until the patient again reports vertical alignment of the two targets. Note the amount of prism and the direction of the base of the prism when the patient reports that the two targets are aligned (see Figure 4–2).

7. The result is the average of values in steps 4 and 6, if they are within 3△ of each other. If the two values are not within 3△ of one another, repeat the measurement, emphasizing the instructions to the patient, and average the two closest values.

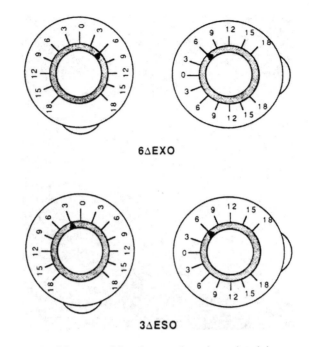

Figure 4–2. Two examples of the position of the Risley prisms during distance lateral phoria measurement.

RECORDING

- Record the size of the deviation in prism diopters and the type of deviation observed.

EXAMPLES

- DLP: ortho
- DLP: 2 Δ exo
- DLP: 4 Δ eso

EXPECTED FINDINGS

- 1Δ XP (±3Δ); 1Δ EP (±1Δ) for presbyopes

Distance Vertical Phoria by von Graefe Technique

PURPOSE To determine the relative vertical position of the visual axes of the eyes at distance when fusion has been broken.

EQUIPMENT

- Phoropter.
- A distance acuity chart that can isolate letters.

SET-UP

- The phoropter should contain the patient's distance correction and be set for the patient's distance PD.
- Display a single letter on the distance chart, one line larger than the patient's best corrected visual acuity in the poorer eye.
- Place the Risley prisms before both eyes. Instruct the patient to close his eyes while you are adjusting the prisms. Set the prism before the left eye at 6Δ base up and set the prism before the right eye at 12Δ base in. The 6Δ base up prism serves as a measuring prism and the 12Δ base in prism serves as a dissociating prism for the vertical phoria test (see Figure 4–3).

  Note: The distance lateral phoria test and the distance vertical phoria test are generally performed sequentially because the set-up for the two tests is the same.

STEP-BY-STEP PROCEDURE

1. Instruct the patient to open both eyes. Ask the patient how many targets he sees and where they are in relation to one another. The patient should see two targets; one up and to the right, one down and to the left. If the patient sees only one target, check to see if one eye is occluded or alternately occlude each eye to help the patient locate each of the images in space or change the amount of base in prism in front of the right eye. If the patient sees two targets, but one is up and to the left and the other is

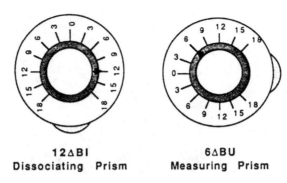

12ΔBI
Dissociating Prism

6ΔBU
Measuring Prism

Figure 4–3. To measure the distance vertical phoria by the von Graefe technique, the Risley prisms are placed in front of the phoropter lens apertures and oriented as shown.

down and to the right, increase the amount of base in prism on the right eye until the targets are seen in the appropriate relationship.

2. Instruct the patient to look at the target to the right.
3. Instruct patient to look at the target to the right, but think about the other, or left one. Tell him that you will make the left target move. Ask him to tell you when the two images or targets are horizontally lined up, one next to the other. Inform him that he should always see double and to continue to look at the target to the right.
4. At about 2Δ per second, reduce the base up prism until the patient reports horizontal alignment of the two targets. Note the amount of prism and the direction of the base of the prism when the patient reports that the two targets are aligned.
5. Continue changing the measuring prism in the same direction (i.e., overshoot the point of horizontal alignment) until the patient sees the two targets as one up and to the left, one down and to the right.
6. Bring the measuring prism back in the other direction until the patient again reports alignment of the two targets. Note the amount of prism and the direction of the base of the prism when the patient reports that the two targets are aligned (see Figure 4–4).
7. The result is the average of values in steps 4 and 6, if they are within 2Δ of each other. If the two values are not within 2Δ of one another, repeat the measurement, emphasizing the instructions to the patient, and average the two closest values.

RECORDING

• Record the size of the deviation in prism diopters and the type of deviation observed. For vertical phorias, you must always identify the eye with the hyper deviation.

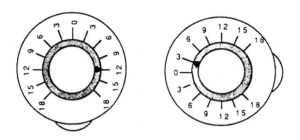

3ΔBU on OS, 3Δ right hyperphoria

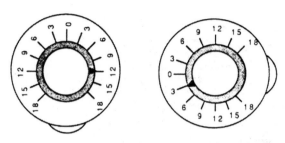

3ΔBD on OS, 3Δ left hyperphoria

Figure 4–4. Two examples of the position of the Risley prisms during distance vertical phoria measurement.

EXAMPLES

- DVP: ortho
- DVP: 2Δ right hyper
- DVP: 1Δ left hyper

EXPECTED FINDINGS

- Ortho (no deviation) is the expected finding.

Horizontal Vergences at Distance

PURPOSE   To measure, through the application of prism, the patient's ability to use horizontal vergence to maintain binocular vision. Prisms that induce retinal disparity are gradually increased in power, forcing the patient's vergence system to compensate for the disparity.

Horizontal Vergences (BI and BO Vergences)

When testing base in (BI) and base out (BO) vergences, the examiner is looking for three subtest findings. These include:

1. *Blur point:* The blur represents the point when the patient can no longer compensate for the prism-induced retinal disparity while maintaining stable accommodation.
2. *Break point:* The break represents the point when the patient, using all vergence sources, can no longer maintain single vision.
3. *Recovery point:* The recovery indicates that the induced retinal disparity has been decreased to the point that the patient can access the vergence system and regain single vision.

EQUIPMENT

- Phoropter.
- A distance acuity chart that can isolate single letters.

SET-UP

- The phoropter should contain the patient's distance correction and PD.
- Expose an isolated letter one line larger than the patient's best corrected visual acuity in the poorer eye.
- The Risley prisms, set to 0, are positioned before both eyes so horizontal prism may be introduced (see Figure 4–5).

STEP-BY-STEP PROCEDURE

1. Instruct the patient to open both eyes and ask him what he sees. He should see one clear image. If the patient sees two targets, end the test and record "diplopia."

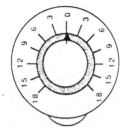 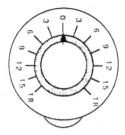

Figure 4–5. To measure the distance horizontal vergences, the Risley prisms are placed in front of the phoropter lens apertures and oriented as shown.

2. Instruct the patient to look at the target and try to keep it clear. Ask the patient to report if:
   a. the target blurs (blur point).
   b. the target becomes double (break point).
   c. the target moves either left or right. This indicates an eye is being suppressed. If this occurs the test is invalid and should be stopped. Record "suppression" and indicate which eye. The eye being suppressed may be determined by asking the patient which direction the target appears to be moving. The target will be moving toward the apex of the prism before the eye *not* being suppressed. For example, if base out vergences are being tested and the patient reports the target is moving left, the right eye is seeing and the left eye is being suppressed. This is known because the apex of the prism over the right eye is pointing to the left, the direction in which the target is moving.
3. Introduce base in prism equally before both eyes at a speed of approximately 1 prism diopter per second. Base in is always tested before base out because base out testing affects accommodation and convergence in a way that may carry over and modify the base in findings.
4. As prism is added note the *total* prism before the two eyes at each point described here: first, when the patient first reports the letter has blurred (blur point); second, when the letter has broken into two (break point). For example, if the patient reported the letter became double when there was 3Δ in front of the right eye and 4Δ in front of the left eye, the break point is 7Δ.
5. Overshoot the break point slightly by adding a little more prism in the same direction.
6. Then instruct the patient to tell you when the target becomes single again.
7. Reduce the prism until the patient reports the target is single again. This is the recovery point. Note the total amount of prism before both eyes.
8. Repeat steps 2 through 7 with base out prism before both eyes.

RECORDING

- Indicate that the test was performed at distance, then record the orientation of the prisms (BI and BO) along with the corresponding results.
- Each result should contain three values, blur, break, and recovery, in prism diopters.
- If no blur point is observed, an "X" is entered.
- If recovery values are in the direction opposite to what you expect (e.g., testing BO but had to go into BI for recovery to occur), record as a negative value.

EXAMPLES

- Distance Vergences:
  BI X/10/4 BO 12/18/8
- Distance Vergences:
  BI: Suppression OD BO: 4/6/22

EXPECTED FINDINGS

- Morgan (adult, clinical population)
  Distance BI: X/7/4 Standard deviation X/3/2
  Distance BO: 9/19/10 Standard deviation 4/8/4
- Saladin and Sheedy (adult, nonclinical population)
  Distance BI: X/8/5 Standard deviation X/3/3
  Distance BO: 15/28/20 Standard deviation 7/10/11
- The numbers provided are population norms. These serve as a general indicator. Precise interpretation of the vergence findings require that they be viewed in relation to other functional test results.
- Typically, there is no blur point for base in vergence testing at distance. Blur on base in testing indicates a relaxation of accommodation and this should not occur if the patient has been properly refracted. However, the patient should be asked to report blur during base in testing because this indicates that the patient is not properly refracted.

Vertical Vergences at Distance

PURPOSE   To measure, through the application of base up or base down prism, the patient's vertical fusional vergence abilities.

Vertical Vergences (Supra- and Infravergences)

When testing supravergence (base down, BD) and infravergence (base up, BU), the examiner is looking for two subtest findings. These are:

1. *Break point:* The break represents the point when the patient has used all his vertical vergence and can no longer maintain single vision.
2. *Recovery point:* The recovery indicates that the retinal disparity induced by the prisms has been decreased to the point that the patient can access the vertical vergence system and regain single vision.

   Note: There is no blur finding for vertical vergence testing because accommodation does not change during vertical vergence movements.

EQUIPMENT

- Phoropter.
- A distance acuity chart that can isolate letters.

SET-UP

- The phoropter should contain the patient's distance correction and be set for the patient's distance PD.
- Expose an isolated letter one line larger than the patient's best corrected visual acuity in the poorer seeing eye.
- The Risley prisms, set to zero, are positioned before *both* eyes so that vertical prism may be introduced (see Figure 4–6).

STEP-BY-STEP PROCEDURE

1. Ask the patient to open both eyes and report what he sees. He should see one clear image.
2. Instruct the patient to look at the letter and to tell you when it doubles.
3. At about 1 prism diopter per second introduce base up prism before the right eye. This measures right infravergence.

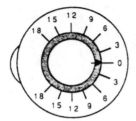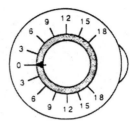

Figure 4–6. To measure the distance vertical vergences, the Risley prisms are placed in front of the phoropter lens apertures and oriented as shown.

> *Note:* Unlike the measurement of horizontal vergences, it is only necessary to move the prism before one eye. A supravergence measured in one eye is equal to an infravergence in the other. The second prism is placed, with no prism power, before the contralateral eye to equalize the quality of the image presented to the two eyes.

4. Note the amount of base up prism before the right eye at the break point.
5. Overshoot the break point slightly by adding a little more prism in the same direction; 2 to 3Δ is usually sufficient.
6. Instruct the patient to tell you when the target becomes single again.
7. Reduce the prism until the patient reports the target is single. This is the recovery point. Note the amount of base up prism before the right eye.
8. Repeat steps 2 through 7 starting with base down prism over the right eye. This measures right supravergence.

RECORDING

- Record the technique and the distance at which it was performed.
- Record the eye over which the prism was introduced.
- Record the orientation of the prisms (BU and BD) or the type of vergence (infra or supra) along with the corresponding results.
  (a) Each result should contain two values, break and recovery.
  (b) If the recovery values are in the direction opposite to what you expect (e.g., testing BU but had to go into BD for recovery to occur), record as a negative value.

EXAMPLES

- Distance vertical vergences: OD infra 4/2, OD supra 2/−1
- Distance vertical vergences: OD BU 6/4, BD 3/1

EXPECTED FINDINGS

- Break: 3Δ to 4Δ
  Recovery: 1.5Δ to 2Δ
- The numbers provided are population norms. These serve as a general indicator. Precise interpretation of the vergence findings require that they be viewed in relation to any vertical heterophoria that may exist.

Near Lateral Phoria by von Graefe Technique

PURPOSE   To determine the relative horizontal position of the visual axes of the eyes at near when fusion has been broken. The von Graefe phoria test can also be used to measure the AC/A ratio.

EQUIPMENT

- Phoropter.
- Near point rod.
- Near point card with a small block of letters approximately 20/30 in size.

SET-UP

- The phoropter should contain the patient's near correction and be set for the patient's near PD.
- Place the near point card in good illumination on the near point rod 40 cm from the patient.
- Place the Risley prisms before both eyes. Instruct the patient to close his eyes while you are adjusting the prisms. Set the prism before the right eye at 12Δ base in and the prism before the left eye at 6Δ base up. The 12Δ base in prism serves as a measuring prism and the 6Δ base up prism serves as a dissociating prism for the lateral phoria test (see Figure 4–7).

STEP-BY-STEP PROCEDURE

1. Instruct the patient to open both eyes. Ask the patient how many targets he sees and where they are in relation to one another. The patient should see two targets, one up and to the right, one down and to the left. If the patient sees only one target, check to see if one eye is occluded or alternately occlude each eye to help the patient locate each of the images in space. If the patient is still unable to see two targets, change the dissociating prism to 6Δ base down on the left eye or change the amount of the

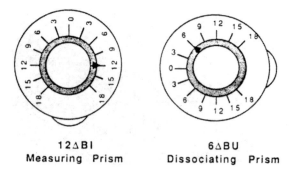

12△BI
Measuring Prism

6△BU
Dissociating Prism

Figure 4–7. To measure the near lateral phoria by the von Graefe technique, the Risley prisms are placed in front of the phoropter lens apertures and oriented as shown.

base in prism in front of the right eye. If the patient sees two targets, but one is up and to the left and the other is down and to the right, increase the amount of base in prism on the right eye until the targets are seen in the appropriate relationship.

2. Instruct the patient to look at the lower target, and to keep it clear.
3. Instruct the patient to look at the lower target, but think about the other, or upper one. Inform him that you will make the upper target move. Ask him to tell you when the two images or targets are vertically lined up, one directly above the other. Tell him that he should always see double, to keep the images clear, and to continue to look at the lower target.
4. At about 2△ per second, reduce the base in prism until the patient reports vertical alignment of the two targets. Note the amount of prism and the direction of the base of the prism when the patient reports that the two targets are aligned.
5. Continue changing the measuring prism in the same direction (i.e., over-shoot the point of alignment), until the patient sees the two targets, one up and to the left, one down and to the right.
6. Bring the measuring prism back in the other direction until the patient again reports vertical alignment of the two targets. Note the amount of prism and the direction of the base of the prism when the patient reports that the two targets are aligned (see Figure 4–8).
7. The result is the average of values in steps 4 and 6, if they are within 3△ of each other. If the two values are not within 3△ of one another, repeat the measurement, emphasizing the instructions to the patient, and average the two closest values.
8. The von Graefe phoria test can be used to measure the gradient AC/A ratio. The near lateral phoria test is repeated through +1.00 or −1.00 over the patient's near correction. The finding is then compared to the phoria

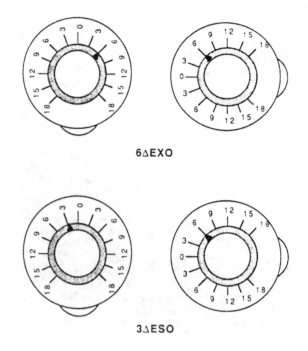

6ΔEXO

3ΔESO

Figure 4–8. Two examples of the position of the Risley prisms during near lateral phoria measurement.

finding through the near correction. The phoria will become more exo or less eso through +1.00 and more eso or less exo through −1.00.

RECORDING

- Record the size of the deviation in prism diopters and the type of deviation observed.
- For the gradient AC/A, record whether the test was done through +1.00 or −1.00, record the phoria finding, and the AC/A ratio (the difference between the two phoria findings).

EXAMPLES

- NLP: ortho
- NLP: 2Δ exo, −1.00 2Δ eso, AC/A 4/1
- NLP: 5Δ eso, +1.00 3Δ exo, AC/A 8/1

EXPECTED FINDINGS

- Near lateral phoria: 3Δ XP (±3Δ); 8Δ XP (±3Δ) for presbyopes
- AC/A: 4/1 (±2Δ)

Near Vertical Phoria by von Graefe Technique

PURPOSE   To determine the relative vertical position of the visual axes of the eyes at near when fusion has been broken.

EQUIPMENT

- Phoropter.
- Near point rod.
- Near point card with a small block of letters approximately 20/30 in size.

SET-UP

- The phoropter should contain the patient's near correction and be set for the patient's near PD.
- Place the near point card in good illumination on the near point rod 40 cm from the patient.
- Place the Risley prisms before both eyes. Instruct the patient to close his eyes while you are adjusting the prisms. Set the prism before the left eye at 6Δ base up and the prism before the right eye at 12Δ base in. The 6Δ base up prism serves as a measuring prism and the 12Δ base in prism serves as a dissociating prism for the vertical phoria test (see Figure 4–9).

STEP-BY-STEP PROCEDURE

1. Instruct the patient to open both eyes. Ask the patient how many targets he sees and where they are in relation to one another. The patient should see two targets, one up and to the right, one down and to the left. If the patient sees only one target, check to see if one eye is occluded or alternately occlude each eye to help the patient locate each of the images in space or change the amount of the dissociating prism to more or less base in prism on the right eye. If the patient sees two targets, but one is up and to the left and the other is down and to the right, increase the amount of

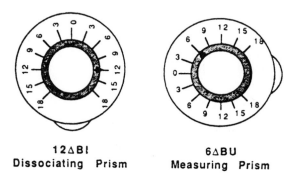

12△BI
Dissociating Prism

6△BU
Measuring Prism

Figure 4–9. To measure the near vertical phoria by the von Graefe technique, the Risley prisms are placed in front of the phoropter lens apertures and oriented as shown.

base in prism on the right eye until the targets are seen in the appropriate relationship.

2. Instruct the patient to look at the target to the right.
3. Instruct the patient to continue to look at the target to the right, but think about the other, or left one. Inform him that you will make the left target move. Ask him to tell you when the two images or targets are horizontally lined up, one next to the other. Tell him that he should always see double and to continue to look at the target to the right.
4. At about 2△ per second, reduce the base up prism until the patient reports horizontal alignment of the two targets. Note the amount of prism and the direction of the base of the prism when the patient reports that the two targets are aligned.
5. Continue changing the measuring prism in the same direction (i.e., overshoot the point of horizontal alignment) until the patient sees the two targets one up and to the left, one down and to the right.
6. Bring the measuring prism back in the other direction until the patient again reports alignment of the two targets. Note the amount of prism and the direction of the base of the prism when the patient reports that the two targets are aligned (see Figure 4–10).
7. The result is the average of values in steps 4 and 6, if they are within 2△ of each other. If the two values are not within 2△ of one another, repeat the measurement, emphasizing the instructions to the patient, and average the two closest values.

RECORDING

- Record the size of the deviation in prism diopters and the type of deviation observed. For vertical phorias, always identify the eye with the hyper deviation.

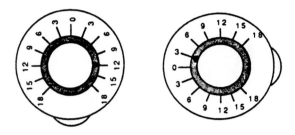

3ΔBU on OS, 3Δ right hyperphoria

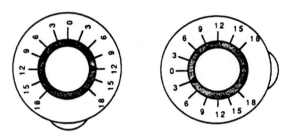

3ΔBD on OS, 3Δ left hyperphoria

Figure 4–10. Two examples of the position of the Risley prisms during near vertical phoria measurement.

EXAMPLES

- NVP: ortho
- NVP: 1 Δ right hyper
- NVP: 3 Δ left hyper

EXPECTED FINDINGS

- Ortho (no deviation)

Horizontal Vergences at Near

PURPOSE To measure, through the application of prism, the patient's ability to use horizontal vergence to maintain binocular vision. Prisms that induce retinal disparity are gradually increased in power, forcing the patient's vergence system to compensate for the disparity.

Note: The following description presumes the reader has read the procedure for horizontal vergences at distance. As distance and near testing are quite similar, some information previously stated is omitted here.

EQUIPMENT

- Phoropter with near point rod.
- Near point card with an isolated vertical line of letters. The lettering on these cards approximates 20/30. A card with a block of letters of comparable size is frequently used.

SET-UP

- The phoropter should contain the habitual or induced near correction and be adjusted for the patient's near PD.
- Place the vergence target under good illumination on the near point rod 40 cm from the patient.
- The Risley prisms, set to zero, should be positioned before both eyes (see Figure 4–11).

STEP-BY-STEP PROCEDURE

1. Instruct the patient to open both eyes and ask him what he sees. He should see one clear image. If the patient sees two targets, instruct the patient to reach out and touch the card. If this does not result in one clear image, end the test and record "diplopia."
2. Instruct the patient to look at the target and try to keep it clear. Ask that the patient report if:
   a. the target blurs (blur point).

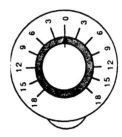 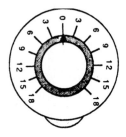

Figure 4–11. To measure the near horizontal vergences, the Risley prisms are placed in front of the phoropter lens apertures and oriented as shown.

     b. the target becomes double (break point).

     c. the target moves either left or right (suppression).

3. Introduce base in prism before both eyes at a speed of approximately 1 prism diopter per second.

4. As prism is added, note the *total* amount of prism before the two eyes when the patient reports the letters have blurred (blur point) and when the line of letters has broken into two (break point).

5. Overshoot the break point slightly by adding a little more prism in the same direction.

6. Instruct the patient to tell you when the target becomes single again.

7. Reduce prism until the patient reports the target is single (recovery point) and note the total amount of prism before both eyes.

8. Repeat steps 2 to 7 with base out prism before both eyes.

RECORDING

- Record the technique and the distance at which it was performed, near or 40 cm.
- Record the orientation of the prisms (BI and BO) along with the corresponding results.
- Each result should contain three values, blur, break, and recovery, in prism diopters.
- If no blur point is observed, an "X" is entered.
- If recovery values are in the direction opposite to what you expect, record as a negative value.

EXAMPLES

- Near Horizontal Vergences
  BI: 8/14/8 BO: 20/24/18
- Near Horizontal Vergences
  BI: Suppression OS BO: 12/16/−4

EXPECTED FINDINGS

- Morgan (adult, clinical population)
  Near BI:13/21/13 Standard deviation 4/4/5
  Near BO:17/21/11 Standard deviation 5/6/7
- Saladin and Sheedy (adult, nonclinical population)
  Near BI:14/19/13 Standard deviation 6/7/6
  Near BO:22/30/23 Standard deviation 8/12/11
- The numbers provided are population norms. These serve as a general indicator. Precise interpretation of the vergence findings require that they be viewed in relation to other functional testing.

Vertical Vergences at Near

PURPOSE   To measure the patient's vertical fusional vergence abilities, through the application of base up or base down prism. The following description presumes the reader has read the procedure for vertical vergences at distance. As distance and near testing are quite similar, some information previously stated is omitted.

EQUIPMENT

- Phoropter with a near point rod.
- A near point card with an isolated line of horizontal letters. The lettering on these cards approximates 20/30. A card with a block of letters of comparable size is frequently used.

SET-UP

- The phoropter should contain the patient's habitual or induced near correction and be set for the patient's near PD.
- Place the near vergence target under good illumination on the near point rod at 40 cm.
- The Risley prisms, set to zero, should be positioned before both eyes so that vertical prism may be introduced (see Figure 4–12).

STEP-BY-STEP PROCEDURE

1. Ask the patient to open both eyes and report what he sees. He should see one clear image.
2. Instruct the patient to look at the line of letters and to tell you when it doubles.
3. At about 1 prism diopter per second introduce base up prism before the right eye (right infravergence).
4. Note the amount of base up prism before the right eye at the break point.
5. Overshoot the break point slightly by adding a little more prism in the same direction.
6. Instruct the patient to tell you when the target becomes single again.

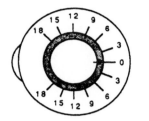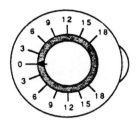

Figure 4–12. To measure the near vertical vergences, the Risley prisms are placed in front of the phoropter lens apertures and oriented as shown.

7. Reduce the prism until the patient reports the target is single. This is the recovery point. Note the amount of base up prism before the right eye.
8. Repeat steps 2 through 7 starting with base down prism over the right eye (right supravergence).

RECORDING

- Record the technique and the distance at which it was performed (distance or near).
- Record the eye over which the prism was introduced, the orientation of the prisms (BU and BD), and the corresponding results. Each result should contain two values, break, and recovery.
- If recovery values are in the direction opposite to what you expect, record the value as a negative value.

EXAMPLES

- Vertical vergences (near) OD: infra 4/2, supra 2/−1
- Vertical vergences (near) OD: BU 6/4, BD 3/1

EXPECTED FINDINGS

- Break: 3Δ to 4Δ
- Recovery: 1.5Δ to 2Δ
- The numbers provided are population norms. These serve as a general indicator. Precise interpretation of the vergence findings require that they be viewed in relation to any vertical heterophoria that may exist.

Fusional Vergence Facility at Near

PURPOSE   To test the ability of the patient's fusional vergence system to respond to rapid changes in disparity over time. This test is especially helpful in diagnosing binocular problems in symptomatic patients with normal fusional vergences.

EQUIPMENT

- 12Δ base out and 3Δ base in mounted in a flipper device.
- Near target: vertical line of small letters.
- Illumination source.
- Timepiece with second hand.

SET-UP

- The patient wears his habitual near correction.
- The patient holds the near target at 40 cm in good illumination.
- Brightly illuminate the near point card.

STEP-BY-STEP PROCEDURE

1. Place the 12Δ base out lenses in front of the patient's eyes and ask him to report when the print becomes single and clear.
2. As soon as the print becomes single and clear, flip the lenses to the 3Δ base in position.
3. Repeat steps 1 and 2, noting the number of full cycles that the patient completes in 60 seconds. A full cycle consists of both the BI and BO lenses.

RECORDING

- Record the number of cycles completed in 60 seconds.

EXAMPLE

- Fusional facility at N: 4 cycles per minute

EXPECTED FINDINGS

• Fusional facility at N: 15 cycles per minute

Negative Relative Accommodation/Positive Relative Accommodation (NRA/PRA)

PURPOSE   To test the patient's ability to increase and decrease accommodation under binocular conditions when the total convergence demand is constant. Under these conditions, changes in accommodative convergence are compensated for by changes in fusional vergence. The results of the NRA/PRA contribute to the functional analysis. They are part of the near refraction to determine an add for a presbyope.

EQUIPMENT

- Phoropter.
- Near point card.
- Near point rod.
- Illumination source.

SET-UP

- The phoropter contains the patient's habitual correction or the best distance prescription from his most recent refraction if the patient is a nonpresbyope. If the patient is presbyopic, the patient's tentative near prescription is placed in the phoropter.
- Put the near point card on the near point rod at 40 cm under bright illumination.
- Set the phoropter to the patient's near PD. Make sure that both of the patient's eyes are unoccluded.

STEP-BY-STEP PROCEDURE

1. Direct the patient's attention to letters one or two lines larger than his best near VA on the near point card. Because the endpoint of the test occurs

when the letters become blurry, ascertain that the letters are clear at the beginning of the test. If the letters are not clear, add plus sphere power, +0.25 D at a time, until the patient reports that the letters are clear. This becomes the *tentative near prescription*. If the letters remain blurry despite the addition of plus, the NRA/PRA cannot be performed.

2. Do the NRA. Add plus lenses binocularly, +0.25 D at a time, until the patient reports the first sustained blur. *First sustained blur* means that the patient notices that the letters are not as sharp and clear as they were initially, even if the patient can still read them.
3. Note the total amount of plus added.
4. Return the lenses in the phoropter to the value at which you began the test, either the patient's distance prescription or the tentative near prescription.
5. Again make certain that the letters are clear to the patient.
6. Do the PRA. Add minus lenses binocularly, −0.25 D at a time, until the patient reports the first sustained blur. Note the total amount of minus added.

RECORDING

- Record the amount of plus added for the NRA and the amount of minus added for the PRA, relative to the starting point of either the distance refraction or the tentative near prescription. Record the tentative add (the amount of plus added to the distance refraction to arrive at the tentative near prescription), when using the NRA/PRA as part of the near refraction of the presbyope.

EXAMPLES

- NRA/PRA: +2.25/−2.50
- NRA/PRA +1.00/−1.00 through tentative add +1.25

EXPECTED FINDINGS

- In the nonpresbyope: NRA: +2.00 (±0.50); PRA −2.37 (±1.00)
- In the presbyope, the NRA and PRA vary widely. However, the sum of the add and the NRA should not exceed +2.50 D. When the presbyopic add is appropriate, the NRA and PRA should have the same absolute value.

Accommodative Facility

PURPOSE   To measure the patient's ability to make rapid and accurate accommodative changes under monocular or binocular conditions. Accommodative facility testing is part of a full functional analysis. The findings help to distinguish primary accommodative from primary binocular anomalies.

INDICATIONS

Accommodative facility as described here is done only on nonpresbyopes.

EQUIPMENT

- +2.00/−2.00 lenses mounted in a flipper device.
- Near target (printed material containing letters one or two lines larger than the patient's near visual acuity in his poorer seeing eye).
- Eye patch.
- Polaroid glasses.
- Polaroid bar reader.
- Illumination source.
- Timepiece with second hand.

SET-UP

- The patient wears his *distance* correction.
- Have the patient hold the near target at 40 cm in good illumination.
- The patient wears the Polaroid glasses over his habitual correction during the binocular but not the monocular part of this test.
- Place the bar reader over the near target during the binocular but not the monocular part of this test.

STEP-BY-STEP PROCEDURE

1. Make sure that both of the patient's eyes are unoccluded, and he is wearing the Polaroid glasses.

2. Place the +2.00 lenses in front of the patient's eyes and ask him to report when the print clears.
3. As soon as the print clears, flip the lenses to their -2.00 position.
4. Repeat steps 1 and 2, noting the number of full cycles that the patient completes in 60 seconds. A full cycle consists of both +2.00 and -2.00 lenses. Throughout steps 1 to 3, keep telling the patient to be certain that he can see all of the letters through all of the bars of the bar reader (see Figure 4–14). If the patient is unable to see through all the bars, he is suppressing one eye. Binocular facility testing cannot be done on this patient. Determine which eye is being suppressed (see Figure 4–15). Proceed to step 6.
5. If the patient clears 8 or more cycles in 60 seconds, record the actual number of completed cycles. If the patient clears fewer than 8 cycles in one minute, go to step 6.
6. Remove the Polaroid glasses and the bar reader. If the patient passes the binocular accommodative facility testing, the test is complete. If the patient fails the binocular accommodative facility testing, proceed to steps 7 and 8 below to test facility monocularly.
7. Patch the patient's left eye and repeat steps 2 and 3 on his right eye. Note the number of full cycles the patient completes in 60 seconds.
8. Then patch the patient's right eye and repeat steps 2 and 3 on his left eye. Note the number of full cycles the patient completes in 60 seconds.

RECORDING

- Record the number of cycles completed in 60 seconds for both eyes together and, if applicable, for each eye monocularly.
- If the patient is able to complete fewer than the expected number of cycles per minute (cpm) on any portion of the test, record the actual cpm and indicate whether he had greater difficulty clearing the plus lenses, the minus lenses, or both.
- If suppression occurred during the binocular portion of the test, record which eye suppressed.

EXAMPLES

- Accom. Fac. OU 4 cpm, slow on plus, cleared minus easily/OD 12 cpm, OS 11 cpm
- Accom. Fac. OU 3 cpm (failed minus)/OD 4 cpm (failed minus), OS 3 cpm (failed minus)
- Accom. Fac. OU suppression OD after 1 cycle/OD 8 cpm, OS 7 cpm

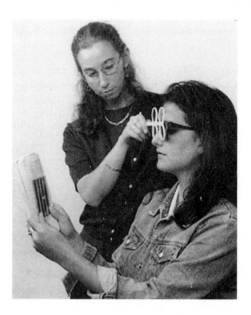

Figure 4–14. A patient is shown during binocular accommodative facility testing.

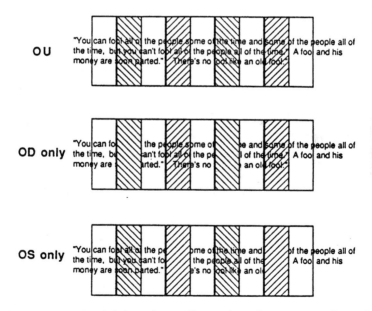

Figure 4–15. Text as seen through the bar reader. "OU" illustrates when neither eye is suppressed. "OD only" illustrates when the left eye is suppressed and only the right eye can see the text. "OS only" illustrates when the right eye is suppressed and only the left eye can see the text.

EXPECTED FINDINGS

- Children 8 to 12 years old: 5 cpm binocularly, 7 cpm monocularly
- Adults 13 to 30 years old: 10 cmp binocularly, 11 cpm monocularly
- The monocular findings should be within 4 cpm of one another for each eye.

Dynamic Retinoscopy: Monocular Estimation Method (MEM)

 PURPOSE To objectively measure the accommodative response to the near working distance. This technique is useful in the diagnosis of binocular anomalies and for predicting the efficacy of some forms of therapeutic intervention.

EQUIPMENT

- Retinoscope.
- MEM retinoscopy card.
- Trial lens set or lens rack.

SET-UP

- The MEM card should be attached to the retinoscope with the beam of the retinoscope passing through the hole in the center of it (see Figure 4–16).
- The test is performed under normal room illumination.
- The patient should wear his habitual near correction.
- The test is performed under binocular viewing conditions.

STEP-BY-STEP PROCEDURE

1. Position yourself so
   a. the MEM card is at the patient's customary working distance (CWD). When examining children, Harmon's Distance (the distance from the patient's elbow to his knuckles) is frequently used as an alternative to the CWD.
   b. you are on the patient's midline and the patient's eyes are slightly depressed, thereby more closely simulating a normal reading posture.
2. The streak of the retinoscope should be oriented vertically and positioned on the bridge of the patient's nose.

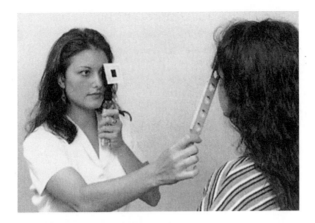

Figure 4–16. An examiner performing MEM retinoscopy.

3. Ask the patient to read the letters or words on the card. With children it is often useful to have them read out loud.
4. While the patient is reading, *quickly* guide the streak across the patient's right eye and evaluate the reflex for with or against motion or for neutrality. Be sure to observe the reflex in the center of the pupil rather than at the edge.
5. Estimate the dioptric value required to neutralize the observed motion. (With—plus; Against—minus).
6. Confirm the estimate by *quickly* (<1 second) interjecting a lens of the estimated power into the patient's line of sight while evaluating the reflex. If the estimate is correct, neutrality will be observed.
   Note: It is critical that the lens be interjected quickly, the reflex evaluated, and the lens removed quickly. Prolonged exposure to the lens is likely to induce a change in the accommodative response resulting in invalid data.
7. Repeat steps 2 through 6 for the left eye.

RECORDING

- Record the technique used (MEM).
- Record the lens power required to attain neutrality for the OD and the OS.

EXAMPLES

- MEM OD   +0.50
       OS   +0.75

EXPECTED FINDINGS

- +0.25 to +0.50

Dynamic Retinoscopy: Bell Retinoscopy

PURPOSE   To measure the linear magnitude of the accommodative lag using a mobile target and a retinoscope. This procedure allows the examiner to directly view the patient's response to changes in the stimulus to accommodation. This technique is useful in the diagnosis of binocular anomalies and for predicting the efficacy of some forms of therapy.

EQUIPMENT

- Retinoscope.
- Bell retinoscopy target. Current practice suggests that either a reflectant chrome or clear Lucite sphere be used. The actual target is not the sphere but rather the reflected or transmitted image in the sphere.
- Yardstick.

STEP-UP

- The test is performed under normal room illumination.
- The patient should wear his habitual or induced near correction.
- The test is performed under binocular viewing conditions.
- The patient holds one end of the yardstick against his cheek while the examiner sets the other end over either his shoulder or his ear.
- The examiner should be positioned at eye level and at a distance where the retinoscope is 20 in from the patient (see Figure 4–17).

STEP-BY-STEP PROCEDURE

1. Position the target against your forehead directly above the retinoscope.
2. Ask the patient to look at the image in the sphere and to keep it clear.
3. Observe the initial retinoscopic reflex in the right eye using a vertical streak. Typically, with motion is observed indicating an accommodative lag. It may be useful to screen for astigmatic error by rotating the streak.

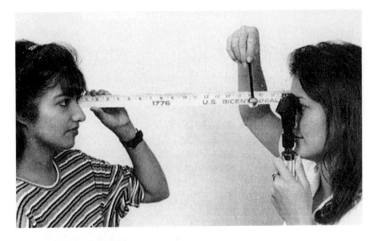

Figure 4–17. An examiner performing bell retinoscopy.

4. If with motion is seen as expected, begin to move the sphere toward the patient while you remain stationary.
   Note: If against motion is seen at the outset, the examiner may use +0.50 probe lenses. If the patient has a need for plus at near, the addition of these lenses may stimulate a relaxation of the accommodation creating a shift to with motion.
5. Continue moving the target toward the patient until the motion changes from with to against motion. Look at the yardstick and mentally note this distance.
6. Continue moving the target toward the patient for an additional 2 to 3 in and then reverse direction, moving the sphere away from the patient and toward you.
7. Continue to monitor the retinoscopic reflex and note the distance at which the reflex changes from against to with motion.
8. Repeat steps 3 through 7 for the left eye.

RECORDING

- Record the technique used.
- For each eye record the distance at which the initial with motion changed to against motion and when the against then returned to with motion.
- If the retinoscopic reflex was initially against, record this and the patient's response to the probe lenses.

EXAMPLES

- Bell Retinoscopy: OD 15"/17"
                       OS 14"/17"
- Bell Retinoscopy: Against motion/no change with +0.50

EXPECTED FINDINGS

Normal findings for Bell Retinoscopy are 17 to 14 in for the change to against motion and 15 to 18 in for the reverse shift to with motion.

Amplitude of Accommodation: Minus Lens to Blur

PURPOSE
To measure the amplitude of accommodation monocularly by using minus lenses to increase the stimulus to accommodation.

INDICATIONS

This test is done when other tests, such as the push-up amplitude, suggest that a nonpresbyopic patient has a reduced amplitude of accommodation.

EQUIPMENT

- Phoropter.
- Near point card.
- Near point rod.
- Illumination source.

SET-UP

- The phoropter contains the patient's best distance correction from the most recent refraction.
- Place the near point card at 40 cm on the near point rod under bright illumination.
- Remember that the test is done monocularly only.

STEP-BY-STEP PROCEDURE

1. With the patient seated behind the phoropter, occlude his left eye.
2. Instruct the patient to look at a row of letters one or two lines larger than his best near visual acuity. For most nonpresbyopes, 20/30 letters are appropriate.
3. Add minus lenses −0.25 D at a time, allowing 5 to 10 seconds for the patient to clear the letters. Continue to add lenses until the patient reports that he can no longer clear the target and keep it clear. The first sustained blur marks the endpoint of this test.

4. The amount of minus added to the patient's prescription plus 2.50 D (the accommodative demand for a near point card at 40 cm) is the total amplitude of accommodation.
5. Repeat steps 2 through 4 on the left eye with the right eye occluded.

RECORDING

- Record the amplitude of accommodation in diopters for each eye separately.
- Record the method of testing used.

EXAMPLES

- Amp OD 7 D OS 7 D (minus lens method)
- Amp OD 3.5 D OS 3.5 D (minus lens method)

EXPECTED FINDINGS

The amplitude of accommodation as measured by the minus lens to blur method is approximately 2.0 D less than that measured by the push-up method (see Donders' Table).

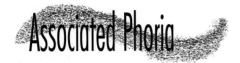

Associated Phoria

PURPOSE To measure the amount of prism required to neutralize a misalignment of the visual axis under binocular viewing conditions. The associated phoria may be manifested either horizontally or vertically.

INDICATIONS

The associated phoria test is of great value in determining the amount of prism to prescribe for patients with vertical imbalances. It is a valuable diagnostic procedure for binocular problems in general, although its value may be greatest for the presbyopic population. The associated phoria is a single data point on the forced vergence curve.

EQUIPMENT

- Associated phoria targets generally come in three designs:
  a. without a central fusional stimulus.
  b. with a central fusional stimulus.
  c. with a peripheral fusional stimulus (see Figure 4–18).
  Depending on the manufacturer, the target may have separate nonius lines for the vertical versus horizontal function. Others are unified as one target.
- Phoropter with polarizing filters.
  Note: The associated phoria may also be measured out of the phoropter using polarized glasses over the patient's correction and a prism bar.

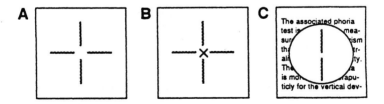

Figure 4–18. Three types of associated phoria targets. **A.** Without a central or peripheral stimulus to fusion. **B.** With a central fusional stimulus. **C.** With a peripheral fusional stimulus.

SET-UP

- The phoropter should contain the patient's PD and the induced or habitual correction for the distance being tested.
- The target should be placed at the appropriate testing distance. For near this may be at either 40 cm or the patient's customary working distance.
- The target should be well illuminated.
- The polarizers should be positioned in front of both eyes.

STEP-BY-STEP PROCEDURE

1. Instruct the patient to look at the target and ask him what he sees (see Figure 4–19).
2. If the patient reports he sees two lines (½ the target), the patient is suppressing and the test is over. Determine which eye is suppressing and record the results.
3. If the patient sees four lines, test for the existence of a vertical fixation disparity. Ask the patient if the horizontal lines form a perfect line, if they are exactly aligned with one another, or if one line looks higher than the other.
   a. If the horizontal lines appear aligned, go to step 6.
   b. If the horizontal lines are not aligned, a vertical fixation disparity exists (see Figure 4–20). Continue with step 4.

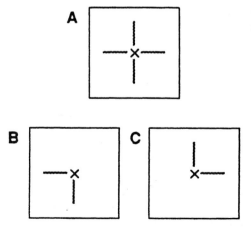

Figure 4–19. What the patient sees. **A.** The complete target. **B.** The lines seen by the left eye. **C.** The lines seen by the right eye.

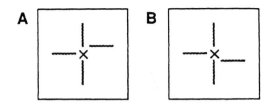

Figure 4–20. The target as it appears if a vertical fixation disparity exists. **A** indicates a left hyper fixation dispar-ity, and **B** depicts a right hyper fixation disparity as seen by the patient.

4. Determine the direction of the patient's vertical associated phoria.
   a. If the right line is too high, use base up prism in front of the right eye or base down prism in front of the left eye.
   b. If the left line is too high, use base down prism in front of the right eye or base up prism in front of the left eye.
5. Determine the minimum amount of prism to achieve alignment of the hor-izontal nonius lines. This prism value is the vertical associated phoria.
6. Test for the existence of a horizontal fixation disparity. Ask the patient if the vertical lines form a perfect line, if they are exactly aligned with one another, or if one line looks off center.
   a. If the vertical lines appear aligned, there is no horizontal associated phoria and the test is ended.
   b. If the vertical lines are not aligned, a horizontal fixation disparity ex-ists. Go to step 7.
7. Determine the direction of the patient's horizontal associated phoria (see Figure 4–21).
   a. If the top line is to the left, this is a crossed or exo fixation disparity. Measure the horizontal associated phoria by using base in prism over either the right eye or the left eye to align the nonius lines.
   b. If the top line is to the right, this is an uncrossed or eso fixation dis-parity. Measure the horizontal associated phoria by using base out prism over either the right eye or the left eye to align the nonius lines.
8. Measure the size of the associated phoria by determining the minimum amount of prism needed to achieve alignment of the vertical nonius lines. This prism value is the horizontal associated phoria.

RECORDING

- Record the technique used and at what distance the test was done.
- Record the amount and direction of the prism required to achieve alignment.
- If a vertical associated phoria exists, specify the eye over which the prism was placed.

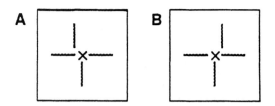

Figure 4–21. The target as it appears if a horizontal fixation disparity exists. **A** indicates an exo fixation disparity, while **B** depicts an eso fixation disparity as seen by the patient.

EXAMPLES

- Associated phoria: ortho/ortho, D and N
- Associated phoria: 2Δ BO/2Δ BD OD at N
- Associated phoria: Suppression OS

Maddox Rod Phoria

To measure the lateral and vertical phoria at distance and at near.

INDICATIONS

The Maddox rod phoria test is an alternative to the von Graefe phoria technique. It is used when the patient is unable to see two targets on the von Graefe test or when the phoria test must be done in space rather than behind the phoropter. Because this test can be done in free space with the patient wearing glasses, it is particularly useful for ruling out a prism-induced vertical phoria due to a patient's head tilt behind the phoropter lenses.

EQUIPMENT

- Penlight for near testing and muscle light for distance testing.
- Maddox rod (red or white).
- Prisms (Risley prisms, prism bars, or hand held prisms).

SET-UP

The Maddox rod phoria test can be done at distance and at near, using the phoropter and Risley prisms, or in space, using a hand held Maddox rod and loose prisms or a prism bar.

Set-up for Testing in the Phoropter

- The examiner turns on the muscle light for distance testing or the examiner holds the penlight at 16 in for near testing.
- The patient's distance correction and distance PD are placed in the phoropter for distance testing. The patient's near correction and near PD are placed in the phoropter for near testing.
- The Maddox rod is placed over the patient's right eye as follows:
  a. for measuring the lateral phoria, the grooves on the Maddox rod are oriented horizontally. The patient sees a vertical streak.
  b. for measuring the vertical phoria, the grooves on the Maddox rod are oriented vertically. The patient sees a horizontal streak (see Figure 4–22).
- The Risley prism is placed over the patient's right eye as follows:

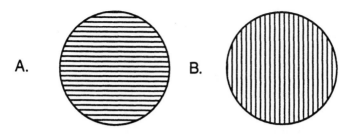

Figure 4–22. The orientation of the Maddox rod for phoria testing. **A** shows the orientation for lateral phoria testing and **B** shows the orientation for vertical phoria testing.

   a. for measuring the lateral phoria, the prism is oriented base in with sufficient prism to move the streak to the right of the spot of light.

   b. for measuring the vertical phoria, the prism is oriented base up with sufficient prism to move the streak below the spot of light.

Set-up for Testing in Space

- The examiner turns on the muscle light for distance testing or the examiner holds the penlight at 16 in for near testing.
- The patient wears his distance glasses for distance testing. The patient wears his near correction for near testing.
- The patient holds the Maddox rod over his right eye as follows:
  - a. for measuring the lateral phoria, the grooves on the Maddox rod are oriented horizontally. The patient sees a vertical streak.
  - b. for measuring the vertical phoria, the grooves on the Maddox rod are oriented vertically. The patient sees a horizontal streak.
- The examiner holds the prism bar over the patient's right eye as follows:
  - a. for measuring the lateral phoria, the prism is oriented base in with sufficient prism to move the streak to the right of the spot of light.
  - b. for measuring the vertical phoria, the prism is oriented base up with sufficient prism to move the streak below the spot of light.

STEP-BY-STEP PROCEDURE

1. Instruct the patient to look at the light but to be aware of the red or white line.
2. For the lateral phoria measurement, reduce the base in prism until the patient reports that the streak is in the center of the light. Note the amount of prism and the direction of the base.
3. For the vertical phoria measurement, reduce the base up prism until the

patient reports that the streak is in the center of the light. Note the amount of prism and the direction of the base.

RECORDING

- Record D for distance and N for near.
- Record the lateral and vertical phorias separately.
- Record the size of the deviation in prism diopters.
- Record the direction of the deviation.
- Indicate the type of Maddox rod used (red or white).

EXAMPLES

- DLP c red MR ortho; DVP c red MR ortho
- NLP c red MR 6Δ exo; NVP c red MR 2Δ R hyper

Modified Thorington Phoria

PURPOSE   To measure the lateral and vertical phoria at near.

INDICATIONS

The Modified Thorington phoria test is an alternative to the von Graefe test for the near lateral and vertical phoria measurements. It can be done with the patient behind the phoropter or in free space.

EQUIPMENT

- Penlight.
- Maddox rod.
- Thorington card. The spacing of the targets on this card is such that, at a 40-cm viewing distance, the separation between targets represents one prism diopter. There is a small hole in the center of the card. A penlight is held behind this hole to provide the light source.

SET-UP

- The patient wears his habitual near correction.
- The patient holds the Maddox rod over his right eye as follows:
  a. for measuring the lateral phoria, the grooves on the Maddox rod are oriented horizontally. The patient sees a vertical streak. The Thorington card with the horizontal rows of targets is used.
  b. for measuring the vertical phoria, the grooves on the Maddox rod are oriented vertically. The patient sees a horizontal streak. The Thorington card with the vertical rows of targets is used.
- The Thorington card is held at 40 cm with a penlight behind the hole in the center of the card.

STEP-BY-STEP PROCEDURE

1. Instruct the patient to look at the light in the center of the card.
2. Instruct the patient to tell you the location of the streak relative to the light: to the left, to the right, or through the light for the lateral phoria (see Fig-

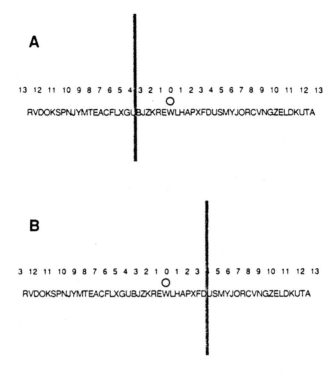

Figure 4–23. Two examples of the patient's view during the Modified Thorington test for near lateral phoria measured with the Maddox rod on the patient's right eye. **A.** The red line is between 3 and 4 to the left of the 0. This is a crossed diplopia response indicating a 3.5Δ exophoria. **B.** The red line is through the 4 to the right of the 0. This is an uncrossed diplopia response indicating a 4Δ esophoria.

ure 4–23); above, below, or through the light for the vertical phoria (see Figure 4–24).

    For the horizontal phoria, if the streak is through the light, the patient has no deviation (*orthophoria*). If the streak is to the right of the light, the patient has an *esophoria*. If the streak is to the left of the light, the patient has an *exophoria.*

    For the vertical phoria, if the streak is through the light, the patient has no deviation (orthophoria). If the streak is above the light, the patient has a left hyperphoria. If the streak is below the light, the patient has a right hyperphoria.

3. To determine the size of the phoria, ask the patient to tell you the target closest to which the streak passes.
4. A chart for testing the phoria at 10 feet is available using the procedures described above.

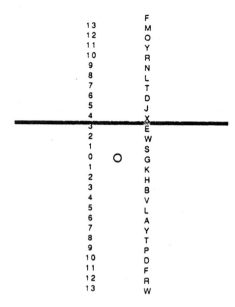

Figure 4–24. An example of the patient's view during the Modified Thorington test for near vertical phoria measured with the Maddox rod on the patient's right eye. The red line is between 3 and 4 above the 0 indicating a 3.5Δ left hyperphoria.

RECORDING

• Record the size and the direction of the phoria.

EXAMPLE

• NLP/NVP by Modified Thorington: NLP 6Δ exo/NVP 2Δ left hyper

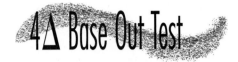

4Δ Base Out Test

PURPOSE   To confirm or rule out the presence of a small central scotoma.

INDICATIONS

A small central suppression zone should be suspected in a patient with a slight reduction in visual acuity (20/25 to 20/40) in one eye and mildly reduced stereopsis (30 to 80 seconds of arc). Monofixation syndrome secondary to a small angle strabismus is the most likely cause of this central suppression. Macular diseases affecting the foveal area will create a similar clinical presentation.

EQUIPMENT

- Loose 4Δ prism.
- A distance visual acuity chart that can isolate letters.

SET-UP

- The patient wears his best distance correction.
- The room illumination must be sufficient to allow the examiner to observe the patient's eye movements.
- The examiner must be in a position to see the patient's eyes easily without interfering with the patient's view of the target.
- Isolate a single letter, one line above best VA in the patient's poorer eye, on the distance visual acuity chart.

STEP-BY-STEP PROCEDURE

1. Instruct the patient to fixate continually on the target even if it appears to move, and to attempt to keep the target single at all times.
2. Hold the 4Δ prism between your thumb and forefinger so it will be positioned base out when placed in front of the patient's better seeing eye. *Note*: Always test the patient's better seeing eye first. If you are testing the patient's right eye, the prism should be held in your left hand with

its base pointing to your left. If you are testing the patient's left eye, the prism should be held in your right hand with its base pointing to your right.

3. Quickly insert the prism in front of the better seeing eye while watching the opposite eye for movement. A normal response is a concomitant movement outward, then an inward refixation movement. Keep the prism in front of the eye for several seconds to allow time for the refixation movement. Step 3 may be repeated as often as necessary to ascertain the movement of the poorer seeing eye.

4. Turn the prism so it will be positioned base out for the poorer seeing eye. Quickly insert the prism in front of the poorer seeing eye while watching the better seeing eye for movement. A normal response is a concomitant movement outward, then an inward refixation movement of the better seeing eye. Keep the prism in front of the eye for several seconds to allow time for the refixation movement. Step 4 may be repeated as often as necessary to ascertain the movement of the better seeing eye.

Note: Because atypical responses to the 4Δ Base Out Test have been reported in the literature, other tests of central suppression should be used in addition to this test when the results are variable or atypical.

RECORDING

- Write "4Δ base out test" or "4BO."
- Record "positive" if the test results indicate suppression of an eye. Indicate which eye is suppressing.
- Record "negative" if the test results do not indicate suppression.

EXAMPLES

- 4BO—positive, OD suppressing
- 4BO—negative, no suppression either eye

EXPECTED RESULTS

- Normal result (indicating no suppression of either eye). When the prism is placed in front of the right eye, the left eye will make a concomitant outward movement as predicted by Hering's law. The patient will then see double, so the left eye will make an inward refixation movement to avoid diplopia. When the prism is placed over the left eye, the right eye will make an outward movement followed by an inward refixation movement (see Figure 4–25).
- Abnormal result (indicating suppression of the poorer seeing eye). When the prism is placed over the better seeing eye, the opposite eye will make a con-

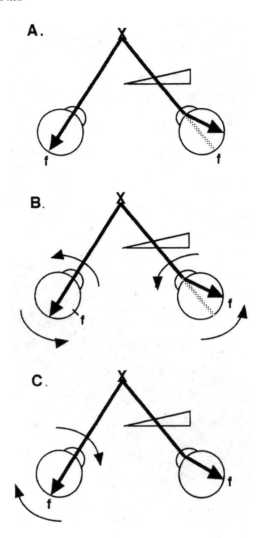

Figure 4–25. Movement of the eyes during the 4Δ Base Out test when the patient does not have a suppression scotoma. **A.** The prism placed over the patient's right eye, shifting the retinal image and causing the patient to see double. **B.** To avoid diplopia, the right eye moves inward to regain foveal fixation. The left eye makes a concomitant outward movement. **C.** To avoid diplopia, the left eye makes an inward refixation movement to regain foveal fixation.

comitant outward movement consistent with Hering's law. However, because the eye without the prism is suppressing, the patient does not see double. Therefore, the eye does not refixate to avoid diplopia. When the prism is placed in front of the suppressing eye, it will not be aware of the retinal image shift. There will be no movement of either eye (see Figure 4–26).

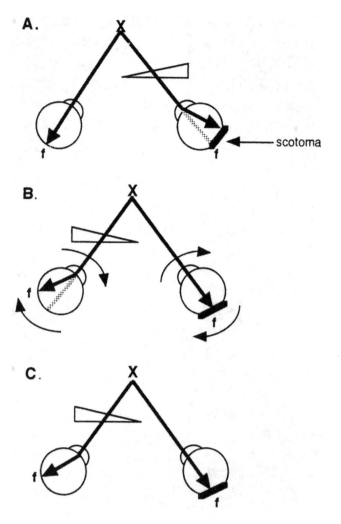

Figure 4–26. Movement of the eyes during the 4△ Base Out test when the patient has a suppression scotoma in his right eye. **A.** When the prism is placed over the patient's right eye, the retinal image shifts but is still located within the suppression zone. The patient does not see double so neither eye moves. **B.** When the prism is placed over the patient's left eye, the retinal image shifts and the left eye moves inward to regain foveal fixation. The right eye makes a concomitant outward movement. **C.** The retinal image in the right eye is still located within the suppression zone, so there is no refixation movement of the right eye.

4△ Base Out *at a glance*

PROCEDURE	NORMAL RESULT WHEN THERE IS NO CENTRAL SUPPRESSION SCOTOMA	RESULT WHEN THERE IS A CENTRAL SUPPRESSION SCOTOMA OF THE RIGHT EYE	RESULT WHEN THERE IS A CENTRAL SUPPRESSION SCOTOMA OF THE LEFT EYE
Place 4△ BO on OD	OD moves in OS moves out and then in	OD does not move OS does not move	OD moves in OS moves out but does not move in
Place 4△ BO on OS	OS moves in OD moves out and then in	OS moves in OD moves out but does not move in	OS does not move OD does not move

5

OCULAR HEALTH ASSESSMENT

Daniel Kurtz, OD, PhD

CHAPTER AT A GLANCE

INTRODUCTION TO OCULAR HEALTH ASSESSMENT

Ocular health assessment is usually performed at the end of the examination because pupillary dilation and the bright illumination required for many of the procedures may alter other test results. By this point in the examination, the examiner should have a fairly clear indication of the patient's ocular health status. The case history provides many clues about the health of the eyes. Symptoms such as haloes around lights, flashes of light, or eye pain imply potentially serious problems. The patient may have a medical condition that has associated ocular manifestations, or he may be taking a systemic medication that produces ocular side effects. Many of the entrance tests such as pupillary testing, color vision testing, and extraocular motility testing screen primarily for ocular health problems. The patient's best-corrected visual acuity is an excellent indicator of the health of the eye. If visual acuity is 20/20 or better, the macula and optic nerve are functioning well, and the media along the visual axis are clear. If visual acuity is not 20/20 and functional etiologies such as amblyopia have been ruled out, an ocular health problem is the likely cause.

The main route or the core testing portion of the ocular health examination is designed to effectively and efficiently screen for disease or potential problems in each of three major areas:

1. the anterior segment of the eye
2. the posterior segment of the eye
3. the neurological elements of the eyes and the visual system (including screening for glaucoma). To enhance examination of the neurological status of the patient, see also Chapter 8, Cranial Nerve Screening.

If the main route uncovers unusual findings or if the patient's symptoms or case history suggest an ocular health problem, side trips or problem-specific testing are incorporated into the examination (see Figure 5–1). There are numerous problem-specific tests available, and that number continues to grow as new technology and instrumentation become available. It is beyond the scope of this book to include all these techniques. The techniques chosen for inclusion in this text allow the examiner to assess a wide range of common ocular problems without the need for expensive, high-technology equipment.

The main route suggested in this section is not meant to be rigidly defined. Individual examiners may prefer to modify this portion of the examination based on their own professional judgment or patient population. For

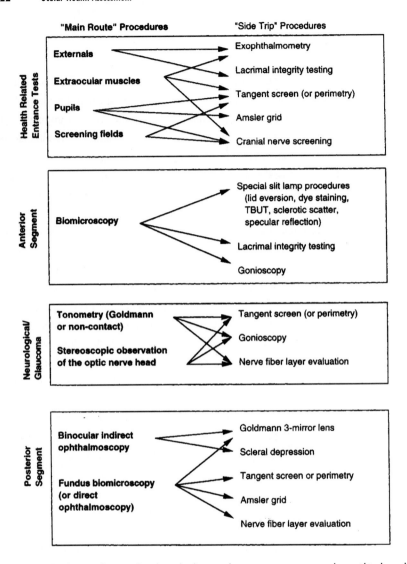

Figure 5-1. This diagram illustrates the relationship between the main route or core procedures within the ocular health assessment examination and the side trip or problem-specific procedures. The main route procedures are in bold print on the left and the side trips are in plain print on the right.

instance, an examiner whose patient population is primarily geriatric may include the Amsler grid test in his main route to routinely screen for macular disease.

When contemplating the tests to include in the core examination, it is important to determine whether or not the patient's eyes will be dilated.

Pupillary dilation greatly enhances the examiner's ability to observe certain ocular structures, such as the crystalline lens, the vitreous, and the peripheral retina. Pupillary dilation makes possible a number of techniques that are difficult or impossible to perform on the undilated eye. These procedures include binocular indirect ophthalmoscopy, fundus biomicroscopy, and Goldmann 3-mirror lens evaluation of the retina. The standard of optometric care now recommends that all comprehensive ocular examinations include examination of the ocular fundus with pupillary dilation.

When incorporating dilation into the examination, careful consideration must be given to the sequence of testing. Many of the pharmaceutical agents used for dilation affect the accommodative mechanism of the eye, so that all tests requiring accurate focusing must be completed prior to instillation of the dilating drops. Pupillary testing must also be completed before dilation, because the pupils will be unable to constrict after dilation. Biomicroscopy should be performed to evaluate the integrity of the anterior segment of the eye, and the anterior chamber angle depth must be estimated via the van Herick technique to determine if it is safe to dilate. If the angle depth is less than 1/4:1 according to the van Herick method, then gonioscopy should be performed to more accurately assess the angle and the safety of dilation. Finally, the patient's intraocular pressure (IOP) must be measured prior to dilation.

All techniques that are enhanced by pupillary dilation should be deferred until after dilation occurs. These include evaluation of the crystalline lens and anterior vitreous with the biomicroscope, and assessment of the posterior segment. Figure 5–2 presents a suggested examination sequence for a comprehensive examination when the patient's pupils are to be dilated.

A number of techniques described in this section involve instruments that are placed in direct contact with ocular surfaces or fluids. It is critical that these instruments be disinfected following the guidelines set forth by the Centers for Disease Control (CDC). It is recommended that instruments be soaked for at least 10 minutes in one of the following solutions: 3% hydrogen peroxide, 70% ethanol or isopropyl alcohol, or 0.5% sodium hypochlorite (1:100 dilution of common household bleach). Scrupulous care is required to wash off all disinfecting solutions before the instrument comes in contact with the eye or tear fluid. The examiner should observe universal health precautions whenever a procedure involves touching a patient: vigorous hand washing with soap and hot water or a germicidal hand-washing solution is appropriate before and after every patient encounter to prevent the spread of infection.

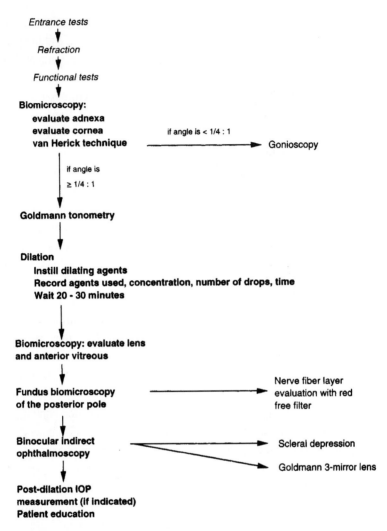

Figure 5–2. Flow diagram illustrating a suggested sequence of tests for the ocular health assessment when the patient's pupils are being dilated. The first three groups (in italics) are not part of the health assessment, but are included to remind the examiner that these tests must be completed prior to dilating the patient's pupils. The procedures on the right are problem-specific techniques that are performed only when indicated.

The procedures presented in this chapter are grouped according to their primary purpose. Techniques for evaluating the anterior segment of the eye are presented first. Procedures for observing the posterior segment are next. Tests used to assess the neurological elements of the eye, including screening for glaucoma, are at the end of the chapter and in Chapter 8.

Biomicroscopy (Slit Lamp)

PURPOSE   To evaluate the health of the anterior segment of the eye as far poster-
            ior as the anterior portion of the vitreous humor. The slit lamp is used
            in conjunction with auxiliary lenses to view the anterior chamber angle
            and the ocular fundus. The slit lamp is essential in the evaluation of
            contact lenses on the eye.

EQUIPMENT

- Biomicroscope (slit lamp).

BASIC COMPONENTS OF A SLIT LAMP

Although slit lamps vary considerably from manufacturer to manufacturer, there
are a number of components common to all slit lamps.

Illumination Arm

The illumination arm houses the illumination system. The angle of the arm can be
varied from 0° to 90° from the straight ahead position. The following components
are located on the illumination arm:

- *Slit controls:* There are two size controls, one to vary the slit width and another
  to vary the slit height. There is also a control that varies the orientation or tilt of
  the beam.
- *Click stop:* The click stop changes the position of the reflecting mirror to alter
  the angle of the beam with respect to the viewing system. When the mirror is
  "in click stop," the focus of the slit beam will be coincident with the focus of
  the viewing system. This is known as the "confocal" quality of the biomicroscope.
- *Filters:* The filters are used to vary the appearance of the slit beam. Most slit
  lamps include a cobalt blue filter, a green or red-free filter, and at least one neutral density filter.

Microscope Arm

The microscope arm houses the viewing system, composed of the objective and
ocular lenses. The angle of the microscope arm can be varied, although it is nor-

mally kept in the straight ahead position. The following components are located on the microscope arm:

- *Oculars:* The oculars are adjustable to compensate for the examiner's refractive error. The distance between the oculars is variable and can be adjusted to match the examiner's PD.
- *Magnification changer:* The magnification changer allows magnification to be adjusted either in a stepwise fashion or in a continuous fashion (zoom system).

Slit Lamp Position Controls

- *Joystick/elevation knob:* These may be two separate controls or a single control. They are found on the instrument base. The joystick controls the forward movement, and therefore the focus, of the slit lamp. It also controls the left-to-right movement of the slit lamp. The elevation knob controls the height of the microscope.

SET-UP

- The patient removes his optical correction.
- The room illumination is dim.
- Disinfect the forehead rest and the chin rest.
- Adjust the height of the instrument table to a comfortable position for both the patient and the examiner.
- Set the reflecting mirror in the click stop position.
- Instruct the patient to place his chin in the chin rest and his forehead gently against the forehead rest.
- Adjust the chin rest to align the patient's outer canthus with the demarcation line on the upright support of the headrest.
- Set the magnification on a low setting ($6\times$ or $10\times$). Remove all filters from the illumination system.
- Instruct the patient to close his eyes. Turn on the instrument. Using the patient's eyelashes for fixation, focus each ocular by closing one eye at a time and rotating the eyepiece. Always begin with the eyepiece on the highest plus setting (as far counterclockwise as possible) and rotate it clockwise until the image first clears.
- Open both of your eyes and set the slit lamp to your PD by adjusting the separation of the oculars. If the PD is set properly, you should obtain a binocular view when looking through the oculars.
- Use one hand to operate both the joystick (to align and focus the microscope) and the elevation knob (to align the microscope) and the other hand to operate the slit controls, to vary the angle between the lamp and the microscope, and to manipulate the patient's eyelids.

STEP-BY-STEP PROCEDURE

The anterior segment of the eye is usually examined in an anterior-to-posterior sequence. The structures are generally examined in the following order: lids and lashes, conjunctiva, tear film, cornea, anterior chamber angle, iris, and lens. During a routine slit lamp examination the right eye is usually examined first, followed by the left eye.

LIDS AND LASHES
1. Use diffuse illumination with the illumination arm set approximately 30° from the straight ahead position.
2. Set the magnification on a low setting (6× or 10×).
3. Instruct the patient to close his eyes. Starting at the temporal canthus, scan across the upper lid and lashes.
4. Instruct the patient to open his eyes. Scan from nasal to temporal across the lower lid and lashes, observing the tear meniscus, the lid apposition to the globe, and the openings of the Meibomian glands.

CONJUNCTIVA
5. Narrow the beam to a wide parallelepiped, with the illumination arm set approximately 30° from the straight ahead position.
6. Keep the magnification on a low setting (6× or 10×).
7. Instruct the patient to open his eyes and to look up.
8. Inform the patient that you are going to touch his lower lid. Place your index finger close to the patient's lower lash margin and evert the lower lid. Scan the inferior palpebral and bulbar conjunctiva looking for elevations, depressions, or discolorations. Evaluate the openness of the inferior punctum. You should be scanning from temporal to nasal at this point.

TABLE 5–1. TYPE OF SLIT BEAM, ANGLE OF THE ILLUMINATION ARM FROM THE STRAIGHT AHEAD POSITION, AND MAGNIFICATION USED TO EVALUATE VARIOUS OCULAR STRUCTURES DURING THE ROUTINE SLIT LAMP EXAMINATION

Ocular Structure	Type of Slit Lamp Beam	Angle of Illumination Arm	Magnification
Lids/lashes	Diffuse	30°	Low
Conjunctiva	Wide parallelepiped	30°	Low
Cornea	Narrow parallelepiped	30–45°	Medium
Anterior chamber			
Angle depth	Optic section	60°	Medium
Aqueous	Conical beam	30°	High
Iris	Wide parallelepiped	30–45°	Medium
Lens	Narrow parallelepiped	20–30°	Medium

9. Instruct the patient to look down.
10. Inform the patient that you are going to touch his upper lid. Place your thumb close to the upper lash margin and elevate the lid. Scan across the superior bulbar conjunctiva.
11. Instruct the patient to look first to the left and then to the right, while you scan the nasal and temporal bulbar conjunctiva.
12. If indicated, evert the upper lid at this time (see section on special slit lamp procedures).

CORNEA AND TEAR FILM

13. Decrease the beam to a narrow parallelepiped, approximately 1 to 3 mm wide. Set the illumination arm approximately 30° to 45° from the straight ahead position (see Figures 5–3 and 5–4).
14. Set the magnification on a medium setting (16× or 20×).
15. Instruct the patient to look straight ahead. At this point the illumination arm is angled temporally, so it is often convenient to estimate the depth of the temporal anterior chamber by the van Herick technique now (see steps 19 to 26 below). Then, scan across the central portion of the cornea looking for any opacities or irregularities. When you reach the apex of the cornea, swing the illumination arm to the other side, set it at the proper angle, and continue scanning. It may be necessary to back up slightly after shifting the illumination arm, so you do not miss scanning part of the cornea. If appropriate, when you have scanned to the nasal aspect of the cornea, measure the nasal anterior chamber by the van Herick method.
16. Instruct the patient to look down. Elevate the upper lid with your thumb, and scan across the superior one third of the cornea. Remember to shift the illumination arm when you reach the corneal apex.

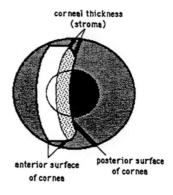

Figure 5–3. Diagram of a corneal parallelepiped. Note the three dimensional effect obtained when the parallelepiped is properly focused.

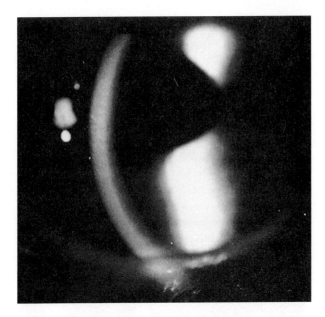

Figure 5–4. Photograph of a corneal parallelepiped.

17. Instruct the patient to look up. Pull down the lower lid with your index finger if necessary, and scan across the inferior one third of the cornea. Remember to shift the illumination arm when you reach the corneal apex.
18. If indicated, specular reflection should be performed at this time (see section on special slit lamp procedures).

Depth of the Anterior Chamber Angle by the van Herick Technique

If you have not done so already, measure the depth of the anterior chamber angle at this time.

19. Set the illumination arm 60° to the temporal or nasal side of the patient's line of fixation. As an alternative, the illumination arm can be set 30° to one side and the microscope 30° to the other side, yielding a 60° angle between the lamp and the microscope.
20. The magnification should remain on a medium setting (16× or 20×).
21. Narrow the beam to an optic section (see Figures 5–5 and 5–6).
22. Instruct the patient to look straight ahead.
23. Focus the light sharply on the cornea at the very edge of the temporal limbus.
24. Compare the width of the "shadow" formed on the iris (representing the depth of the anterior chamber) to the width of the optic section (representing the thickness of the cornea) (see Figures 5–7 and 5–8).

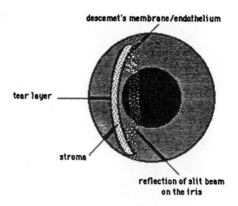

Figure 5–5. Diagram of a corneal optic section.

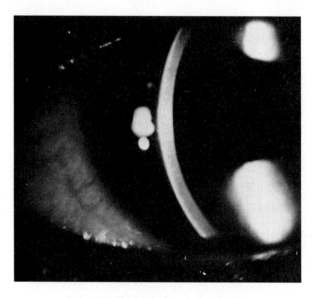

Figure 5–6. Photograph of a corneal optic section.

Note: The shadow is actually a dark interval between the light on the cornea and the light on the iris that represents the optically empty aqueous in the anterior chamber.

25. If the angle width is less than 1/4:1, gonioscopy should be performed to evaluate the angle more thoroughly.
26. If the microscope arm was moved for this procedure (see step 19), return it to the straight ahead position before proceeding.

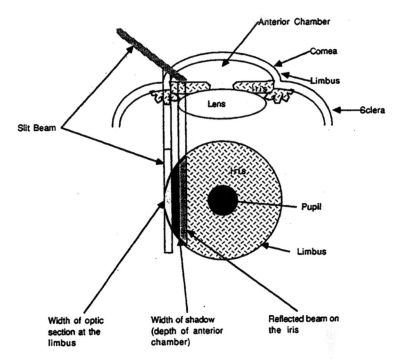

Figure 5–7. Diagram of the set-up for estimating the depth of the anterior chamber angle using the van Herick technique. The width of the "shadow" or dark interval (representing the depth of the anterior chamber) is compared to the width of the optic section (representing the thickness of the cornea).

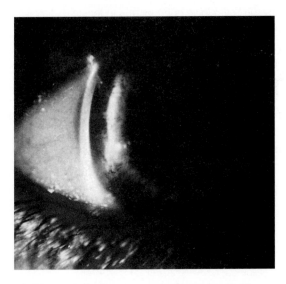

Figure 5–8. Photograph of the van Herick technique. An optic section is positioned at the temporal limbus. The width of the "shadow" is greater than the width of the optic section, so the anterior chamber angle is estimated as >1:1.

IRIS

27. Increase the slit width to a wide parallelepiped (approximately 3 mm), and set the illumination arm 30° to 45° from the straight ahead position.
28. Keep the magnification on a medium setting (16× or 20×).
29. Instruct the patient to look straight ahead.
30. Scan across the iris surface, looking for irregularities. Note the pupillary light reflex. The pupil should constrict when the slit lamp beam reaches the pupillary margin.

Crystalline Lens

31. Narrow the angle of the illumination arm to about 10° to 20° from the straight ahead position.
32. Keep the magnification on a medium setting (16× or 20×).
33. Reduce the slit beam to a narrow parallelepiped.
34. Slowly move the slit lamp closer to the patient until the light is directed through the pupil and becomes sharply focused on the anterior surface of the lens (see Figure 5–9). Scan the front of the lens. Then move the biomicroscope closer to the patient to examine the deeper layers of the lens. Focus on the posterior surface of the lens. Look for any opacities, irregularities, or discolorations within the lens. Swing the illumination arm to the opposite side, set at the proper angle, and again examine the lens from the anterior to the posterior surface. If any opacity is noted, narrow the beam to an optic section to locate its precise depth within the crystalline lens.

RECORDING

- Record for each eye separately.
- List each structure evaluated and record your observations for each.
- Record any abnormalities or pertinent negatives.
- Drawings and photographs are recommended in cases where they enhance descriptions.

EXAMPLE

OD		OS
Clear	Lids	Clear
Clear	Lashes	Flaky
Clear	Conjunctiva	Concretions, inferior palpebral

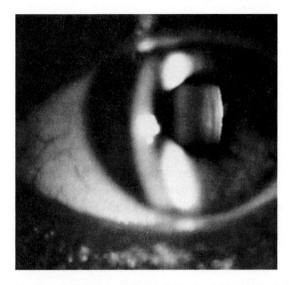

Figure 5–9. Photograph showing a parallelepiped of the lens through a nondilated pupil.

Small opacity, anterior stroma at limbus 3 o/c	Cornea	Arcus inferiorly
1/2:1	Angle	1/2:1
Flat	Iris	Flat; nevus at 3:00 periph.
Clear	Lens	Epicapsular stars

BIOMICROSCOPY *at a glance*

PURPOSE	TECHNIQUE
Prepare the slit lamp	Focus the oculars Adjust the PD Check click stop Magnification on low
Prepare the patient	Adjust table height so patient is comfortable Adjust chin rest to proper height
Scan the lids and lashes	Diffuse beam Illumination arm at 30° Low magnification
Scan the conjunctiva	Narrow parallelepiped Illumination arm at 30° Low magnification Hold lids and direct the patient's gaze as needed

BIOMICROSCOPY *at a glance (cont.)*

PURPOSE	TECHNIQUE
Scan the cornea	Narrow parallelepiped Illumination arm at 30–45° Medium magnification Scan three times—superior, central, inferior cornea—holding lids and directing patient's gaze as needed
Estimate the depth of the anterior chamber angle	Optic section Illumination arm at 60° Medium magnification Focus at the temporal limbus Compare depth of anterior chamber to thickness of cornea
Scan the iris	Wide parallelepiped Illumination arm at 30–45° Medium magnification
Scan the lens	Narrow parallelepiped Illumination arm at 20–30° Medium magnification

SPECIAL SLIT LAMP PROCEDURES

The following procedures are not considered to be part of the routine slit lamp evaluation, but are incorporated into the examination when indicated. For the special slit lamp procedures, the set-up is the same as that outlined for biomicroscopy.

Examination of the Anterior Chamber

PURPOSE   To check for the presence of cells and flare in the aqueous.

INDICATIONS

Indicated when you suspect or wish to rule out an active iritis or anterior uveitis, based on the patient's symptoms, history, or other examination findings.

STEP-BY-STEP PROCEDURE

1. This procedure is usually done at the completion of the routine slit lamp examination because of the need to adjust a number of controls on the slit lamp.
2. Reduce all the room illumination. Wait a few minutes until you are dark adapted.
3. Set the illumination arm 30° from the straight ahead position.
4. Adjust the magnification to a high setting ($25\times$ or $40\times$).
5. Create a conical beam by adjusting the width of the beam to a narrow parallelepiped and adjusting the vertical slit control to the shortest setting.
6. Instruct the patient to look straight ahead and to blink whenever he needs to.
7. Direct the beam into the pupil. Move the slit lamp forward and back, alternately focusing from the cornea to the anterior surface of the lens. Whenever the slit lamp is focused in between the cornea and the lens, direct your attention to the anterior chamber to look for the presence of cells or flare in the aqueous.

RECORDING

- The results of this procedure are included in the slit lamp recording section, under "anterior chamber."
- Record for each eye separately.

- If the anterior chamber is clear, record "no cells or flare" or "no C or F."
- If the anterior chamber is not clear, record your observations. The number of cells and the amount of flare may be graded on a scale of 1 to 4, or as minimal, moderate, or severe. You may also indicate the number of cells seen.

EXAMPLES

- OD   OS
  no cells or flare   AC   moderate flare, no cells
- OS   OD
  grade 2+ flare   AC   clear, no C or F
  minimal cells

Eversion of the Upper Lid

PURPOSE   To allow observation of the palpebral conjunctiva of the upper lid.

INDICATIONS

Indicated for all contact lens patients or prior to fitting a patient with contact lenses to establish the baseline condition of the palpebral conjunctiva. Indicated if the patient has a red eye or if the patient's symptoms, history, or other examination findings suggest a foreign body under the upper lid.

ADDITIONAL EQUIPMENT

- Sterile cotton swab.
  Note: Make sure your hands are recently washed before performing this procedure.

STEP-BY-STEP PROCEDURE

1. With the patient positioned in the slit lamp, instruct the patient to look down.
2. Grasp the patient's eyelashes or upper lid at the lid margin between your thumb and index finger. Gently pull the lid down and away from the globe.
3. With your free hand, insert the cotton tip of the swab at the posterior (upper) margin of the tarsal plate in the center of the lid. An alternate technique is to use the index or middle finger of either hand in place of the swab.
4. Gently press down on the swab while pulling the lid margin out and upward. Once the lid is everted, tether it firmly against the superior orbital rim with your thumb or index finger.
5. Remove the cotton swab and reposition the slit lamp to view the superior palpebral conjunctiva. The illumination arm should be set approximately 30° from the straight ahead position and the beam should be adjusted to a wide parallelepiped.
6. Scan the superior palpebral conjunctiva, looking for elevations, depressions, foreign bodies, or injection.

RECORDING

- The results for this procedure are recorded in the slit lamp recording section under "palpebral conjunctiva."
- Record for each eye separately.
- There is no need to indicate that lid eversion was done. By recording observations for the superior or upper palpebral conjunctiva, it is assumed that you everted the patient's lid.

Corneal or Conjunctival Staining

PURPOSE To evaluate the integrity of the corneal or conjunctival epithelium.

INDICATIONS

Ophthalmic dyes are used when slit lamp evaluation of the cornea indicates that the corneal epithelium may be disrupted. This procedure is also indicated when the patient has signs or symptoms suggesting corneal disease.

ADDITIONAL EQUIPMENT

- Sodium fluorescein strips.
- Rose Bengal or lissamine green strips.
- Sterile saline solution.
  Note: Lissamine green and rose Bengal reveal similar staining patterns, but lissamine green produces less stinging or irritation upon instillation and is tolerated better than rose Bengal by most patients.

STEP-BY-STEP PROCEDURE

1. Wet the end of the strip with a drop of sterile saline solution.
2. Instruct the patient to look to the left or to the right. As shown in Figure 5–10, pull down the lower lid and touch the moistened end of the strip to the patient's temporal bulbar conjunctiva, such that if the patient blinks when the strip touches his eye, the strip will not rub across his cornea.
3. Instruct the patient to blink several times to spread the dye over the corneal and conjunctival surfaces.
4. Reposition the patient in the slit lamp.
5. Set the illumination arm 30° from the straight ahead position. Adjust the slit to a wide parallelepiped and set the magnification to the medium setting.
6. Insert the cobalt blue filter if using fluorescein dye. Rose Bengal or lissamine green stain is observed without the use of filters.
7. Scan the cornea and conjunctiva looking for areas of staining. Fluorescein staining appears bright green when viewed with the cobalt blue filter. Rose

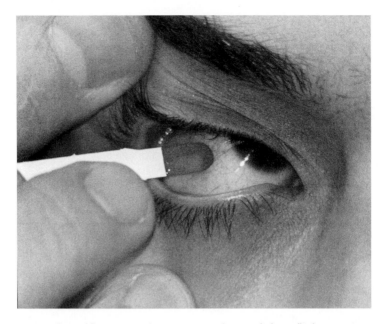

Figure 5–10. Instillation of fluorescein into the patient's eye. As the patient looks nasally, the examiner supports the upper lid, pulls down the lower lid, and touches the moist end of the fluorescein strip to the temporal bulbar conjunctiva.

Bengal staining appears deep pink in white light. Lissamine green staining appears pale green in white light.

8. Carefully note the location and the pattern of staining. Many standardized scales and standardized sets of photographs now exist for assessing and grading the degree and location of staining in the eye. It is recommended that the reader select one such scale and use it consistently in clinical practice so as to make evaluation of staining consistent upon repeated measures on the same patient or between patients.

RECORDING

- The results for this procedure are recorded in the slit lamp recording section under "cornea" or "conjunctiva."
- Record for each eye separately.
- Indicate the ophthalmic dye used.
- If the results are normal, record "no staining." If there is staining, indicate the amount and the pattern of the staining. Illustrations are extremely helpful (see Figure 5–11).

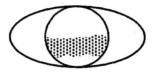

Figure 5–11. Illustration recording moderate punctate staining of the interpalpebral zone of the cornea. This pattern of staining is usually associated with dry eye conditions.

EXAMPLES

- OD   OS
  no staining with RB   Cornea   mild punctate staining with
                                       RB inf. cornea

- OD   OS
  large area of coalesced   Cornea   no staining with NaFl
  staining with NaFl,
  central cornea

Specular Reflection Technique

PURPOSE   To evaluate the corneal endothelium.

INDICATIONS

The use of specular reflection is indicated when other examination findings suggest corneal endothelial dysfunction.

STEP-BY-STEP PROCEDURE

1. Adjust the slit beam to a medium width parallelepiped.
2. Begin with the magnification on low or medium (10× or 16×).
3. Focus the parallelepiped on the cornea with the illumination arm set approximately 30° from the straight ahead position.
4. Using the joystick, adjust the position of the microscope or change the angle of the illumination arm until the slit beam intersects the reflection of the light filament on the cornea. This is the point at which the angle of reflection is equal to the incident angle of the light. When properly set up, you will see an area of bright glare from the front surface of the cornea. This will be visible through one ocular only.

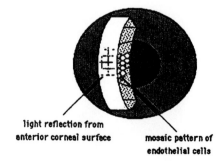

light reflection from
anterior corneal surface

mosaic pattern of
endothelial cells

Figure 5–12. Diagram showing the use of specular reflection for observing the corneal endothelium. When high magnification (25× or 40×) is used, the mosaic pattern of the endothelial cells can be visualized within the reflected light on the posterior aspect of the parallelepiped.

5. Increase the magnification to the highest setting (25× or 40×).
6. Adjust the focus of the slit lamp so that it is sharply focused on the corneal endothelium. Exact focus is critical. Observe the mosaic pattern of the endothelial cells (see Figure 5–12).
7. To observe other areas of the endothelium, it is necessary to move the entire slit lamp and readjust the illumination arm.

RECORDING

- The results of this procedure are listed in the slit lamp recording section under "cornea." It is not necessary to indicate that specular reflection was used.
- Record your observations for each eye separately.

Sclerotic Scatter Technique

PURPOSE   To evaluate the cornea for areas of localized corneal edema. Sclerotic scatter is used primarily to observe corneal edema caused by firm contact lenses.

INDICATIONS

Sclerotic scatter is indicated in all rigid contact lens wearers. It should be performed immediately after the lenses have been removed, because corneal edema may dissipate quickly.

STEP-BY-STEP PROCEDURE

1. Adjust the slit beam to a narrow parallelepiped.
2. Push the microscope to one side so you are able to directly observe the cornea along the patient's line of sight without looking through the oculars of the slit lamp.
3. Adjust the slit beam to a narrow parallelepiped, and set the illumination arm approximately 45° from the patient's line of sight.
4. Focus the slit beam at the patient's temporal limbus. When the beam is properly positioned, you will see a halo of light at the nasal limbus (see Figures 5–13 and 5–14).

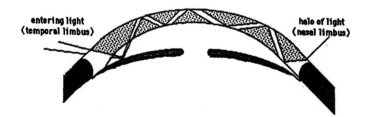

Figure 5–13. Diagram of sclerotic scatter, showing the path of the light as it travels through the cornea. If the cornea is clear, the light entering at the temporal limbus will be totally internally reflected and emerge at the nasal limbus, producing a limbal glow. If the cornea is edematous or opacified, the light will be scattered rather than reflected, and haziness will be observed.

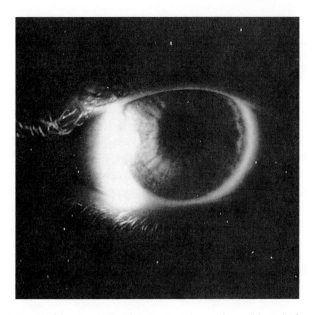

Figure 5–14. Photograph of the set-up for the sclerotic scatter technique. The parallelepiped is focused on the temporal limbus, creating a halo of light at the nasal limbus.

5. Observe the patient's cornea against the dark background of the pupil, looking for haziness.

RECORDING

- The results of this procedure are listed in the slit lamp recording section under "cornea." It is not necessary to indicate that sclerotic scatter was used.
- Record your observations for each eye separately.
- The haziness caused by localized corneal edema is referred to as central corneal clouding (CCC). It is usually graded on a scale of 1 to 4, or quantified as mild, moderate, or severe.

EXAMPLE

OD		OS
no edema	Cornea	grade 1+ CCC

Instillation of Drops

PURPOSE   Pharmaceutical agents in the form of eye drops are routinely instilled in a patient's eyes to anesthetize the cornea or to dilate the pupil. Many ocular therapeutic pharmaceutical agents are in drop form and may be instilled in the same manner.

EQUIPMENT

- Bottle containing eye drops.
- Tissues.

SET-UP

- The patient is seated and given a tissue.
- Dim room illumination may prevent excess lacrimation.

STEP-BY-STEP PROCEDURE

1. Inform the patient that you are going to instill drops in his eyes and that the drops may cause temporary stinging. If you plan to instill dilating drops, the patient should be informed of the adverse effects of dilation. He should give his consent before you proceed.
2. Remove the bottle cap and hold it in the palm of your hand without touching the inside surface. Hold the bottle between the thumb and index finger of your dominant hand.
3. Instruct the patient to lean his head back and look up to the ceiling. Provide a fixation target if necessary.
4. Using the middle finger of the hand holding the bottle or the index finger of your opposite hand, gently pull down or evert the lower lid of the patient's right eye as shown in Figure 5–15. This creates a pocket in the inferior cul-de-sac to hold the drop immediately following its instillation. Occasionally, it may be necessary to hold the patient's upper lid in addition to everting his lower lid. Then, it is appropriate to use one hand to hold the lids and the other hand to hold the bottle.

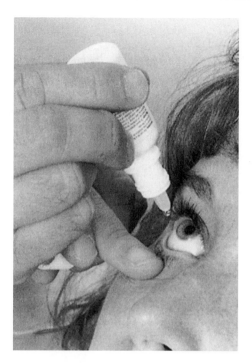

Figure 5–15. Instillation of drops into the patient's right eye. While the patient looks up, the examiner pulls down the inferior lid to form a pocket where the drop is instilled.

5. Position the bottle tip close to the patient's eye, but far enough away that the patient's lashes will not touch the tip even if he blinks (1 to 2 cm).
6. Squeeze the bottle to allow a single drop to fall into the patient's inferior cul-de-sac.
7. Repeat steps 3 to 6 for the left eye if indicated.
8. Instruct the patient to close his eyes and gently wipe the excess fluid from his eyes with a tissue.
9. If you experience great difficulty in controlling the eyelids sufficiently to permit instillation of drops (e.g., in small children), you may use the following technique:
   a. do not attempt to open the patient's eyes, but allow him to keep his eyes gently shut;
   b. recline the patient into a supine position;
   c. place two drops of the agent on the inner canthus where the upper and lower lids meet;
   d. instruct the patient to open his eyes slowly. The hydrostatic pressure of the patient's tears will pull the drops into the eye in sufficient quantity to work.

RECORDING

- Record the pharmaceutical agent used including its concentration, how many drops were instilled into each eye, and the time of day.

EXAMPLES

- Dilated with 1 drop 1% tropicamide, 1 drop 2.5% phenylephrine OD only @ 9:45 AM
- 1 drop 1% cyclopentolate OD & OS @ 11:35 AM

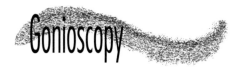
Gonioscopy

PURPOSE   To observe and evaluate the anterior chamber angle.

INDICATIONS

Gonioscopy is indicated prior to pupillary dilation when the anterior chamber angle is less than 1/4:1 by the van Herick technique. Other indications include glaucoma or suspected glaucoma of either the open-angle or closed-angle variety, any condition that predisposes the patient to iris neovascularization, syndromes associated with glaucoma (e.g., pigment dispersion or pseudoexfoliation), a history of blunt trauma to the eye, or any suspicious iris lesions. Gonioscopy is contraindicated in the presence of corneal penetrating injury or hyphema.

EQUIPMENT

- Goldmann 3-mirror lens or 4-mirror gonioscopy lens, cleaned and disinfected.
- Biomicroscope.
- Gonioscopy fluid or other highly viscous lubricant.
- Topical anesthetic (e.g., 0.5% proparacaine).
- Sterile saline irrigating solution.
  Note: Numerous indirect (mirrored) gonioscopic lenses are available, varying in size, shape, and number of mirrors. The Goldmann 3-mirror lens is commonly used because it is versatile, allowing for observation of the entire retina as well as the anterior chamber angle. The procedure described here assumes use of the 3-mirror lens but, with minor modifications, will apply to all indirect gonioscopy lenses.

SET-UP

- Adjust the slit lamp so it is comfortable for both the patient and the examiner.
- Focus the oculars, set the PD, remove all filters, and set the magnification on the lowest setting.
- Adjust the slit beam to a medium width parallelepiped and set the illumination arm of the biomicroscope in the straight ahead position (zero degrees).
- Prepare the gonioscopy lens by filling the concave face of the lens with 2 to 3 drops of gonioscopy fluid. Take care to avoid bubbles in the solution. The first

drop from the bottle should be dropped onto a tissue. The bottle should be stored upside down.

• Rule out conditions that would contraindicate gonioscopy, such as severe corneal trauma or a red eye of infectious etiology.

• Instill a single drop of a topical anesthetic into the eye to be examined. If both eyes are to be examined, instill the anesthetic into both at the start of the test.

STEP-BY-STEP PROCEDURE

Insertion of the 3-Mirror Lens

1. Position the patient in the slit lamp. It is helpful to lower the chin rest slightly, so the patient's lateral canthus falls slightly below the alignment mark. This ensures that the slit beam can reach the gonioscopy mirror when the mirror is in the superior position.

2. Grasp the gonioscopy lens in your dominant hand between your thumb and index finger. Hold it in such a way that when it comes to rest on the patient's eye, the thumbnail-shaped mirror will be located in the 12 o'clock position.

3. Instruct the patient to look down and grasp the patient's upper lid firmly with your nondominant hand.

4. Instruct the patient to look up and pull down the patient's lower lid with the middle or fourth finger of the hand holding the lens. At the same time, firmly tether his upper lid against the superior rim of his orbit.

5. Insert the lower edge of the lens into the inferior cul-de-sac (see Figure 5–16). Rock the lens toward the patient until the entire lens is firmly in contact with the globe as shown in Figure 5–17. Look through the central lens of the Goldmann 3-mirror to tell when the lens is in contact with the globe.

6. Instruct the patient to *slowly* look down until he is fixating straight ahead. Then slowly release the patient's lids. Continue holding the lens throughout the entire procedure, but do not push the lens forward against the patient's cornea.

7. Check that the thumbnail-shaped mirror is located in the 12 o'clock position. If it is not, rotate the lens until this mirror comes to that position. This permits you to observe the inferior angle first. The inferior angle is usually the most open and the most pigmented, so it is easier to identify the angle structures.

Insertion of the 4-Mirror Gonioscopy Lens

1. Position the patient in the slit lamp. It is helpful to lower the chin rest slightly, so the patient's lateral canthus falls slightly below the alignment

GONIOSCOPY *at a glance*

PURPOSE	TECHNIQUE
Prepare slit lamp	Adjust oculars, set PD Low magnification Illumination arm at 0° Medium width parallelpiped
Prepare goniolens	Fill meniscus with 2 to 3 drops of gonio fluid
Prepare patient	Scan anterior segment Instill topical anesthetic
Insert goniolens	Hold lens in dominant hand Hold patient's upper and lower lids Insert lower edge of lens in cul-de-sac, rotate lens to contact cornea Patient fixates straight ahead Release lids
Observe anterior chamber angle	Position goniomirror at 12 o'clock Position slit beam in mirror Focus on angle structures, increase magnification if needed Rotate lens 90°, rotate slit, focus Rotate lens through 360°, focusing in all four quadrants
Remove goniolens	Patient looks up Apply pressure against lower lid at edge of lens to break suction Clean and disinfect lens Irrigate patient's eye with sterile saline solution

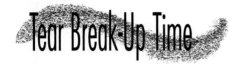

Tear Break-Up Time

PURPOSE To measure the stability of the tear film.

INDICATIONS

Tear break-up time (TBUT) should be measured when you suspect a lacrimal insufficiency based on the patient's symptoms or the slit lamp evaluation. A baseline TBUT should be measured prior to fitting a patient with contact lenses. The TBUT must be performed prior to instillation of a topical anesthetic or dilating agent because these may alter the composition of the tear film.

EQUIPMENT

- Biomicroscope.
- Sodium fluorescein strips.
- Sterile saline solution.

SET-UP

- Adjust the biomicroscope so it is comfortable for both the patient and the examiner.
- Focus the oculars, adjust the PD, and set the magnification on the lowest setting (6× or 10×).
- Insert the cobalt blue filter and set the illumination arm approximately 30° from the straight ahead position. Open the slit to a wide parallelepiped.

STEP-BY-STEP PROCEDURE

1. Moisten the end of a fluorescein strip with one drop of sterile saline.
2. Instruct the patient to look to the left or to the right. As shown in Figure 5–10, pull down the lower lid and touch the moistened end of the strip to the patient's temporal bulbar conjunctiva, such that if the patient blinks when the strip touches his eye, the strip will not be dragged across his cornea.
3. Instruct the patient to blink several times to spread the dye over the corneal

and conjunctival surfaces and then to keep his eyes open looking straight ahead.

4. Position the patient in the slit lamp and focus on the patient's cornea. The tear film will appear green due to the fluorescein.
5. Scan the entire cornea looking for dry areas, which will appear as dark spots or streaks. Count the number of seconds between the last blink and the first appearance of these dry spot formations.
6. Repeat steps 4 and 5 two more times and average the results. Note the position of the first dry spots. Observe if the tear film consistently breaks up in a specific location.
7. Instill fluorescein in the patient's left eye as in steps 1 to 3.
8. Repeat steps 4 to 6 on his left eye.

RECORDING

- Record the results for each eye separately.
- Record the average of the three trials in seconds.

EXAMPLE

- TBUT: OD 15 seconds; OS 12 seconds.

EXPECTED FINDINGS

- The normal TBUT is between 15 and 45 seconds. A break-up time longer than 20 seconds is not diagnostically significant.
- A TBUT less than 10 seconds is indicative of an unstable tear film.
- If the tear film consistently breaks up in the same location, it probably indicates a defect in the corneal epithelium rather than a tear deficiency.

Schirmer Tests: Schirmer #1 Test and Basic Lacrimation Test

PURPOSE   To evaluate the integrity of the lacrimal secretion system. The Schirmer #1 test measures the amount of total tear secretion within a 5-minute period. Total secretion is the sum of basal secretion and reflex secretion. In the basic lacrimation test, a topical anesthetic is used to eliminate reflex secretion, so only the amount of basal secretion within a 5-minute period is measured.

INDICATIONS

The Schirmer tests are indicated when a lacrimal deficiency is suspected based on the patient's symptoms or the slit lamp findings.

EQUIPMENT

- Two Schirmer test strips.
- Topical anesthetic (e.g., 0.5% proparacaine).
- Millimeter ruler (or millimeter scale on the Schirmer box).

SET-UP

- Before removing the Schirmer strips from their cellophane wrapping, fold the rounded ends of the strips so they will be creased at the notch.
- Remove the strips from the cellophane wrapper, taking care not to touch the rounded ends.
- Dim the room illumination.
- Perform the test with the patient in the upright, seated position.

STEP-BY-STEP PROCEDURE

Schirmer #1 Test
1. Instruct the patient to look up.
2. Gently pull down the lower lid of the right eye.

3. Place the folded, notched end of a Schirmer strip over the lower lid margin at its lateral third. Avoid touching the cornea with the Schirmer strip (see Figure 5–22).
4. Insert the second Schirmer strip in the left eye in the same manner.
5. Instruct the patient to keep his eyes open and continue to look up. He may blink freely, although excessive blinking may result in significant reflex tearing.
6. Remove the Schirmer test strips after 5 minutes, unless the entire strip wets before the end of the time period.
7. Mark the wet portion of the strip. Measure the amount of wetting from the notch in millimeters.

Basic Lacrimation Test
1. Instill one drop of topical anesthetic in each of the patient's eyes.
2. Wait for the reactive hyperemia and reflex tearing to subside, then gently blot the excess fluid from the patient's inferior cul-de-sac.
3. Repeat steps 1 through 7 under Schirmer #1 test.

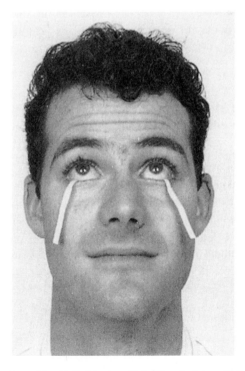

Figure 5–22. Schirmer strips positioned in the lateral one third of the patient's lower lid. The patient is instructed to look up to avoid contact between the strips and the cornea.

RECORDING

- Record the data for each eye separately.
- Record the test used (Schirmer #1 or basic lacrimation).
- Record the amount of wetting (in mm) on the Schirmer strip and the amount of time (in minutes) the strip was left in the eye.

EXAMPLES

- Schirmer #1 test: OD 30 mm/3 min.
- Basic lacrimation test: OS 10 mm/5 min.

EXPECTED RESULTS

- Although there is some disagreement about the interpretation of Schirmer tests, it is generally believed that wetting less than 10 mm in 5 minutes on either the Schirmer #1 test or the basic lacrimation test is significant. Wetting less than 5 mm in 5 minutes is considered diagnostic of lacrimal insufficiency.
- If there is 25 mm of wetting or more in a 5-minute period on the Schirmer #1 test, it indicates excessive reflex tearing. The basic lacrimation test should be performed.

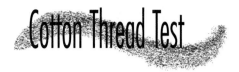
Cotton Thread Test

PURPOSE   To evaluate the integrity of the lacrimal secretion system.

INDICATIONS

The cotton thread test is indicated when a lacrimal deficiency is suspected based on the patient's symptoms or the slit lamp findings.

EQUIPMENT

- Cotton thread designed for lacrimal testing (e.g., Phenol red thread).
- Millimeter ruler (or millimeter scale on the box that the threads come in).
- Timepiece accurate to the second.

SET-UP

- Wait at least 5 minutes after the instillation of any eye drops. Anesthetic is not needed to perform this test.
- Remove the threads from the cellophane wrapper, taking care to preserve their sterility by not allowing them to touch anything.
- Unbend the ends of the threads so they can be easily hooked over the lower lid and in contact with the lower palpebral conjunctiva.
- The eyes are tested one at a time.
- Perform the test with the patient in the upright, seated position.

STEP-BY-STEP PROCEDURE

1. Instruct the patient to look up.
2. Gently evert the lower lid of the right eye.
3. Place the bent end of one thread over the lower lid margin at approximately one third of the distance from the lateral to the nasal canthus. Avoid touching the cornea with the thread.
4. Instruct the patient to keep his eyes open, to look straight ahead, and to blink normally.
5. After exactly 15 seconds remove the test thread by everting the lower eyelid and lifting upward on the thread.

6. Measure the full length of the wet portion of the thread from its very tip, in millimeters, disregarding the bend.
7. Repeat steps 3 through 6 for the left eye.

RECORDING

- Record the data for each eye separately.
- Record "cotton thread test."
- Record the amount of wetting (in mm) on the thread. If a length of time other than 15 seconds was used, also record the duration of the test.

EXAMPLES

- cotton thread test: OD 15 mm   OS 10 mm

EXPECTED RESULTS

- Wetting of 10 to 20 mm is considered normal

Fluorescein Clearance Test (or "Dye Disappearance Test")

PURPOSE   To evaluate the rate at which new tears replace existing tears in the eye.

INDICATIONS

The fluorescein clearance test is indicated when a lacrimal deficiency or possible blockage of the lacrimal drainage system is suspected based on the patient's symptoms or the slit lamp findings.

EQUIPMENT

- Four Schirmer test strips per eye being tested. In most patients it is only necessary to test one eye.
- Burton lamp or other UV light source.
- Sterile saline solution.
- Accurate timepiece.
- Fluorescein strips.

SET-UP

- Before removing the Schirmer strips from their cellophane wrapping, fold the rounded ends of the strips so they will be creased at the notch.
- Remove one strip from its cellophane wrapper, taking care not to touch the rounded ends.
- Dim the room illumination.
- Wet a fluorescein strip with sterile saline.
- Perform the test with the patient in the upright, seated position.

STEP-BY-STEP PROCEDURE

1. Instruct the patient to look to his left or right and gently pull down the lower lid of the right eye.

2. Touch the wetted fluorescein strip to the bulbar conjunctiva. The goal is to instill 5 μL of solution into the tear film.
3. Place the folded, notched end of a Schirmer strip over the lower lid margin at its lateral third. Avoid touching the cornea with the Schirmer strip (see Figure 5–22).
4. Remove the first Schirmer strip after 60 seconds and replace it with another.
5. Instruct the patient to keep his eyes open and continue to look up. He may blink freely, although excessive blinking may result in significant reflex tearing.
6. Remove the second Schirmer test strip after 10 minutes and replace it with another.
7. Remove the third Schirmer strip 20 minutes after the initial instillation of fluorescein and replace it with the final strip, which is removed 30 minutes after the start of the test.
8. As you remove each strip, examine it under the blue light for the presence of fluorescein.

RECORDING

- Record the eye tested.
- Record the presence or absence of fluorescein at each time interval from the beginning of the test.

EXAMPLES

- Fluorescein clearance test: OD 1 min + fl, 10 min + fl, 20 min neg fl, 30 min neg fl
- Fluorescein clearance test: OD 1 min + fl, 10 min + fl, 20 min + fl, 30 min + fl

EXPECTED RESULTS

- In patients with normal tear production and turnover, no fluorescein should be detectable at the 20- or 30-minute test.
- When fluorescence is present at the 20- and 30-minute tests, it is clear evidence of an aqueous tear deficiency
- For other types and causes of dry eye, an intermediate percentage of patients will show fluorescence at the 20- or 30-minute test, and interpretation of the results is ambiguous.

Jones #1 (Primary Dye) Test

PURPOSE   To determine the patency of the lacrimal excretory system, from the punctum to the inferior meatus of the nose.

INDICATIONS

The Jones #1 test should be performed when the patient complains of tearing, particularly unilateral tearing, or if the slit lamp evaluation shows pooling of the tears or punctal stenosis. This test can only be performed on one eye at each visit, and must be done prior to Goldmann tonometry or other tests requiring bilateral instillation of fluorescein.

EQUIPMENT

- Sodium fluorescein strips.
- Sterile cotton-tipped applicator.
- White tissue paper.
- Burton lamp or other UV light source.

SET-UP

- Wet a fluorescein strip with a couple of drops of sterile saline.
- Instruct the patient to look up, gently pull down his lower lid, and instill a moderate amount of fluorescein into the inferior cul-de-sac. The equivalent of 1 to 2 drops of liquid is required. Instill fluorescein into the symptomatic or suspect eye only.
- Instruct the patient to blink firmly three or four times.

STEP-BY-STEP PROCEDURE

Method #1 (Traditional Jones #1 Test)
1. Wait 2 minutes after instillation of the fluorescein.
2. Insert a sterile cotton-tipped applicator into the nose under the inferior meatus, located approximately 4 to 5 cm into the nose along the floor of the nasal canal.

3. Remove the applicator and check the cotton tip for the presence of fluorescein. If fluorescein is not grossly visible, observe the cotton tip under the UV light for fluorescence.

Method #2 (Modified Jones #1 Test)

1. After instilling the fluorescein and having the patient blink, wipe away the excess fluorescein.
2. Wait approximately 6 minutes, then instruct the patient to gently blow his nose on a piece of white tissue.
3. Examine the tissue for the presence of fluorescein. If fluorescein is not grossly visible, examine the tissue under the UV light.

Method #3 (Fluorescein Appearance Test)

1. After instilling the fluorescein and having the patient blink, wipe away the excess fluorescein.
2. Wait 15 to 30 minutes and examine the back of the patient's throat with the UV light for the presence of fluorescein.
3. If fluorescein is not present, continue checking for up to 90 minutes after instillation of the fluorescein. In the large majority of patients, fluorescein will be present within 30 to 60 minutes.

RECORDING

- Indicate which testing method was used (Jones #1, modified Jones #1, or fluorescein appearance test) and which eye was tested.
- The Jones test is recorded as "positive" if fluorescein appears on the cotton applicator, tissue, or in the throat. A positive result indicates that the lacrimal excretory system is not obstructed.
- The Jones test is recorded as "negative" if fluorescein is not present.
- The above terminology may be confusing, because for most tests "positive" indicates that an abnormality is present. It may be less confusing to simply record the presence or absence of fluorescein.

EXAMPLES

- Jones #1 test: OD negative
- Fluorescein appearance test OD: no fluorescein after 90 min

Direct Ophthalmoscopy

PURPOSE   To evaluate the health of the posterior segment of the eye. The direct ophthalmoscope is also useful to detect certain anomalies in the anterior segment of the eye.

EQUIPMENT

• Monocular direct ophthalmoscope.

SET-UP

• Adjust the examining chair so the patient's eyes are slightly lower than your eye level.
• Instruct the patient to remove his corrective lenses and look at a non-accommodative fixation target straight ahead or slightly above the horizontal at distance.

STEP-BY-STEP PROCEDURE

1. Hold the handle of the ophthalmoscope in your right hand and align the aperture in front of your right eye to examine the patient's right eye. Brace the head of the ophthalmoscope against your face or glasses. Use your index finger to turn the lens wheel.

2. Position your ophthalmoscope about 10 to 15 cm from the patient's eye, about 15° temporal to his line of sight. Using the spot beam with a +8 to +10 diopter lens, focus on the patient's iris. Check the optical clarity of the media by moving the ophthalmoscope about 30° in each direction (back and forth and up and down). Observe the orange reflex of the fundus within the pupil for dark areas indicative of media opacities.
   Note: this is similar to the use of the direct ophthalmoscope for the Bruckner test.

3. Slowly reduce the plus power and move closer to the patient until your hand holding the ophthalmoscope touches his face. Continue reducing plus power slowly until the features of the ocular fundus come into focus.

4. Locate the optic nerve head ("disc"). The optic nerve head should be visible when you are positioned approximately 15° temporal to the patient's visual axis.

5. Examine the disc: margins, rim tissue (color and contour), cup size, and depth. Determine the cup-to-disc (C/D) ratio for both its horizontal and vertical dimensions. This step is critical. Check the veins as they exit from the cup for spontaneous venous pulsation (SVP).

6. Examine the region adjacent to the disc.

7. Examine the fundus out to the midperiphery by following blood vessels from the optic nerve head in each of four directions: superior, nasal, inferior, and temporal. Instruct the patient to look up, down, right, and left while examining the corresponding quadrant. Evaluate the vasculature, looking carefully at arteriovenous (AV) crossings. Estimate the ratio of the thickness of the arteries to the thickness of the veins (A/V ratio). Evaluate the retinal background, noting the color and evenness of the pigmentation.

8. Move so you are positioned along the patient's line of sight and examine the macula. As an alternative, instruct the patient to look directly at the middle of the ophthalmoscope light and examine the macula. The former method is preferred, because the latter method may introduce constriction of the pupil due to the near response of the pupil. Determine if the color of the macula is homogenous and look for the presence of a foveal reflex.

9. Repeat steps 2 through 8 on the patient's left eye, holding the ophthalmoscope in your left hand and using your left eye.

RECORDING

- Record your observations for each eye separately.
- Observations should be noted for each of the following: media, disc margins, disc color, C/D ratio (indicating the horizontal and vertical measurements separately), vasculature (including A/V ratio and presence or absence of SVP), macula (including presence or absence of foveal reflex), and background. Abnormalities and pertinent negatives should be noted.
- Drawings or diagrams of what you have seen are recommended when they will enhance descriptions.

EXAMPLE

OD		OS
clear	media	clear
0.3 H and V	C/D	0.3/0.5 H/V
pink	color	pink
distinct, flat	margins	blurry superiorly, flat
A/V 2/3, + SVP	vasculature	A/V 2/3], + SVP
clear, + FR	macula	pigment mottling, no FR
clear	background	clear, tessellated

Binocular Indirect Ophthalmoscopy

PURPOSE   To evaluate the health of the posterior segment of the eye. Binocular indirect ophthalmoscopy allows examination of the entire ocular fundus through a dilated pupil. It is the instrument of choice for screening of the peripheral retina.

EQUIPMENT

- Binocular indirect ophthalmoscope (BIO) with power supply.
- Hand held condensing lens. Lens powers range from +14 D to +33 D. The +20 D lens is most commonly used.
- Dilating agents (e.g., 0.5% or 1% tropicamide and 2.5% phenylephrine or 1.0% hydroxyamphetamine).

SET-UP

Preparing the Patient

- Prior to dilating the patient, you must obtain best-corrected visual acuity and intraocular pressure, and you must estimate the depth of the anterior chamber angle. In addition, you should perform any other tests whose findings are necessary to understand the patient's problems and that cannot be properly done on the dilated eye.
- Dilate the patient's pupils approximately 30 minutes prior to the time of the examination.
- Adjust the patient to a reclining position so he is facing upward and his face is parallel to the floor and slightly below your waist level.
  Note: Some examiners prefer to perform binocular indirect ophthalmoscopy with the patient sitting up. However, when the patient is reclined, it is easier for the examiner to control the patient's lids and to obtain views of the far peripheral retina, particularly of the inferior fundus. The procedure described below assumes the patient is reclined but, with minor modifications, may apply to a patient who is seated.

Preparing the BIO and Condensing Lens

- Position the BIO on your head, adjusting the headbands to provide an even distribution of weight and a comfortable fit. The forehead strap should be positioned directly above your eyebrows.

- Position the oculars as close to your eyes (or your glasses) as possible. When properly positioned, the oculars should have a slight degree of pantoscopic tilt. Adjusting the position of the oculars is accomplished by loosening the set screw(s) on the bracket that attaches the illumination system to the headband.
- Adjust the PD to allow you to achieve binocular viewing. Adjustment of the PD is accomplished either by sliding the individual oculars or by turning a screw located next to or below the oculars. Close your left eye and hold out your thumb at eye level, 40 to 50 cm away. Adjust the right ocular until your thumb is centered in your field of view. Close your right eye and adjust the left ocular in the same manner. If the PD is properly adjusted for you, you should see singly when both eyes are opened.
- Turn on the power supply and set the intensity of the light by positioning the rheostat at or below the halfway setting. Adjust the position of the light on the BIO by turning the horizontal rod or set screw that controls the mirror angle. The light should be positioned in the upper half of your field of view while looking at your thumb at a 40 to 50 cm viewing distance.
- Hold the condensing lens in your dominant hand between your thumb and index finger. The lens is held with the more convex surface facing the examiner. Most lenses have a ring or dot marking either the more convex or the less convex surface.
- Tilt the lens slightly so it is approximately parallel to your face. The lens may also be tilted slightly along the horizontal or vertical axis to reduce reflections from the lens surface.

STEP-BY-STEP PROCEDURE

Obtaining a Stationary View

1. Instruct the patient to fixate in the direction you wish to view (e.g., instruct the patient to look up to examine the superior retina).
2. Use one of your hands to hold the patient's upper lid and the other hand to hold the patient's lower lid. Use the middle finger of your dominant hand (the hand holding the condensing lens) to grasp one of the patient's lids. This allows you to rest your hand on the patient's face to steady the lens.
3. Position your head so the light from the BIO is centered in the patient's pupil.
4. Holding the condensing lens at arm's length from you and approximately 2 cm from the patient's eye, position the lens so it intersects the beam of light and is centered in front of the patient's pupil. If the lens is properly positioned, you will see a blurred image of the red fundus reflex through the lens.

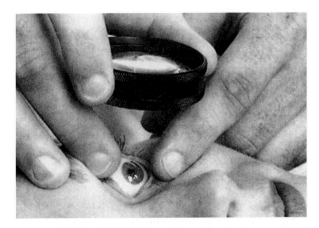

Figure 5–23. Proper placement of the condensing lens to achieve a full image in the lens. Note that the hand holding the lens is being steadied against the patient's face.

5. Slowly pull the lens away from the patient's eye, keeping the red reflex centered in the lens, until the entire lens is filled with the reflex. If you are using a +20 D lens, it should be approximately 4 to 5 cm away from the eye at this point. You should have a clear view of the retina through the condensing lens (see Figure 5–23).

Scanning the Retina

To view the entire retina, you must be able to scan with the BIO in addition to obtaining stationary views. Scanning means that you must move both yourself and the condensing lens while maintaining a view of the ocular fundus.

6. First obtain a stationary view as described in steps 1 through 5.
7. Move from the waist or hips, both back and forth and side to side. As you move, keep all components of the optical system (examiner's line of sight, center of the condensing lens, center of the patient's pupil) aligned. You will lose the retinal image if proper alignment is not maintained. Remember to keep the condensing lens at arm's length and approximately 4 to 5 cm from the patient's eye. As you move, keep the lens tilted so it is roughly parallel to your face.

Conducting a Systematic Examination

The authors recommend that you view the peripheral retina first and the posterior pole last to enhance the patient's comfort during the examination. Encourage the patient to blink whenever necessary but to keep his eyes open between blinks. Do not hold the examining light in one place for longer than 8 seconds at a time.

8. To examine the patient's right eye, begin by standing on the patient's right side.

9. Beginning with the superior retina, obtain overlapping views in eight positions: superior, superior nasal, nasal, inferior nasal, inferior, inferior temporal, temporal, and superior temporal. Instruct the patient to look in the direction you wish to view and stand 180° away. For example, to view the nasal retina of the patient's right eye, instruct the patient to look directly to his left while you stand on the patient's right, or temporal, side. You will need to walk clockwise around the patient during examination of the right eye to maintain this relationship. The patient should not look as far to the side as he is able, but only toward the direction you indicate.

10. In each of the eight positions, first obtain a stationary view of the equatorial region. Then, scan toward the peripheral retina, then back toward the posterior pole and then to the left and to the right.

11. After completing the examination of the peripheral retina, instruct the patient to look at your right ear, and obtain a stationary view of the posterior pole.

12. When you have completed the examination of the right eye, you should be standing on the patient's left side.

13. Examine the patient's left eye by repeating steps 9 through 11, walking counterclockwise around the patient. You will be standing on the patient's right side at the completion of the examination.

RECORDING

- Record the presence and size (in disc diameters, DD) of retinal lesions or other unusual variations in the fundus appearance. Indicate the location of the lesions by clock hour and distance (in disc diameters) from the closest retinal landmark. Figure 5–24 illustrates the normal peripheral retinal landmarks. It is helpful to remember that the field of view through a +20 D condensing lens is 8 disc diameters.

- The use of photographs, drawings, or diagrams is recommended to enhance your descriptions.

- Remember that your view through the condensing lens is inverted (upside down and backward). Illustrations and descriptions should be anatomically correct. Indicate where the lesion actually is located on the retina, not where it appears to be located through the condensing lens.

- Record pertinent negatives when applicable, for example, "peripheral retina WNL; no holes, tears, lesions, or detachments."

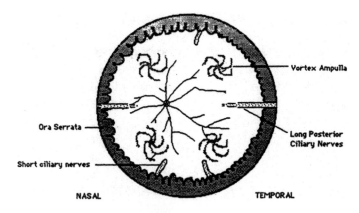

Figure 5–24. Diagram showing peripheral retinal landmarks. The ora serrata is the anterior limit of the retina. The nasal ora serrata is more scalloped in appearance than the temporal portion. The long posterior ciliary nerves, located at 3 and 9 o'clock, divide the retina into superior and inferior halves. The short ciliary nerves, located close to the vertical midline, divide the retina roughly into nasal and temporal halves. The ampullae of the vortex veins mark the equatorial region of the retina. There is one or more ampulla in each quadrant.

EXAMPLES

- OD: area of lattice degeneration at 1:00, 2 DD anterior to the vortex ampulla. No holes, tears, or detachments.
- OS: choroidal nevus with overlying drusen at 4:30, 3 DD from the ONH, 2 DD round, no elevation. Periphery clear; no holes, tears, lesions, or detachments.

Binocular indirect ophthalmoscopy *at a glance*

PURPOSE	TECHNIQUE
Prepare patient	Wait approximately 30 minutes after dilating pupils Recline patient
Prepare BIO	Adjust headband Position oculars Adjust PD Adjust position of light within your field of view Properly position condensing lens in your dominant hand
Obtain stationary view of patient's retina	Hold patient's lids, instruct him to fixate Position BIO light in center of pupil Position condensing lens close to patient's eye, center to see red reflex Pull lens away from eye until entire lens fills with red reflex Tilt lens if necessary to reduce reflections and provide a clearer image
Systematically scan retina	Begin at the superior retina, obtain overlapping views in eight positions At each position, scan from equator to far periphery, then back toward posterior pole Walk around patient, always standing opposite area being observed Obtain a stationary view of posterior pole

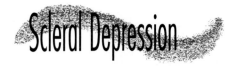

PURPOSE   Scleral depression is used in conjunction with binocular indirect ophthalmoscopy to expand the examiner's view of the far peripheral retina
and to allow three-dimensional viewing of peripheral retinal lesions.

INDICATIONS

Scleral depression is indicated whenever the examiner desires more information
about a peripheral retinal lesion noted during binocular indirect ophthalmoscopy.
It is also indicated when the patient has symptoms, such as flashes or floaters, sug-
gestive of vitreous traction, or a history of recent, direct trauma to the eye.

EQUIPMENT

- BIO.
- Hand held condensing lens.
- Scleral depressor.

SET-UP

- The set-up is the same as for binocular indirect ophthalmoscopy.
- The scleral depressor is held between the thumb and the forefinger of your dominant hand. If you are using the thimble type of depressor, put your index finger
  inside the thimble and use your thumb to stabilize it if necessary.
- Inform the patient that he will feel some pressure from the scleral depressor, but
  it will not be painful.

STEP-BY-STEP PROCEDURE

1. With the BIO, precisely localize the lesion or retinal area that you wish
   to depress.
2. Stand 180° from the area you want to observe. Instruct the patient to look
   toward you.
3. Position the scleral depressor on the patient's lid, tangential to the globe
   and directly over the area to be depressed as shown in Figure 5–25. It is
   helpful to remember that the ora serrata is located approximately 8 mm

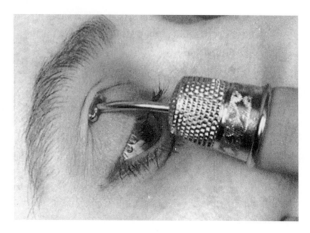

Figure 5–25. The examiner is positioning the scleral depressor on the upper lid behind the patient's superior limbus. Note that the depressor is held tangential to the globe.

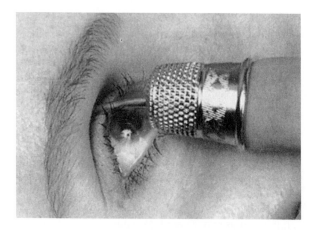

Figure 5–26. The scleral depressor is now properly positioned for depression of the patient's superior peripheral retina. When the depressor is in position, the patient will be instructed to look up.

behind the limbus and the equator is about 6 mm posterior to the ora serrata.

4. Instruct the patient to look away from you, in the direction of the depressor. Keep the depressor positioned tangential to the globe (see Figure 5–26).

5. Obtain a view of the retina through the condensing lens. If your scleral depressor is positioned properly you will see under the tip of the depressor an elevated area slightly paler than the surrounding retina. If you do not observe this elevation, move the depressor more posteriorly or side to

side, always maintaining its position tangential to the globe. Do not press inward on the globe. Very little pressure is required for scleral depression.

6. Once you are certain that the scleral depressor is overlying the area you wish to examine, use a massaging motion along the lid to manipulate the retina and obtain different views of the lesion and the surrounding tissue.

7. If you are using scleral depression to extend your peripheral retinal view rather than observing a specific lesion, repeat steps 3 through 6 for each of the eight positions of gaze during your routine binocular indirect ophthalmoscopy examination.

RECORDING

- Record your observations in the peripheral retinal evaluation section of the patient's record.
- Indicate that scleral depression was performed.
- Record pertinent negatives as well as abnormal findings.

EXAMPLES

- OD: Scleral depression 360°—no holes, tears, or detachments
- OS: Small retinal hole, 2 DD posterior to ora at 2 o/c. Scleral depression shows no subretinal fluid, no traction

Fundus Biomicroscopy

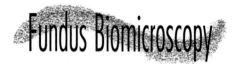

PURPOSE   To evaluate the health of the posterior segment of the eye. A non-contact auxiliary lens is used in conjunction with the biomicroscope to provide an inverted, wide-field, stereoscopic image with excellent resolution. Fundus biomicroscopy is used primarily for viewing the posterior pole. Views of the peripheral retina may be obtained with some lenses.

EQUIPMENT

- Non-contact auxiliary lens.
  Note: Numerous auxiliary lenses for fundus biomicroscopy are available, varying in size, power, field of view, and optical design. The procedure that follows applies to any high-plus condensing lens (e.g., 78 D, 90 D, or Super-field) that provides an indirect view of the fundus (an inverted and reversed aerial image).
- Biomicroscope.
- Dilating agents (0.5% or 1.0% tropicamide and 2.5% phenylephrine or 1% hydroxyamphetamine).

SET-UP

- Disinfect the forehead rest and the chin rest of the biomicroscope.
- Prior to dilating the patient, you must obtain best-corrected visual acuity and intraocular pressure, and you must estimate the depth of the anterior chamber angle. In addition, you should perform any other tests whose findings are necessary to understand the patient's problems and that cannot be properly done on the dilated eye.
- Dilate the patient's pupils approximately 30 minutes prior to the examination.
- Adjust the table height and chin rest of the biomicroscope so the patient is comfortable. Set the illumination arm of the biomicroscope in the straight ahead position (zero degrees). Narrow the beam to a thin slit. Set the magnification on the lowest setting (6× or 10×).
- Hold the auxiliary lens vertically between the thumb and index finger of your left hand to examine the patient's right eye. Hold the lens in your right hand to examine the patient's left eye. As an alternative you may use a lens holder mounted on the upright support of the head rest or an adapter that rests against the patient's eyelids. These are not available for all lenses.

STEP-BY-STEP PROCEDURE

1. Instruct the patient to fixate straight ahead.
2. Center the slit lamp beam in the patient's right pupil and focus on the cornea.
3. Place the lens in front of the patient's eye so the back surface just clears the lashes (approximately 8 mm from the patient's cornea). The distance between the lens and the cornea will vary depending on the power of the auxiliary lens used. If the lens is properly positioned, you will see a blurred red fundus reflex when looking through the oculars of the slit lamp (see Figure 5–27).
4. Using the joystick, focus on the fundus image by slowly moving the slit lamp away from the cornea, keeping the beam centered in the pupil.
5. Once the retinal image is focused, widen the slit lamp beam to observe a greater area of the ocular fundus. The magnification can be changed to the medium or high setting at this time. Use the joystick and the vertical adjustment knob on the slit lamp to scan across the posterior ocular structures. To view a specific portion of the retina, ask the patient to change fixation. It will be necessary to realign the lens.
6. If the reflections from the surface of the lens are interfering with your view, tilt the lens slightly or increase the angle of the illumination arm to approximately 10° from the straight ahead position to reduce the glare.
7. Center the slit lamp beam in the left eye and repeat steps 3 through 6 on the patient's left eye.

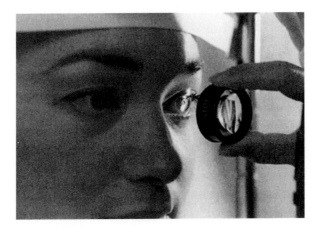

Figure 5–27. Proper positioning of the auxiliary lens for observation of the posterior pole during fundus biomicroscopy.

8. To check for possible irregularities of the macula, narrow the beam to a slit and focus it in the macular area first oriented vertically and then oriented horizontally. Check the slit on the macula for gaps and/or curves. Checking the macula this way is known as the "Watzke-Allen slit beam test," and a positive finding is called a "Watzke sign."

RECORDING

- Record the information obtained during fundus biomicroscopy in the retinal evaluation portion of the patient's record.
- Note in the record which auxiliary lens was used because the view obtained with one lens may appear different than the view obtained with other methods of retinal evaluation.
- Remember that your retinal view is inverted. Descriptions and illustrations should be anatomically correct. If an anomaly is observed, indicate where the lesion is located on the retina, not where it appears through the lens.

Nerve Fiber Layer Evaluation

PURPOSE   To increase the visibility of the retinal nerve fiber layer (NFL), allowing observation of focal defects or diffuse loss of fibers. This procedure is incorporated into the fundus biomicroscopy examination when
indicated.

INDICATIONS

Damage to the NFL may be the first clinical sign of glaucoma, so careful observation of the NFL is indicated for all glaucoma suspects. NFL defects are expected
when there is visible optic nerve damage or visual field loss due to any disease process affecting the NFL.

EQUIPMENT

- Biomicroscope with red-free filter.
- Clear auxiliary lens that will allow for a high resolution, stereoscopic view of
  the posterior pole (e.g., Super-field, 90 D, or 78 D lens).

SET-UP

- Same patient and instrument set-up as for fundus biomicroscopy.
- Insert the red-free filter in front of the slit beam.
- Increase the rheostat setting so the light is as bright as the patient can tolerate.

STEP-BY-STEP PROCEDURE

1. Obtain a clear, stereoscopic view of the posterior pole of the right eye using the step-by-step procedure described for fundus biomicroscopy.
2. Carefully observe the NFL around the optic nerve head (ONH), looking
   for focal defects. Also compare the NFL superior to the NFL inferior to
   the ONH.
3. Repeat steps 1 and 2 for the left eye. Compare the symmetry of the NFL
   between the two eyes.

RECORDING

- Record your observations of the NFL as part of your fundus biomicroscopy examination.
- Note the following for each eye: overall appearance of NFL, presence or absence of focal NFL defects, and symmetry of NFL superior and inferior to the ONH.
- Compare the symmetry of the NFL between the two eyes.

EXPECTED RESULTS

- *Normal findings:* The healthy NFL will appear as fine linear striations overlying the retinal features. The striations are more prominent close to the ONH and are most visible within several disc diameters superior and inferior to the disc.
- *Abnormal findings:* Focal defects will appear as dark slits or wedges within the NFL traveling out from the edge of the disc. The NFL is missing or damaged in these areas, so the underlying retinal features are darker and more distinct. Diffuse defects will present as an overall decrease in striations and increase in the prominence of the retinal details. Diffuse defects are most easily appreciated by comparing the symmetry of the NFL inferior and superior to the disc and between the two eyes.

Retinal Evaluation With the Goldmann 3-Mirror Lens

PURPOSE To allow observation and evaluation of specific areas of the retina. The Goldmann 3-mirror lens is used in conjunction with the biomicroscope, allowing the magnification to be varied and providing a stereoscopic image. It is also useful for examination of the vitreous.

INDICATIONS

The Goldmann 3-mirror lens is not practical as a technique to screen the peripheral retina because of its small field of view. It is used to observe a retinal lesion or unusual variation found during the binocular indirect ophthalmoscopy examination when a more magnified view is desired. The central lens provides a high-resolution, stereoscopic image of the posterior pole.

EQUIPMENT

- Goldmann 3-mirror lens, cleaned and disinfected.
- Biomicroscope.
- Gonioscopy fluid (e.g., 1% or 2% methylcellulose).
- Topical anesthetic (0.5% proparacaine).
- Sterile saline irrigating solution.
- Dilating drops (0.5% or 1% tropicamide and 2.5% phenylephrine or 1% hydroxyamphetamine).
- Sterile saline irrigating solution.
- Tissues.

SET-UP

- Prior to dilating the patient, you must obtain best-corrected visual acuity and intraocular pressure, and you must estimate the depth of the anterior chamber angle. In addition, you should perform any other tests whose findings are necessary to understand the patient's problems and that cannot be properly done on the dilated eye.

- Dilate the patient's pupils approximately 30 minutes prior to the examination.
- Adjust the slit lamp so it is comfortable for both the patient and the examiner.
- Focus the oculars, set the PD, remove all filters, and set the magnification on the lowest setting.
- Adjust the slit beam to a medium width parallelepiped and set the illumination arm of the biomicroscope in the straight ahead position (zero degrees).
- Prepare the lens by filling the concave face of the lens with 2 to 3 drops of gonioscopy fluid. Take care to avoid bubbles in the solution. The first drop squeezed from the bottle should be dropped onto a tissue. The bottle should be stored upside down.
- Scan the anterior segment of the patient's eye with the biomicroscope to rule out conditions that contraindicate use of the 3-mirror lens, such as corneal trauma or a red eye of infectious etiology.
- Instill a single drop of topical anesthetic in the eye to be examined.

STEP-BY-STEP PROCEDURE

Insertion of the 3-Mirror Lens

1. Position the patient in the slit lamp.
2. Hold the 3-mirror lens in your dominant hand between your thumb and index finger.
3. Instruct the patient to look down and grasp the patient's upper lid firmly with your nondominant hand.
4. Instruct the patient to look up and pull down the patient's lower lid with the middle or fourth finger of the hand holding the lens. At the same time, firmly tether his upper lid against the superior rim of his orbit.
5. Insert the lower edge of the lens into the inferior cul-de-sac (see Figure 5–16). Rock the lens toward the patient until the entire lens is firmly in contact with the globe as shown in Figure 5–17. Look through the central lens of the Goldmann 3-mirror to tell when the lens is in contact with the globe.
6. Instruct the patient to *slowly* look down until he is fixating straight ahead. Then slowly release the patient's lids. Continue holding the lens throughout the entire procedure, but do not push the lens forward against the patient's cornea.

Observation of the Posterior Pole

7. Looking outside the oculars, position the slit beam in the central lens.
8. Look through the oculars and focus the slit lamp on the fundus details.

9. Once the image is focused, you may increase the magnification or widen the slit beam to enhance your view. Because you are viewing the posterior pole, the patient may be uncomfortable if you widen the beam or increase the illumination too much.

10. Use the joystick and the elevation adjustment on the slit lamp to scan across the lens image. To observe a specific portion of the posterior pole, redirect the patient's fixation.

Observation of the Peripheral Retina

11. Select the appropriate mirror to use based on the retinal zone you wish to view (see Figure 5–28). Rotate the lens so this mirror is 180° away from the portion of the retina you want to examine.

12. Looking outside the oculars, position the slit beam in the selected mirror. Rotate the slit beam so it is parallel to the position of the mirror. For example, if the mirror is in the nasal or temporal position, the beam should be horizontal.

13. Look through the oculars and focus on the retina. Once the retina is in focus, you can increase the width of the slit beam or increase the magnification to enhance your view. If glare from the mirror or lens surface interferes with your view, it may be eliminated by altering the angle of the illumination arm slightly (5° to 10°).

14. To extend your field of view through the mirror, you can rock the lens slightly. Rocking in the direction of the mirror will allow you to view more anteriorly. Rocking away from the mirror will allow you to observe more posteriorly. You may also instruct the patient to change his fixation. Changes in the patient's fixation or the positioning of the lens should be small to avoid dislodging the lens.

Removal of the 3-Mirror Lens

15. Remind the patient to keep his forehead pressed firmly against the forehead rest, and instruct him to look up.

16. Hold the lens loosely with one hand. With the index finger of your other hand, apply firm pressure against the lower lid at the edge of the lens to break the suction between the lens and the cornea. Do not pull the lens forward! If you have difficulty removing the lens, ask the patient to blink forcefully as you press against the lid. You may also try rocking the lens slightly up or down.

17. Wipe the gonioscopy solution from the lens with a tissue. The lens should then be cleaned with a nonabrasive rigid contact lens cleaner and disinfected following CDC guidelines.

18. If you have used gonioscopy solution, gently irrigate the patient's eye

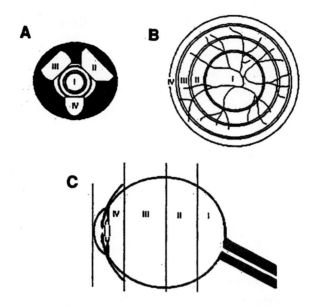

Figure 5–28. A. Diagram of the Goldmann 3-mirror lens. **B.** Fundus diagram indicating the area of the retina observable through each of the 3 mirrors and the central lens. **C.** Diagram of a cross-section of the eye indicating the portion of the eye observable through each of the mirrors.

with sterile saline solution to remove it, because residual solution may cause ocular irritation.

RECORDING

- The Goldmann 3-mirror lens examination is done to enhance retinal evaluation, so the results are recorded with the other retinal findings.
- Note in the record that the 3-mirror lens was used.
- Remember that your view through the mirrors is reversed. Descriptions and illustrations should be anatomically correct. Indicate where the lesion is located on the retina, not where it appears to be through the mirror.

Goldmann Applanation Tonometry

PURPOSE   To measure the intraocular pressure.

EQUIPMENT

- Biomicroscope with Goldmann tonometer and prism.
- Liquid fluorescein combined with a topical anesthetic or 0.5% proparacaine and a fluorescein strip.

SET-UP

Slit Lamp Preparation

- Disinfect the forehead rest and the chin rest of the biomicroscope.
- Make certain that the tonometer prism has been disinfected in accordance with CDC guidelines.
- Adjust the height of the slit lamp table so both the examiner and the patient are comfortable, and the patient is required to lean forward into the forehead rest.
- Adjust the chin rest so the patient is properly aligned.
- Adjust the PD and focus the oculars.
- Set the magnification on the low (10×) or medium (16×) setting.

Patient Preparation

- Evaluate the patient's anterior segment, especially the cornea, to rule out conditions that contraindicate applanation tonometry (e.g., red eye of infectious origin or severely traumatized cornea).
- Prepare the cornea by instilling one drop of anesthetic with liquid fluorescein in the patient's lower cul-de-sac. If you choose to use a topical anesthetic with fluorescein strips, instill a single drop of anesthetic first. Then, wet the fluorescein strip with a drop of sterile saline, instruct the patient to look to the side, control the upper and lower lids so as to limit blinking, and touch the moistened end of the strip to the temporal bulbar or inferior palpebral conjunctiva.
- Insert the cobalt blue filter. Scan across the cornea checking for corneal staining that is present prior to performing tonometry.

Tonometer Preparation

- Position the tonometer arm so the applanation prism is properly aligned in front of the left ocular.

- Rotate the applanation prism to align the zero with the white marking on the prism holder. If the patient's corneal astigmatism exceeds 3 diopters, rotate the prism until the red marking on the prism holder is aligned with the axis mark that corresponds to the patient's minus cylinder axis.
- Open the slit beam to its widest setting. Adjust the illumination arm so the tip of the applanation prism is brightly illuminated with the blue light. The angle of the illumination arm should be 45° to 60° from the straight ahead position.
- Set the measuring dial between 1 and 2 (corresponding to pressure readings of 10 to 20 mm Hg).

STEP-BY-STEP PROCEDURE

1. Reposition the patient in the slit lamp.
2. Instruct the patient to keep his eyes open and to look straight ahead. If the patient has difficulty keeping his eyes open, it may be necessary to hold the patient's upper lid. The upper lid should be held firmly against the patient's orbital rim to avoid pressing against the globe.
3. a. With the tonometer prism positioned slightly inferior to the visual axis, move the tonometer toward the cornea. When the prism is 2 to 3 mm from the cornea, elevate the tonometer to align the prism with the corneal apex and slowly move the joystick forward until the prism is in contact with the cornea. When the prism touches the cornea, the limbus will glow. This can be observed from outside the oculars (see Figure 5–29).
   b. As an alternative, center the prism on the corneal apex to the extent possible and position it approximately 1 mm from the corneal surface. With the prism in this position, when you look in through the slit lamp oculars, you should see a pair of blue or "whitish" reflections in the shape of the tonometer mires. Adjust the position of the prism until these reflections are equal mirror images of one another and centered in the field of view (as if you were aligning the tonometer mires themselves). Then bring the prism into contact with the cornea by rocking it forward with the joy stick. The tonometer mires should be visible and nearly properly aligned.
4. Once the prism is in contact with the cornea, look through the left ocular (the tonometer prism is properly aligned only with the left ocular) and center the semicircles horizontally and vertically as shown in Figure 5–30 by moving the slit lamp up and down and/or left and right.
5. Observe the thickness of the mires to ensure that they are neither too thick nor too thin. Ideal thickness is 1/10 the diameter of the semicircles. Thick mires are an indication of too much fluorescein or excess

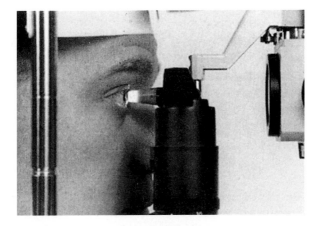

Figure 5–29. Goldmann tonometer with applanation prism in contact with the patient's cornea.

tearing and will cause a false high reading. If you observe excessively thick mires, withdraw the tonometer prism and correct the problem by blotting the excess fluid from the patient's eye with a tissue. Wipe the tonometer tip with a tissue to remove any residual fluorescein before attempting to take a tonometer reading again. Thin mires indicate too little fluorescein and will give a false low reading. If too thin mires are observed, withdraw the tonometer prism and instill more fluorescein in the patient's eye before repeating tonometry (see Figure 5–31).

6. When the mires are of proper thickness and the semicircles are equal in size and centered, turn the pressure dial to obtain the correct reading. The correct position for a pressure reading is when the inner ring of the superior semicircle meets the inner ring of the inferior semicircle. When

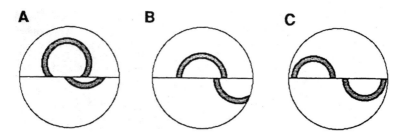

Figure 5–30. A. The upper semicircle is larger than the lower semicircle, indicating that the applanation prism is misaligned vertically on the patient's cornea. The prism must be moved up to center the semicircles. **B.** The lower semicircle is missing its right half, indicating that the applanation prism is misaligned horizontally on the patient's cornea. The prism must be moved to the right to center the semicircles. **C.** The semicircles are full and equal in size, indicating that the applanation prism is properly centered on the patient's cornea.

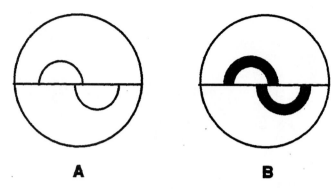

A   **B**

Figure 5–31. A. These mires are too thin, indicating that there is not enough fluorescein in the patient's eye. The pressure reading will be too low if this is not corrected. **B.** These mires are too thick, indicating that there is too much fluorescein or excess lacrimation. The pressure reading will be too high if the problem is not corrected.

the mires are properly aligned and the pressure on the cornea is appropriate for a pressure reading, it is often possible to observe the pulsation of the IOP (see Figure 5–32).

7. As soon as you have obtained an accurate reading of the intraocular pressure, withdraw the tonometer prism from the cornea. Immediately wipe the tonometer tip with a tissue to remove any fluorescein.

8. If the pressure reading is high or if there is a difference of greater than 2 mm between the eyes, a second reading should be taken.

9. When all necessary measures have been taken, reexamine the cornea for significant corneal staining or abrasions.

10. Disinfect the prism following CDC guidelines.

A   **B**   **C**

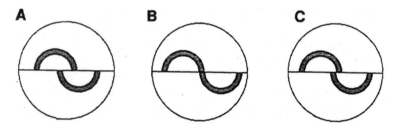

Figure 5–32. When the semicircles are of proper width, equal in size and centered, the pressure dial is adjusted. **A.** The semicircles are overlapping too much, indicating that the pressure dial is set too high. Reduce the reading on the pressure dial. **B.** The semicircles are not overlapping, indicating that the pressure dial is set too low. Increase the reading on the pressure dial. **C.** The semicircles are in the correct position. The inner ring of the upper semicircle is just touching the inner ring of the lower semicircle. The reading on the pressure dial is the patient's intraocular pressure.

RECORDING

- Write "T_A" to indicate that the IOP was obtained by the technique of applanation tonometry.
- The reading for the right eye is recorded above and the reading for the left eye is recorded below.
- Record the time of day the test was performed.

EXAMPLE

T_A—18/23 10:30 AM

EXPECTED FINDINGS

- The average intraocular pressure is 15.5 mm Hg. The normal range is considered to be 8 to 23 mm Hg.
- Pressure readings greater than 23 mm Hg are not automatically assumed to be indicative of glaucoma. Likewise, pressure readings that fall within the normal range do not rule out the possibility of glaucoma. Other examination results, such as optic nerve head appearance and visual fields, must be considered. The age of the patient should also be taken into consideration, because IOP tends to increase with age.
- A difference in pressure readings of more than 2 mm Hg between the two eyes is considered significant.
- Diurnal variations of 3 to 4 mm Hg are considered normal.
- The thinner the cornea, the lower the reading. Patients who have undergone corneal flattening refractive surgery for myopia will exhibit lower tonometer readings after the procedure than before. Preliminary evidence suggests that laser in situ keratomileusis (LASIK) for hyperopia and for astigmatism also results in a lowering of the Goldmann tonometer finding. In the future, measures of IOP by Goldmann tonometry may have to be corrected for the thickness of the patient's cornea.

GOLDMANN APPLANATION TONOMETRY *at a glance*

PURPOSE	TECHNIQUE
Prepare slit lamp	Magnification low or medium Insert cobalt filter
Prepare patient	Scan anterior segment to rule out contraindications Instill topical anesthetic and fluorescein and rescan the cornea.
Prepare tonometer	Position applanation prism Rotate prism to compensate for corneal astigmatism Brightly illuminate tonometer tip Measuring dial set between 1 and 2
Properly position prism on cornea	Ensure contact with cornea by looking for limbal glow Use joystick to move prism until semicircles are equal in size and centered Check the thickness of mires, correct if necessary
Obtain correct intraocular pressure reading	Turn pressure dial until inner rings of the semicircles meet Withdraw prism from the cornea Obtain pressure reading from dial Recheck cornea for staining

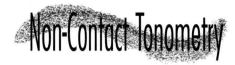

 PURPOSE

To measure the intraocular pressure (IOP). The cornea is applanated by an air pulse, and IOP is measured without direct contact between the eye and the instrument.

INDICATIONS

Tonometry should be performed on all patients. The non-contact tonometer is particularly useful when contact techniques are contraindicated, as in the case of a red eye of infectious origin or a traumatized anterior segment.

Note: Several non-contact tonometers are available. The reader is advised to review the documentation that comes with the particular non-contact tonometer he is using before attempting to perform the procedure. Schematic diagrams of a non-contact tonometer are shown in Figure 5–33 and Figure 5–34.

EQUIPMENT

• Non-Contact Tonometer (NCT).

SET-UP

• Disinfect the forehead rest and the chin rest.
• Turn on the instrument.
• Adjust the level of the table so both the patient and the examiner are comfortable.
• Adjust the height of the chin rest to align the patient's outer canthus with the notch on the upright support of the head rest.
• The headrest override switch should be unlocked. This ensures that a measurement can be obtained only when the patient's forehead is pressed firmly against the headrest.
• Set the auxiliary lens knob to compensate for the patient's refractive error. This knob has five positions. The position facing toward the examiner indicates which lens is in place. The silver bump = plano, the red dot = -3.00, the next position = -10.00, the black dot = $+4.00$ and the adjacent position = $+14.00$.
• Adjust the eyepiece of the instrument to focus the reticle.
• Check the instrument to ensure that it is properly calibrated. This is done by turning the power switch to each of the positions as indicated in Figure 5–35 and pressing the firing button.

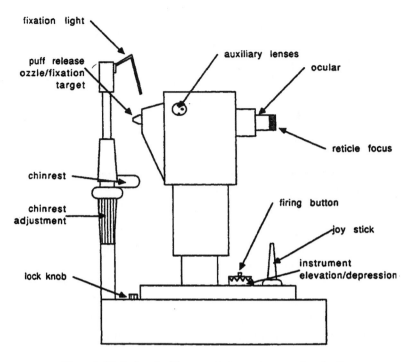

Figure 5–33. A schematic of the non-contact tonometer as seen from the side.

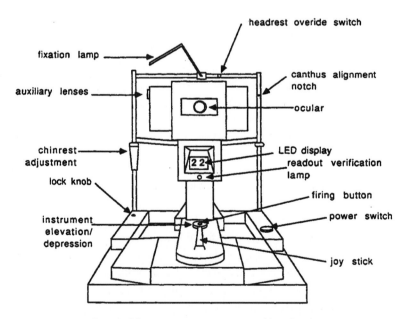

Figure 5–34. A schematic of the non-contact tonometer as viewed from the examiner's perspective.

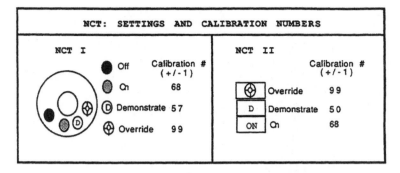

Figure 5–35. There are two power control configurations for non-contact tonometers. Both are shown here with the calibration numbers for each setting identified. It is critical that the instrument be checked for proper calibration if the IOP measurements are to be considered accurate. The instrument is considered calibrated if it reads within 01 of the numbers shown.

STEP-BY-STEP PROCEDURE

1. Inform the patient that the instrument is used to measure the pressure in the eye and that you would like to demonstrate how it works.
2. Put the power knob on D (for demonstrate), or press the D switch, and "puff" the patient's finger. Reassure the patient that it is just air and will not be painful.
3. Instruct the patient to place his chin in the chinrest and his head in the headrest, to press his forehead firmly against the forehead rests, and to close his eyes.
4. Raise the safety lock knob and advance the NCT until the nozzle is 3 to 5 mm from the patient's right eyelid. The height of the NCT may need to be adjusted so the nozzle is centered relative to the apex of the patient's eyelid.
5. Release the safety lock knob and make sure that the forward travel of the instrument is limited such that it cannot touch the patient.
   Note: The patient's forehead must be firmly pressed against the forehead switch during steps 4 and 5. Proper positioning is shown in Figure 5–36.
6. Instruct the patient to open both eyes.
7. From outside the instrument, perform a rough alignment by centering the light beam projected from the nozzle so that it appears centered in the patient's right pupil. The nozzle should be about 6 to 10 mm from the cornea. The alignment may be confirmed by asking the patient if he can see a red dot. This is the patient's fixation target.
   Note: if the patient cannot see the red dot at this time, make sure the auxiliary lens knob is set to the proper position and redo the rough alignment.

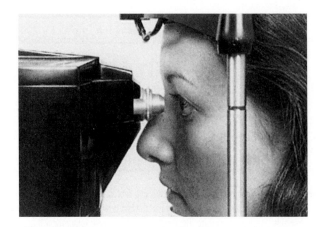

Figure 5–36. An NCT properly positioned and ready to take a reading.

8. Instruct the patient to look at the red dot, to blink at will, but to keep his eyes open between blinks.
   Note: It may be useful to reiterate your instructions to the patient to keep his forehead firmly pressed against the headrest.
9. Look through the eyepiece.
10. Adjust the NCT in and out until you obtain a focused image of a small red dot inside a larger white circle. This image will move around. If it is perfectly stable, the NCT is too far from the patient (see Figure 5–37).
11. Adjust the instrument until the red dot is centered in the black circle of the reticle. This process requires constant readjustment of the instrument.
12. As soon as the red dot is centered and focused, fire by pressing the button in the center of elevating knob.
13. Check the IOP reading. Some NCTs have a light located just below the IOP display. This light will be lighted if the reading is valid. NCTs without this feature will indicate an invalid reading by flashing the reading on and off. A reading of 99 indicates that the patient blinked as the reading was being taken.
14. Obtain three readings within 2 mm Hg of each other.
15. Repeat steps 4 through 14 on the patient's left eye.

RECORDING

- Write "NCT."
- On two lines, one above the other, record the eye that was tested and each of the three readings. The results for the OD are recorded on the top line and the OS on the bottom line. Do not record the average of the readings.
- Record the time of day the measurements were taken.

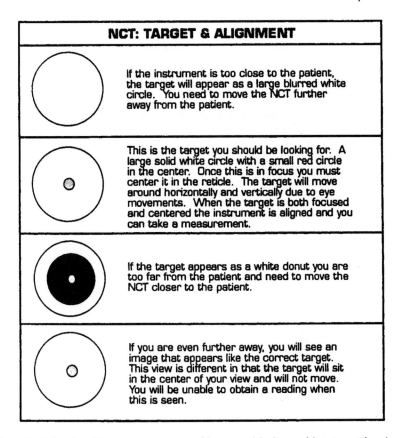

NCT: TARGET & ALIGNMENT

If the instrument is too close to the patient, the target will appear as a large blurred white circle. You need to move the NCT further away from the patient.

This is the target you should be looking for. A large solid white circle with a small red circle in the center. Once this is in focus you must center it in the reticle. The target will move around horizontally and vertically due to eye movements. When the target is both focused and centered the instrument is aligned and you can take a measurement.

If the target appears as a white donut you are too far from the patient and need to move the NCT closer to the patient.

If you are even further away, you will see an image that appears like the correct target. This view is different in that the target will sit in the center of your view and will not move. You will be unable to obtain a reading when this is seen.

Figure 5–37. The relationship between the appearance of the target and the distance of the instrument from the patient is shown.

EXAMPLES

- NCT: OD 15, 16, 15 @ 9:45 AM
          OS 12, 11, 13
- NCT: OD 24, 24, 26 @ 2:15 PM
          OS 16, 15, 18

EXPECTED FINDINGS

- The average intraocular pressure is 15.5 mm Hg. Normal range is considered to be 8 to 23 mm Hg.
- Pressure readings greater than 23 mm Hg are not automatically assumed to be indicative of glaucoma. Likewise, pressure readings that fall within the normal range do not rule out the possibility of glaucoma. Other examination results, such

as optic nerve head appearance and visual fields, must be considered. The age of the patient should also be taken into consideration, because IOP tends to increase with age.

- A difference in pressure readings of more than 2 mm between the two eyes is considered significant.
- Diurnal variations of 3 to 4 mm Hg are considered normal.

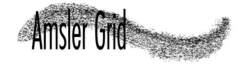

PURPOSE   To assess the integrity of the visual field corresponding to the macular region of the retina.

INDICATIONS

An Amsler grid should be performed whenever macular disease is a possible diagnosis (e.g., when the patient's best corrected VA is reduced, when the patient has an acquired color vision anomaly, or when the macula has any unusual appearance). If only one eye is affected, both eyes should nevertheless be tested. Some authorities include Amsler grid testing among the routine entrance tests, particularly for elderly patients.

EQUIPMENT

- Amsler grid book.
- Occluder.
- Illumination source.

SET-UP

- The patient wears his best near correction and holds the occluder.
- The examiner holds chart #1 at a distance of 30 cm from the patient under bright illumination.

STEP-BY-STEP PROCEDURE

1. Have the patient occlude his left eye, unless one eye sees much better than the other. In that case, test the better-seeing eye first. This will enhance the patient's understanding and thus the reliability of his responses to the test.
2. Say to the patient, "Look at the center white dot. Can you see it? Throughout this test you must continue to look at the white dot, while I ask you some questions about this drawing." If the patient cannot see the white dot, use chart #2.
3. Say to the patient, "While continuing to look at the white dot and without moving your eyes":

    a. "Can you see the four corners?"

    b. "Notice the lines. Are any of them missing pieces? Do any have holes in them? If so, where?"

    c. "Are all the lines straight? Are any wavy, and if so, where?"

    d. "Are all the little squares the same size? If some are larger or smaller, which ones?"

4. Note the patient's response to each of the above questions.

5. Throughout the test watch the patient. Make sure that the nontested eye remains occluded and that the patient maintains fixation on the white dot.

6. Repeat steps 2 to 5 with the other eye occluded.

RECORDING

- If there are no problems, record "Amsler" and the eye tested, followed by WNL, which means "within normal limits."
- If there is a problem, record the eye, the nature of the problem, and its location on the grid.
- If there are problems, attempt to draw what the patient sees or have the patient draw what he sees on an Amsler recording chart (see Figure 5–38).
- It is understood that plate #1 was used unless otherwise noted. If another plate was used, it must be specified.

EXAMPLES

- Amsler   OD WNL/OS WNL
- Amsler   OD WNL OS upper left corner not seen

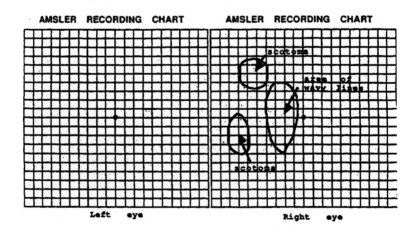

Figure 5–38. The Amsler grid recording chart. A blank form is shown for the left eye. For the right eye, the chart shows positive findings.

• Amsler   OD lines wavy centrally
         OS scotoma 2 to 5° to left 3° above and below fixation

Note: The Amsler grid booklet contains an account of the theory of the test, lists and explains the questions to ask, and briefly gives the indications for the use of all six test plates. The procedure described here pertains only to the first plate. The complete Amsler grid book is available from Keeler Instruments or Hamblin Instruments.

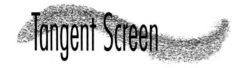

Tangent Screen

PURPOSE   To assess the integrity of the central 30° (radius) of the patient's field of vision.

EQUIPMENT

- *Tangent screen:* a flat, nonreflective, black screen with a small white object attached to the center of the screen to serve as a fixation target. On most tangent screens, the fixation target is surrounded by concentric circles, stitched into the surface of the screen at intervals of 5° when viewed from 1 meter.
- A 1-, 2-, 3-, or 5-mm diameter white test object attached to a black, nonglossy wand.
- Eye patch.

SET-UP

- The tangent screen should be moderately and evenly illuminated (standard illumination is 7 foot-candles). The light should not shine directly into the patient's eyes.
- The patient wears his habitual distance correction.
- Patch the left eye to test the right eye first.
- Have the patient sit with his eye 1 meter from the tangent screen and level with the fixation target.
- The examiner initially stands to the left of the screen. In general, the examiner stands on the side being tested.

STEP-BY-STEP PROCEDURE

1. Show the object to the patient near the fixation point.
2. Tell the patient you are going to test his side vision. Instruct him to tell you when he sees the test object in his side vision and *always to maintain fixation* on the central fixation target. Point to the fixation target during this instruction.
3. Explain to the patient that the disappearance of the object is normal and that he should not be alarmed if it disappears. Tell him to say "gone"

when he no longer sees it, and to say "I see it," or "now" when it comes into view.

4. Always observe the patient, not the screen, to be sure that the nontested eye remains occluded and that the patient directs his gaze at the fixation target at all times.

5. When plotting the visual field, remember to always plot from a location where the target is *not seen* to a location where it *is seen.*

Plot the Temporal Hemifield

6. Plot the blind spot.
   a. Start with the target near the fixation point and move it into the temporal field slightly below the horizontal meridian.
   b. When the patient says "gone," move the target back toward the fixation point until he sees it. Mark this location by sticking a black pin into the tangent screen.
   c. Plot seven more points evenly spaced around the edge of the blind spot.
   d. Move the target slowly all the way around the edge of the blind spot to confirm its borders.

7. Plot the limit of the isopter.
   a. Find the peripheral limit of the visual field, with special emphasis on the vertical and horizontal meridians, looking for meridional steps. This is done by plotting three points on each side of and within 5° of the two vertical and the two horizontal meridians and 1 point each at the 45th, 135th, 225th, and 315th meridians.
   b. If the patient sees the target at the edge of the screen, put a black pin at the edge and move to the next location.
   c. If the patient does not see the target at the edge of the screen, advance it at approximately 2° per second toward the fixation point until he reports that he does see it. Put a black pin at the location where it was first seen.

8. Zigzag the target through Bjerrum's area (the paracentral visual field, 5° to 20° from fixation) in the temporal field, both above and below the horizontal meridian. The healthy patient should see the target throughout Bjerrum's area. If the target disappears or flickers even briefly, retest the point of its disappearance carefully. Map out the full extent of the area of disappearance. Plot from unseen to seen and indicate with a black pin the locations where the target first became visible. This procedure is followed for each place where the target disappeared or seemed to flicker.

9. When the temporal hemifield has been fully tested, move so you are standing in the patient's nasal visual field.

Plot the Nasal Hemifield

Note: Because there is no physiological blind spot in the nasal field, repeat steps 7 and 8 only.

10. Before proceeding to the visual field determination for the left eye, record your findings for the right eye.
11. Patch the patient's right eye and repeat steps 1 through 9 for the left eye.
12. A complete field test requires plotting with at least two different target sizes or test distances; you should repeat the entire field test using another size target. A screening visual field can employ a single isopter.

RECORDING

- Mark the locations of each black pin on the tangent screen by putting small Xs on a standard visual field recording diagram and connect with straight lines.
- Cross-hatch areas of nonseeing, including the blind spot.

EXAMPLE

See Figure 5–39.

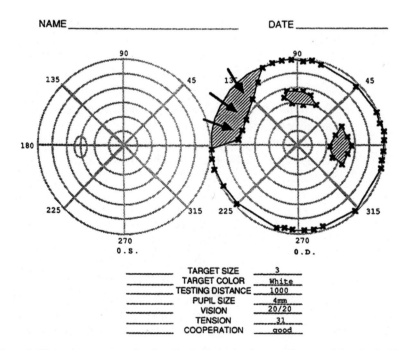

Figure 5–39. A tangent screen recording sheet. For the OS, the chart has not yet been recorded on. For the OD, the chart is filled in and shows a superior nasal step, an arcuate scotoma, and vertical enlargement of the blind spot such as might be found in glaucoma.

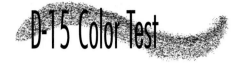

PURPOSE To provide in-depth analysis of color vision defects identified through clinical screening tests.

INDICATIONS

A D-15 color vision test is performed when routine color vision testing or the case history indicates the presence of a color vision anomaly. The D-15 is sensitive to acquired and congenital color vision defects of both the red-green and blue-yellow types.

EQUIPMENT

- D-15 Test, including standard scoring sheet.
- Proper illuminant (MacBeth easel lamp).
- Eye patch.

SET-UP

- The patient wears his habitual near correction.
- Both the examiner and the patient should wear white cotton (photographer's) gloves to protect the colored caps of the test.
- The D-15 box should be open.
- Place the caps color up in a random (scattered) order on the lid closer to the examiner.
- To ensure the validity of the test, work under the proper illuminant, with other light sources in the room turned off.

STEP-BY-STEP PROCEDURE

1. Instruct the patient to place the patch over his left eye to test his right eye.
2. Instruct the patient to rearrange the caps in order of similarity, starting with the reference cap which is glued down and to the patient's left. Tell the patient to do the test quickly, allowing 2 minutes per eye.
3. When the patient has rearranged the caps, close the lid, turn the box over, and open it upside down.

4. The number of each cap is printed on the bottom of the cap and will now be visible.
5. Record the findings for the right eye.
6. Instruct the patient to place the eye patch over his right eye and test his left eye by repeating steps 2 to 5.
7. If any abnormality is found on the first test, retest each eye.

RECORDING

Use the standard recording sheet as shown in Figure 5–40.

- Write down the numbers of the caps in the patient's order in the space where it says "subject's order."
- Connect the dots on the chart according to the numerical order of the caps.
- Make a notation if the patient was unusually slow.

EXPECTED FINDINGS

See Figure 5–40.

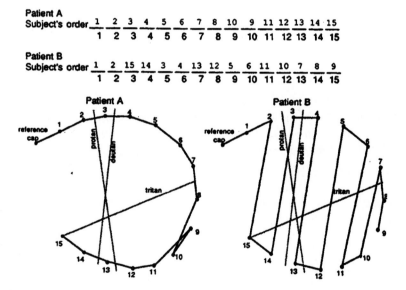

Figure 5–40. Recordings for two patients on the D-15 color vision test. Patient A is normal. The reversal of the order between cap 9 and cap 10 is considered to be within normal limits. Patient B has a strong deuteranomalous color vision defect.

Brightness Comparison Test

PURPOSE   To compare the two eyes with regard to the perceived brightness of an intense light source.

INDICATIONS

Brightness comparison is useful when optic neuropathy in one eye is suspected.

EQUIPMENT

- Transilluminator or binocular indirect ophthalmoscope.
- Occluder.

SET-UP

- The patient sits comfortably in front of the examiner in a dimly lit room.

STEP-BY-STEP PROCEDURE

1. Start by directing the patient to occlude the eye suspected of having pathology.
2. Turn on the transilluminator or BIO to its highest rheostat setting and place it 20 to 50 cm in front of the nonoccluded eye for no more than 5 seconds (see Figure 5–41).
3. Tell the patient that this brightness is rated as 100%. Then have the patient switch the occluder to this eye.
4. Place the light source 20 to 50 cm in front of the other (now nonoccluded) eye for no more than 5 seconds.
5. Ask the patient to rate the brightness of the light seen by this eye on a scale from 1% to 100%, reminding him that the brightness in the other eye was 100%.

RECORDING

- Write "Brightness Comparison."

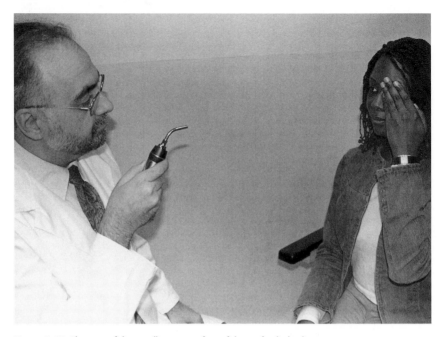

Figure 5–41. Placement of the transilluminator in front of the eye for the brightness comparison test.

- Record the patient's responses as percentages for the OD and for the OS. The first eye tested should be recorded as 100%.

EXAMPLES

- Brightness Comparison: OD 100%; OS 100%
- Brightness Comparison: OD 100%; OS 50%

EXPECTED FINDINGS

- No evidence of pathology: Minimal (10%) to no difference between the eyes.
- A report of less than 90% is consistent with an optic nerve conduction defect in the eye with the lower percentage.

Photostress Recovery Time Test

PURPOSE   To determine the time required for the macula to return to a near-normal level of visual acuity after being exposed to a bright light source for a specified duration of time.

INDICATIONS

Perform the photostress recovery time test when the patient has reduced best-corrected visual acuity in one eye due to suspected macular pathology.

EQUIPMENT

- Direct ophthalmoscope with visuscope (fixation) target.
- Occluder.
- Distance visual acuity chart.
- Timer or watch with second hand.

SET-UP

- The patient sits comfortably facing the visual acuity chart.
- The patient should be relaxed and the room should be free from distractions.
- The examiner sits near the patient to one side.
- Measure and record best-corrected visual acuity prior to the start of this test.

STEP-BY-STEP PROCEDURE

1. Allow the patient to dark adapt both eyes for 1 minute.
2. Have the patient hold the occluder over his left eye.
3. Put the visuscope target in the direct ophthalmoscope and set the rheostat to its brightest position.
4. Hold the ophthalmoscope 2 cm from the patient, look through the ophthalmoscope into the patient's unoccluded eye, and instruct the patient to look at the center of the visuscope target. Monitor the patient's fixation to ensure that he is looking in the proper place (see Figure 5–42)
5. Maintain the light on the patient's macula for 10 seconds.

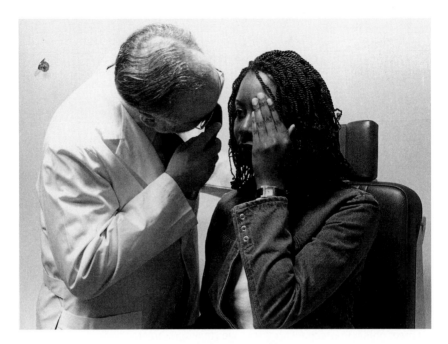

Figure 5—42. Proper position of the examiner to aim the ophthalmoscope at the patient's macula.

6. Withdraw the light, have the patient put on his best optical correction, and present the distance visual acuity chart.
7. Measure the elapsed time in seconds from the removal of the light until the patient is able to read half or more of the letters on the chart one line above his best-corrected visual acuity for that eye.
8. Repeat steps 1 to 7 on the left eye.

RECORDING

- Indicate "photostress (with ophthalmoscope)."
- Record the elapsed time until the endpoint is reached in seconds for the right eye and left eye.

EXAMPLES

- Photostress (with ophthalmoscope): OD 20 secs.; OS 25 secs.
- Photostress (with ophthalmoscope): OD 30 secs.; OS 120 secs.

EXPECTED FINDINGS

- *Normal:* 60 seconds or less in each eye. No greater than 6-second difference between the two eyes.

- *Abnormal:* Greater than 60 seconds in an eye; greater than 6-second difference between the two eyes. A delayed photostress recovery time suggests a macular disorder involving the photoreceptors, the retinal pigment epithelium, and/or the choriocapillaris.

Red Desaturation Test

PURPOSE To test the integrity of the optic nerve by testing the eye's sensitivity to the color red.

INIDICATIONS

To confirm or rule out pathology of one of the optic nerves.

EQUIPMENT

- Two red-capped bottles (such as those containing tropicamide or cyclopentolate). *Note:* be sure that each bottle has a cap of equal color red before starting the test.
- Occluder.

SET-UP

- The patient sits comfortably in front of the examiner in a normally illuminated room.

STEP-BY-STEP PROCEDURE

Comparison Between the Two Eyes

1. Have the patient occlude the eye suspected of optic neuropathy to test the better-seeing eye first.
2. Hold one of the red-capped bottles 40 cm from the patient and instruct him to look at it (see Figure 5–43).
3. Tell the patient that the red cap is worth "100%" or "$1.00-worth" of redness. Give the patient time to process this instruction.
4. Now occlude the better-seeing eye and have the patient look at the same object with the eye suspected of having optic neuropathy.
5. Ask the patient to rate the redness perceived by the suspect eye on a scale of 1% to 100% or from 1 cent to 1 dollar.

Comparing the Central to the Peripheral Visual Field

1. Have the patient occlude the eye suspected of optic neuropathy to test the better-seeing eye first.

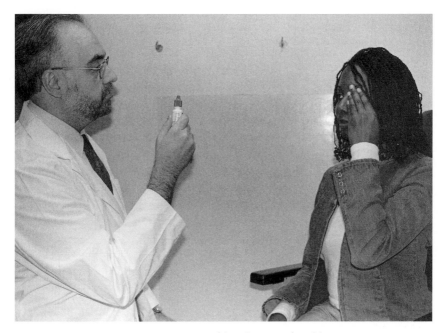

Figure 5–43. Proper presentation of the red cap to test for red desaturation.

2. Hold two red-capped bottles 15 cm apart at a distance of 40 cm from the patient.
3. Have the patient fixate either bottle such that the other bottle falls in his temporal visual field (see Figure 5–44).
4. Ask the patient to tell you which bottle appears more red: the bottle directly in front of him or the bottle in his side vision.
5. Repeat the steps 2 to 4 with the better-seeing eye occluded and record the patient's response.

RECORDING

- Write "Red Desaturation."
- To compare the eyes, record the patient's responses for both the right eye and left eye.
- To compare central and peripheral visual fields, indicate which target the patient saw as redder: the central or the peripheral. Record separately for each eye.

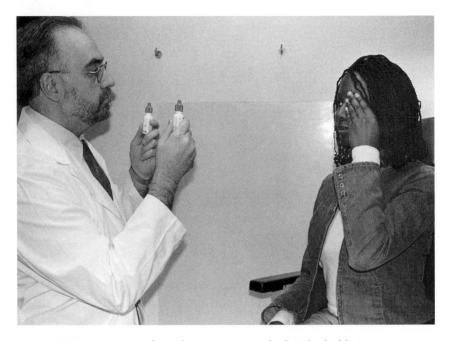

Figure 5–44. Proper presentation of two red caps to compare central and peripheral red desaturation.

EXAMPLES

- Red Desaturation: OD 100%; OS 100%. Central target redder OD and OS.
- Red Desaturation: OD $1.00/OS 50 cents. Central target redder OD; Peripheral target redder OS.

EXPECTED FINDINGS

- *Normal:* Minimal (10%) to no difference when the two eyes are compared. The central target should appear redder in each eye.
- *Abnormal:* Greater than 10% difference between the two eyes. If the peripheral target appears redder, it suggests the presence of a central scotoma.

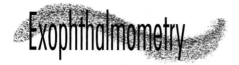

Exophthalmometry

PURPOSE To measure the position of the eyeball in the orbit to rule out proptosis or protrusion (exophthalmos) or recession (enophthalmos) of the eyes relative to the orbital structures.

INDICATIONS

Exophthalmometry is indicated when the external examination suggests an asymmetry in the size of the palpebral apertures, a bilateral increase in aperture size, or an enophthalmos or exophthalmos of one or both eyes. It is done routinely on patients with Graves' disease to monitor the progress of any exophthalmos associated with their condition.

EQUIPMENT

- Hertel and/or Luedde exophthalmometer.
- Distance fixation target located directly in front of the patient.

SET-UP

- Seat the patient so that his eyes are level with the examiner's eyes.

STEP-BY-STEP PROCEDURE

Hertel Exophthalmometer

1. Ask the patient to close his eyes while the instrument is being positioned.
2. Loosen the set screw on the right side of the exophthalmometer's base. The base should now slide freely.
3. Position the left side of the base so that the curved foot plate is resting firmly against the patient's right lateral orbital rim. The inner edge of the foot plate should be at the lateral canthus.
4. Slide the base in or out to position the right side of the base against the patient's left lateral rim as described in step 3.
5. Once the base is properly positioned, tighten the set screw to prevent the base from sliding.

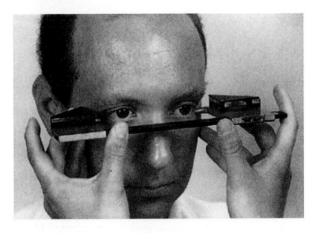

Figure 5–45. Hertel exophthalmometer properly positioned for measuring. Note that the base is held parallel to the floor and the patient is instructed to look straight ahead.

6. Hold the exophthalmometer in both hands, resting your fingers on the patient's face to stabilize it. The instrument base must be parallel to the floor as shown in Figure 5–45.
7. Instruct the patient to open both eyes wide and to fixate on the distance target.
8. To measure the proptosis of the patient's right eye, close your left eye, look into the instrument's left mirror, and move your head from side to side until you are at the measuring position. The measuring position is determined in one of two ways, depending on the particular instrument:
   a. If there are two red vertical lines in the mirror, the measuring point is the position at which the two red lines coincide (see Figure 5–46).
   b. If there are no red lines, the measuring point is the position at which the zero edge of the scale is aligned with the inside edge of the mirror (see Figure 5–47).
9. Determine where the patient's corneal apex intersects the scale. This is the exophthalmometry reading in millimeters.
10. To measure the patient's left eye, close your right eye, look through the right mirror, and repeat steps 8 and 9.
11. Remove the instrument and note the base reading.
12. If subsequent measurements are taken at a later date, the base is preset on the measurement previously used. This ensures that the measurements are made from the same reference point.

Luedde Exophthalmometer
1. Instruct the patient to open both eyes wide and to fixate on the distance target.

A   **B**

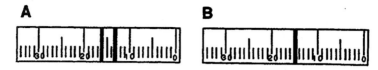

Figure 5–46. A. This is not the proper measuring position, because the two red lines are not overlapping. **B.** When the examiner moves his head, the two red lines will appear to overlap at some point. The measurement is taken from this position.

A   **B**

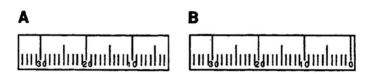

Figure 5–47. A. This is not the proper measuring position, because the 0 is not visible on the right side of the scale. **B.** When the examiner moves his head, the 0 will be aligned with the right edge of the mirror. The measurement is taken from this position.

2. Position the exophthalmometer so that its concave end nests into the orbital rim of the patient's right eye at its outer canthus. Align the instrument so its long axis is parallel to the patient's line of sight both vertically and horizontally. Press the exophthalmometer gently but firmly into the outer canthus.
3. View the corneal apex by looking through the exophthalmometer perpendicular to its long axis to avoid parallax. Read off the position of the corneal apex in mm relative to the orbit.
4. Reposition the exophthalmometer at the lateral canthus of the patient's left eye, Attempt to press the instrument into position with the same force used for the right eye. Repeat step 3.

RECORDING

1. Hertel exophthalmometry readings are recorded as three numbers:
   - Proptosis measurement for the right eye.
   - Proptosis measurement for the left eye.
   - Base reading.
   These numbers may be recorded separately, or as a fraction where the numerator is the proptosis measurements (OD– OS) and the denominator is the base measurement.
2. Luedde exophthalmometer readings are recorded as single numbers for each eye.

3. When recording exophthalmometry findings indicate which type of exophthal-mometer was used.

EXAMPLES

- OD 21, OS 19, base 110—Hertel
- OD 16, OS 21, base 105—Hertel
- OD 17, OS 22—Luedde

EXPECTED FINDINGS

- The average reading is 15 to 17 mm for all adults.
- The range of normal results is approximately 11 to 21 mm for Caucasians and 12 to 24 mm for African-Americans.
- A difference of 2 mm or more between the two eyes is considered significant.
- An increase in the reading of 2 mm or more over time is considered significant.

6

CONTACT LENSES

Ronald K. Watanabe, OD

CHAPTER AT A GLANCE

INTRODUCTION TO THE CONTACT LENS EXAMINATION

There are over 35 million contact lens wearers in the United States alone. Virtually all vision care providers will encounter contact lens wearers on a regular basis. Consequently, it is essential to know how to examine the contact lens patient to ensure that his lenses are fitting properly and providing good quality vision and comfort. This chapter describes the basic contact lens procedures necessary in the fitting and evaluation of commonly encountered contact lens types. Specialty lenses, such as therapeutic or keratoconus lenses, are beyond the scope of this chapter and are not addressed specifically. However, many of these basic procedures apply to these lens types as well.

The contact lens examination is an integral part of the core ocular examination. Although a number of side trips will be required due to the special concerns of contact lens wearers, it is important not to forget the main route. Contact lens patients have the same need for evaluation of functional vision, refractive status, and ocular health as other patients. It is therefore important to consider the procedures described in this chapter a regular part of your examination, just as your patient considers his contact lenses a regular part of his daily routine.

The contact lens examination should flow efficiently within the core ocular examination. For this to occur, you must consider which tests can be performed while the patient is wearing his lenses and which require that the patient remove his lenses. Those tests requiring habitual correction, such as visual acuity, entrance tests, and some functional tests, are more appropriately performed while the patient is wearing lenses. After the lenses are removed, keratometry, refraction, and ocular health assessment can be performed.

A recommended sequence of examination procedures is illustrated in Figure 6–1. This flowchart assumes that the patient is seated in the chair for a comprehensive eye examination and currently wearing contact lenses. The sequence is designed for efficient examination flow for the typical contact lens patient. It may be necessary to modify the test sequence for some patients. For instance, if the patient habitually removes his contact lenses for prolonged periods of reading or other near work, you should delay near point testing until after the patient removes his lenses.

This chapter begins with the contact lens case history, which is incorporated into the general case history. The contact lens external examination

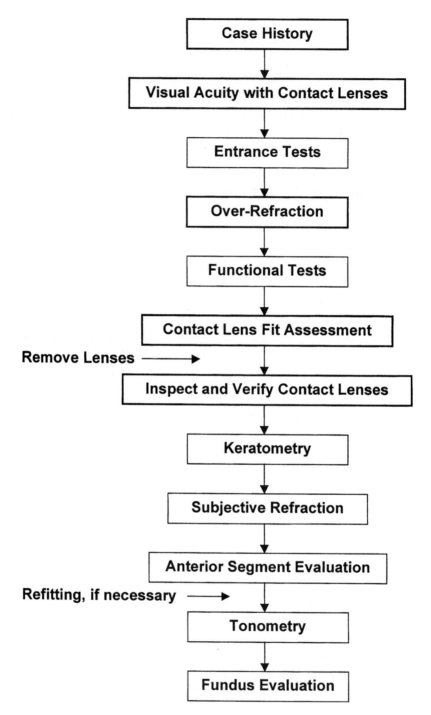

Figure 6–1. Flowchart of the general eye examination incorporating the procedures for contact lens evaluation.

includes procedures to help in the initial fitting of contact lenses. Inspection and verification, insertion and removal, and fit assessment are discussed for both gas permeable and soft lenses. Finally, the over-refraction procedure is explained. The order in which these procedures are presented is the preferred sequence to be followed during a contact lens fitting examination. This sequence will need to be varied during the general eye examination, as illustrated in the flowchart.

This chapter uses techniques and procedures that are described in other chapters. It is unique also in that many of the contact lens–related procedures can be integrated into the core ocular examination. This reinforces the concept that, in most cases, contact lenses are a routine part of primary eye care and not a separate subspecialty. The chapter is organizationally different from other chapters, at times omitting the "recording" or the "expected" findings sections. This is because the contact lens procedures described tend to be either equipment dependent or they do not result in a measurement.

All of the procedures help the practitioner to evaluate a patient's contact lenses. By ensuring that a patient's lenses are fitting properly and that they are not causing any adverse physiological reactions or mechanical effects on the anterior segment, good quality vision is maintained for contact lens patients for many years.

Contact Lens Case History

As discussed in Chapter 1, the case history is one of the most important components of the optometric examination. Without a detailed interview to ascertain the patient's contact lens status, future management will be difficult. The contact lens case history fits into the framework of the general case history and should be thought of as a component of, not separate from, the general case history. It can be done at the beginning of the case history if the chief complaint concerns contact lenses, or it can be done during the correction history portion.

The interview portion of the case history begins with a question as to the patient's reason for his visit. This often elicits the patient's desire to obtain a replacement pair of contact lenses, most likely due to decreasing vision or comfort. Further questions addressing any current symptoms or problems the patient is experiencing with his contact lenses should be asked. In the absence of symptoms, open-ended inquiries about his subjective vision and comfort should be presented.

The questionnaire portion of the case history includes questions concerning the patient's current lens type, wearing time, care and compliance, and past contact lens experience. A summary of the patient's past experience, current status, and future goals completes the contact lens case history.

CONTACT LENS CASE HISTORY QUESTIONS

I. Interview
   A. "What is the reason for your visit today?"
   B. "Describe your vision with your contact lenses."
   C. "Describe your comfort with your contact lenses."
   D. "Are you having any problems with your contact lenses?"
   E. "Do you experience redness, irritation, itchiness, pain, discharge, tearing, or dryness when wearing your lenses?"

II. Questionnaire
   A. Current lens type "What type of lenses do you wear now?"
   B. Soft versus gas permeable.
   C. Conventional versus frequent replacement versus disposable.
   D. Specialty lens type: toric, bifocal, etc.
   E. Wearing time

1. "What is your average wearing time per day?"
2. "How long have you worn your lenses today?"
3. "How often do you wear your lenses (how many days per week)?"
4. "Do you wear your lenses as daily wear or extended wear?"
5. "If extended wear, how many days in a row do you wear your lenses?"

F. Care and compliance
   1. "Describe your current lens care regimen, including the solution brand."
   2. "Have you used other types of care regimens in the past?"
   3. "How often do you replace your contact lenses?"
   4. "When was your last contact lens progress evaluation?"

G. Past contact lens experience
   1. "For how long have you worn contact lenses?"
   2. "Have you worn other types of lenses in the past? Were you successful or unsuccessful? Why did you discontinue that type of lens?"
   3. "Have you had any contact lens–related problems in the past: dry eye, red eye, GPC, infection, ulcer?"

Contact Lens External Examination

PURPOSE To obtain baseline measurements that aid the contact lens fitter in se-
lecting initial contact lens parameters, or assess the appropriateness of
currently prescribed contact lenses.

Note: It is not necessary to perform the external examination for contact
lens wearers as a separate sequence. Some measurements may be obtained in conjunction with other procedures. For example, pupil diameter is obtained during the general pupils procedure.

EQUIPMENT

- PD ruler with pupil gauge.
- Penlight may facilitate certain measurements.

SET-UP

- There is no specific set-up.

STEP-BY-STEP PROCEDURE

The external examination consists of six subprocedures.

Lid Position

1. Instruct the patient to view a distant target. Discourage squinting or wide-
   eyed staring.
2. Observe the points at which the upper and lower lids cross the edge of the
   cornea for each eye.

   Note: An upper lid that covers part of the superior cornea is most suitable
   for a lid attachment gas permeable lens fit. A lower lid that covers part of
   the inferior cornea may require a smaller lens diameter to prevent a gas
   permeable lens from resting on the lid.

Palpebral Aperture Size

1. Instruct the patient to view a distant target. Discourage squinting or wide-
   eyed staring.
2. Place a PD ruler vertically in front of the patient's right eye.
3. Measure the maximum vertical aperture size in millimeters.

4. Repeat for the left eye.

   Note: Both gas permeable and soft lens diameters depend somewhat on this measurement in that a larger aperture may require a larger contact lens diameter, and vice versa.

Corneal Diameter (Horizontal Visible Iris Diameter)

1. Instruct the patient to view a distant target.
2. Place a PD ruler horizontally in front of the patient's right eye as close to the cornea as is safe.
3. Measure the corneal diameter from limbus to limbus to the nearest 0.5 mm.
4. Repeat for the left eye.

   Note: A larger corneal diameter will often require a larger contact lens diameter.

Pupil Diameter

1. Instruct the patient to view a distant target.
2. Hold the PD ruler horizontally in front of the patient's right eye so that the pupil gauge covers half the pupil.
3. Slide the gauge across until the pupil gauge diameter matches the pupil diameter. If a pupil gauge is not available, use a PD ruler to measure the diameter. In dim illumination, it may be necessary to hold a penlight obliquely from the temporal side to visualize the pupil.
4. Measure the pupil diameter in bright, dim, and average lighting conditions.
5. Repeat for the left eye.

   Note: A large pupil in dim illumination may require a contact lens with a large optic zone.

Lid Tension

1. During upper lid eversion, a subjective assessment of lid tension can be obtained.
2. Set up the patient in a slit lamp and instruct the patient to look down.
3. Grasp the lashes of the right upper lid and pull outward.
4. The tension can be rated as tight, normal, or loose.
5. Repeat for the left eye.

   Note: A tight lid is more likely to pull a contact lens upward or push it downward, and a loose lid may lead to an inferior position due to lack of support.

Blink Quality

1. While observing the patient's eyes, note the completeness of the blink and the blink rate. This should be assessed without the patient's knowledge and can be done while talking with the patient.

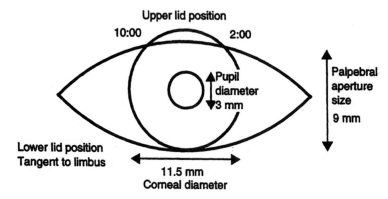

Figure 6–2. Diagram of external measurements: lid position, palpebral aperture size, corneal diameter, and pupil diameter.

Note: Incompleteness of the blink may create a dry eye when contact lenses are worn.

RECORDING

- For lid position, draw and describe the lid position.
- For palpebral aperture size, corneal diameter, and pupil diameter, record your measurements.
- For lid tension and blink quality, describe your observations.

EXAMPLE (see Figure 6–2)

- Lid position: upper lid at 10:00 and 2:00; lower lid tangent to limbus
- Palpebral aperture size: 9 mm
- Corneal diameter: 11.5 mm
- Pupil diameter: 3 mm (bright), 4 mm (normal), 6 mm (dim)
- Lid tension: normal
- Blink quality: full, normal blink rate

EXPECTED FINDINGS

- Lid position: The upper lid covers the superior limbus from 10:00 to 2:00. The lower lid is less than 1 mm below the inferior limbus.
- Palpebral aperture size: ranges from 8 to 11 mm
- Corneal diameter: ranges from 10.5 to 12.5 mm; average 11.5 mm
- Pupil diameter: ranges from 2 to 8 mm, depending on lighting conditions
- Lid tension: moderate tension with good elasticity
- Blink quality: full, complete blinks, 10 to 15 blinks per minute

CONTACT LENS EXTERNAL EXAMINATION *at a glance*

MEASUREMENT	EXPECTED FINDINGS
Lid position	Upper lid: 10:00 and 2:00 Lower lid: Less than 1 mm below the inferior limbus
Palpebral aperture size	8–11 mm
Corneal diameter	10.5–12.5 mm
Pupil diameter	2–8 mm, depending on lighting
Lid tension	Moderate with good elasticity
Blink quality	Full and complete 10–15 blinks per minute

INSPECTION AND VERIFICATION OF GAS PERMEABLE CONTACT LENSES

PURPOSE   To confirm that the contact lens lab has fabricated a patient's lenses as you have specified. To provide insight into why a lens is performing successfully or unsuccessfully. To determine or confirm the parameters of a pair of lenses worn by your patient. To confirm when a patient unknowingly switches his lenses. To monitor parameter changes during lens modification.

Note: Inspection and verification of gas permeable contact lenses require unique equipment for each parameter. This section is organized by parameter and the procedures to evaluate each parameter.

INSPECTION AND VERIFICATION OF GAS PERMEABLE CONTACT LENSES *at a glance*

PARAMETER	INSTRUMENT
Base curve radius	Radiuscope Keratometer with Lensco-Meter
Back vertex power	Lensometer
Optical quality	
Lens diameter	V-channel gauge (lens diameter only) Measuring magnifier (7× to 10×)
Optic zone diameter	Measuring magnifier (7× to 10×)
Center thickness	Center thickness gauge
Edge configuration	Stereo microscope Biomicroscope Measuring magnifier
Surface quality	Stereo microscope
Surface wettability	Biomicroscope Measuring magnifier

Base Curve Radius: Radiuscope

EQUIPMENT

- Radiuscope (see Figure 6–3).

SET-UP

- Clean the lens with a daily cleaner. Rinse with tap water to remove any loose debris from the lens surface.
- Blot the lens dry with a soft, lint-free cloth or tissue prior to measuring the base curve.

STEP-BY-STEP PROCEDURE

Adapted from the *American Optical Manual*.

1. Place a drop of water in the depression on the concave lens holder. Place the contact lens in the depression with the concave surface facing upward so that this surface remains dry.
2. Place the lens holder in its support stage on the instrument so that it is level.
3. Set the illumination control to 50% of the maximum illumination, or to a level that provides a reasonably bright image when you look into the eyepiece.
4. Check the aperture selector of the illuminator to be certain that the large aperture is in place.
5. Observe the green light coming from the objective and move the stage until the green beam appears to be centered on the contact lens.
6. Completely raise the objective of the microscope using the coarse adjustment knob.
7. Look into the eye piece and bring the scale on the right side of the field of view into sharp focus using the scale focusing knob.
8. Lower the objective slowly using the coarse adjustment knob, until you see light come into focus forming a spoke patterned target. Move the

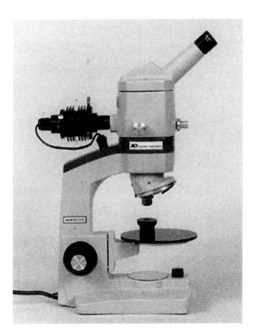

Figure 6–3. The radiuscope.

stage horizontally and vertically until the target is centered in the field of view (see Figure 6–4).

9. Continue to lower the objective. At one point, the filament of the lamp will come into focus. Disregard this image and continue lowering the objective with the coarse adjustment knob.

10. The spoke patterned target will appear again. Bring the image of the target into sharp focus using the fine adjustment knob.

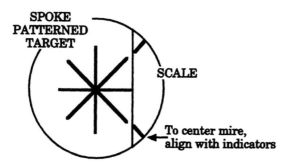

Figure 6–4. Spoke patterned target centered in the field of view of the radiuscope.

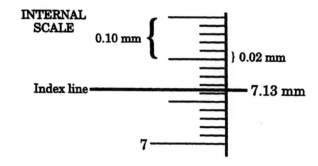

Figure 6–5. Example of radiuscope reading. Interpolation is required to obtain the measurement of 7.13 mm.

11. Use the index adjustment knob to move the index line to zero. You may not be able to move the index line to zero. In this case, set the index line to the nearest whole number.
12. Raise the objective until the original spoke pattern comes back into focus. Bring the image of the target into sharp, clear focus using the fine adjustment knob.

RECORDING

- If your original index line setting was zero, read the radius of curvature directly from the scale at the position of the index line. If your index line was set at +1, that must be added to the scale reading. For example, if the scale reads 6.54 mm and the index line was originally set at +1, the actual base curve radius of the contact lens is 7.54 mm.
- Each number on the scale represents 1 mm. The scale is divided into 0.10-mm increments, indicated by the longer lines. The shortest lines represent 0.02-mm increments. Interpolation is required to read 0.01-mm increments (see Figure 6–5).
- Record the base curve radius in millimeters to the nearest 0.01 mm.

Base Curve Radius: Lensco-Meter

EQUIPMENT

- Keratometer with Lensco-Meter mounted to the upright support.

SET-UP

- Clean the lens with a daily cleaner. Rinse with tap water to remove any loose debris from the lens surface.
- Blot the lens dry with a soft, lint-free cloth or tissue prior to measuring the base curve.

STEP-BY-STEP PROCEDURE

1. Mount the Lensco-Meter holder to the headrest of the keratometer. One end has a screw that can be tightened onto the upright support of the headrest. Position it so that the end of the holder is roughly where a patient's eye would be during keratometry.
2. Select the steel ball with a depression on one end and a knob on the other. Place the contact lens in the depression so that its concave side is facing out. One small drop of a viscous contact lens solution holds the lens in place. If this does not provide adequate adherence of the lens to the steel ball, toothpaste or double-sided tape can be used.
3. Place the steel ball onto the end of the magnetized holder. Position the steel ball so that the concave surface of the contact lens is directly facing the center of the keratometer (see Figure 6–6).
4. Turn on the keratometer and measure the horizontal and vertical curvatures as in conventional keratometry (refer to Chapter 3).

RECORDING

- Convert the dioptric readings to radius of curvature in millimeters using a conversion chart, or by dividing the dioptric value obtained into 337.5.

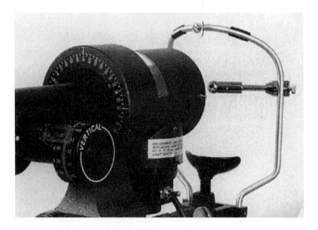

Figure 6–6. Lensco-Meter mounted to the headrest of the keratometer.

- Add a 0.03-mm correction factor for concave surfaces to your result to obtain the base curve radius measurement.
- Record the base curve radius in millimeters to the nearest 0.01 mm.

EXAMPLE

- Keratometry measurement = 45.00 D
  Conversion: 337.5/45.00 = 7.50 mm
  Base curve radius = 7.50 + 0.03 mm = 7.53 mm

Back Vertex Power and Optical Quality

EQUIPMENT

• Lensometer.

SET-UP

• Clean the lens with a daily cleaner. Rinse with tap water to remove any loose debris from the lens surface.
• Blot the lens dry with a soft, lint-free cloth or tissue prior to measuring the back vertex power.

STEP-BY-STEP PROCEDURE

1. Rotate the spring-loaded lens holder away from the lens stop. Clean any ink or debris from the lens stop with a tissue. Turn on the lensometer.
2. Holding the contact lens by the edges, place the back (concave) surface of the lens against the lensometer stop. Make sure that the lens is centered (see Figure 6–7). Do not apply excessive pressure to the lens as it may warp and give you a falsely toric power.
3. Take a measurement as if you were measuring a pair of spectacles. Note the spherical power, amount of prism, and any toricity. Toricity in a presumed spherical lens can indicate warpage or distorted optics, or it can indicate that you are squeezing the lens too much while you are holding it in place.
4. Observe the sharpness of the mires. A cloudy, distorted, or double mire image indicates optical distortion (see Figure 6–8).

RECORDING

• Record the back vertex power in diopters to the nearest 0.12 D.

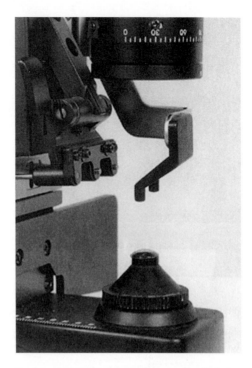

Figure 6–7. Gas permeable contact lens positioned on the lensometer stop for back vertex power measurement.

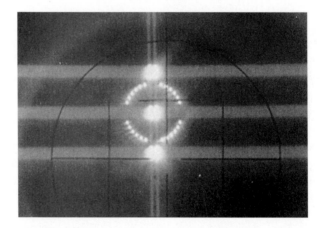

Figure 6–8. Cloudy, distorted lensometer mires due to poor optical quality of a gas permeable contact lens.

Lens Diameter and Optic Zone Diameter

EQUIPMENT

- Measuring magnifier (7× or 10×).
- V-Channel gauge (for overall lens diameter only).

SET-UP

- Clean the lens with a daily cleaner. Rinse with tap water to remove any loose debris from the lens surface.
- Blot the lens dry with a soft, lint-free cloth or tissue prior to measuring the lens diameter and optic zone diameter.

STEP-BY-STEP PROCEDURE

Measuring Magnifier

1. Place the clean, dry lens concave side down on the end of the magnifier.
2. Hold one edge of the lens against the magnifier with your index finger.
3. Hold the magnifier up to a light source and view through the magnifier (see Figure 6–9).
4. Move the lens with your index finger so that one edge is at the zero position and the lens is centered over the scale. While the lens is in this position, note the position of the opposite lens edge and read the overall lens diameter measurement directly off the scale.
5. Move the lens laterally so that one edge of the optic zone is aligned at the zero mark.
6. Note the position of the opposite edge of the optic zone, and read the measurement directly off the scale.
   Note: If you find it difficult to see the edge of the optic zone, the magnifier can be rocked back and forth at the edge of a light source to obtain a

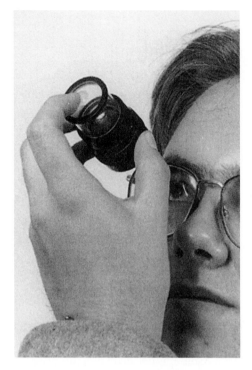

Figure 6–9. Lens diameter, optic zone diameter, and surface quality assessed with the measuring magnifier.

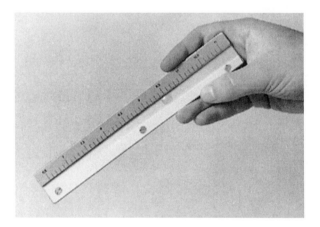

Figure 6–10. V-Channel gauge used to determine overall lens diameter. The measurement, taken at the center of the lens, is 9.5 mm.

better perspective. There is usually a change in the shadowing of the lens at the edge of each zone.

V-Channel Gauge

1. Place the lens concave side down into the wide end of the channel.
2. Tilt the gauge so that the narrow end tilts down, allowing the lens to slide down the channel.
3. Tap the gauge slightly on a table top until the contact lens is resting against the edges of the channel. Do not force the lens further down into the channel.
4. Take the reading from the center of the lens, or at the point of touch (see Figure 6–10).

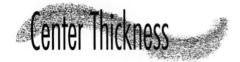

EQUIPMENT

- Center thickness gauge.

SET-UP

- If the center thickness gauge is not set to zero and requires a small adjustment, reset the gauge to zero by turning the dial face.
- For a large adjustment, reset the gauge to zero by loosening the screw at the bottom of the device, resetting, and retightening.

STEP-BY-STEP PROCEDURE

1. Open the device by pressing the lever.
2. Place the contact lens between the pins.
3. Slowly release the lever so that the pins gently hold the center of the lens.
4. The thickness is read directly off the scale. Each increment is 0.01 mm (see Figure 6–11).

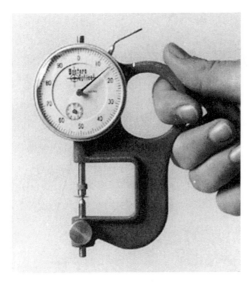

Figure 6–11. Center thickness gauge demonstrating a gas permeable contact lens center thickness of 0.15 mm.

Edge Configuration

EQUIPMENT

- Stereo microscope.
- Biomicroscope.
- Measuring magnifier.

SET-UP

- No specific set-up is required.

STEP-BY-STEP PROCEDURE

Stereo Microscope

1. Place the lens in a holding device, or hold the lens between thumb and index finger, such that the lens edge is directed toward the observer.
2. Center the lens under the objective lens (see Figure 6–12).

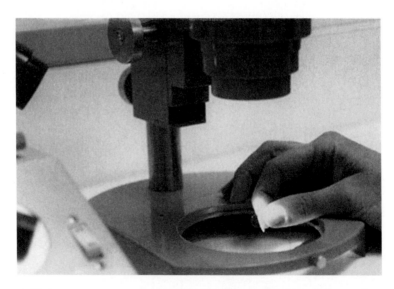

Figure 6–12. Stereo microscope set up to evaluate the edge configuration of a gas permeable contact lens.

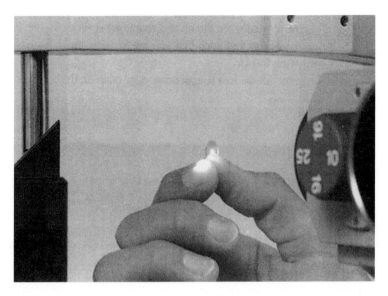

Figure 6–13. Using the biomicroscope to evaluate the edge configuration of a gas permeable contact lens.

3. Bring the edge into focus.
4. Rotate and tilt the lens to appreciate edge contour, thickness, and polish.

Biomicroscope
1. Set the slit lamp to low magnification and wide parallelepiped.
2. Hold the lens between thumb and index finger such that the lens edge is directed toward the observer.
3. Hold the lens in the path of the slit beam and focus on the lens edge (see Figure 6–13).
4. Rotate and tilt the lens to appreciate edge contour, thickness, and polish.

Measuring Magnifier
1. Turn the measuring magnifier around so that the reticule is toward your eye.
2. Hold the lens between thumb and forefinger several millimeters from the ocular lens such that you are viewing the lens profile (see Figure 6–14).
3. Rotate and tilt the lens to appreciate edge contour, thickness, and polish.

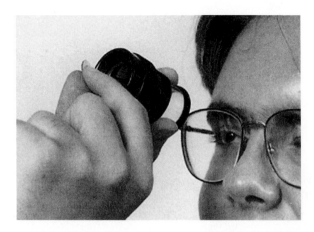

Figure 6–14. Measuring magnifier turned around to evaluate the edge configuration of a gas permeable contact lens.

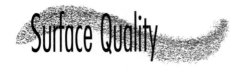

EQUIPMENT

- Stereo microscope.
- Biomicroscope.
- Measuring magnifier.
- Contact lens tweezers.

SET-UP

- Clean the lens with a daily cleaner. Rinse with tap water to remove any loose debris from the lens surface.
- Blot the lens dry with a soft, lint-free cloth or tissue prior to inspecting the lens surface.
- If using a biomicroscope, set to low magnification and wide parallelepiped.

STEP-BY-STEP PROCEDURE

1. Hold the lens with contact lens tweezers such that the surface is facing the objective lens of the stereo microscope or biomicroscope.
2. Bring the lens surface into focus by moving the lens back and forth, or by focusing the instrument (see Figure 6–15).
3. Inspect the lens surface at low and medium magnification.
4. If using the measuring magnifier, place the lens on the end of the magnifier. Look through the ocular toward a light source.
5. Carefully look for films, spots, scratches, or chips (see Figure 6–16).

RECORDING

- If the surface is clean with no deposits, cracks, or chips, record the surface as "clean."
- If deposits, cracks, or chips are present on the lens surface, draw and describe your findings.

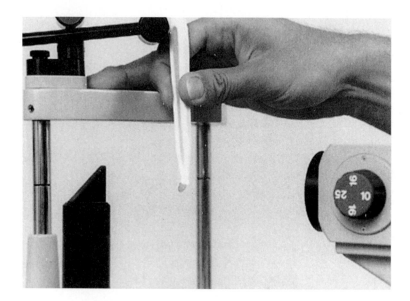

Figure 6–15. Gas permeable contact lens surface inspection using the biomicroscope.

EXAMPLES

- Protein film: can range from a clear, transparent, thin film (mild deposition) to a semi-opaque, white, hazy film (severe deposition).
- Lipid deposits: greasy, shiny, smeary deposits that change by rubbing. Often seen in a fingerprint pattern, they are easily seen under low magnification.
- Cracking and crazing: small lattice-type cracked appearance to lens surface. Can be cracks in a protein film or the lens surface itself.

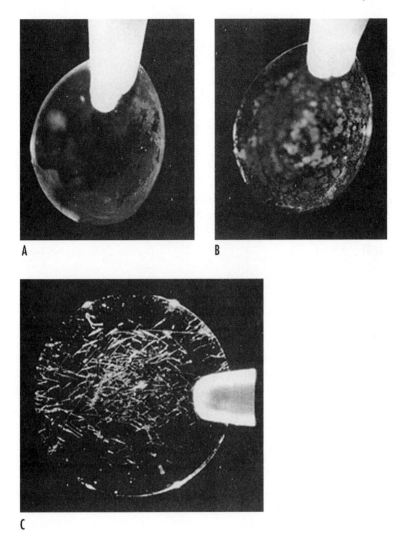

Figure 6–16. Examples of gas permeable contact lens surface deposits and abnormalities. **A.** Protein film. **B.** Lipid deposits. **C.** Cracking and crazing.

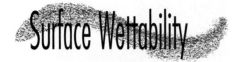

Surface Wettability

Note: Unlike the previous parameters, surface wettability is assessed with the contact lens on the eye.

EQUIPMENT

• Biomicroscope.

SET-UP

• Adjust the biomicroscope so that it is comfortable for the patient.
• Set the magnification to the lowest setting (6× or 10×).
• Set the illumination to a medium parallelepiped at low to moderate intensity.
• If this assessment is to be performed immediately after lens insertion, wait 15 minutes to allow for lens stabilization.

STEP-BY-STEP PROCEDURE

1. Set up the slit lamp to create specular reflection off the anterior contact lens surface.
2. Instruct the patient to blink.
3. Observe the tear film on the front surface of the contact lens.
4. Assess the tear break-up time over the contact lens surface. This is the lens drying time.

RECORDING

• Draw and describe areas of rapid tear break-up or nonwetting.

EXAMPLE

• Areas of rapid tear disruption indicate poor wettability due to deposits, polish residues, or damaged lens surface (see Figure 6–17).

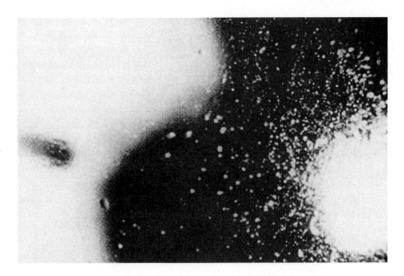

Figure 6–17. Tear disruption and drying on the surface of a gas permeable contact lens.

Insertion, Removal, and Recentering of Gas Permeable Contact Lenses

PURPOSE   To insert or remove a patient's gas permeable contact lenses. To recenter a lens onto the cornea when it has become dislodged.

INDICATIONS

There are several situations when the examiner must be able to insert, remove, or recenter a patient's gas permeable contact lenses. New contact lens patients will be unable to perform these tasks themselves. Patients with poor manual dexterity or new wearers who are still learning these skills will also have difficulty with these tasks.

EQUIPMENT

- Gas permeable contact lens cleaner and wetting solution.

SET-UP

- Prior to handling lenses, wash your hands with a soap that does not contain lotions or fragrances. Dry your hands with a lint-free towel.
- Clean the lens surface with a daily cleaner. Rinse with tap water or saline solution to remove any surface debris. Condition the lens surface by rubbing a few drops of wetting solution onto the lens. This will promote in-eye wetting.

STEP-BY-STEP PROCEDURE

Insertion
1. Place the lens on the tip of your index or middle finger. Make sure your hands are free of excess water.
2. Direct the patient's gaze upward. Firmly grasp and retract the patient's lower eyelid with the middle or fourth finger of the hand holding the contact lens. Grasp the lid as close to the lid margin as possible.

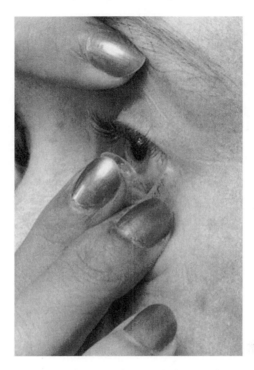

Figure 6–18. Insertion of a gas permeable contact lens.

3. Direct the patient's gaze downward. Retract the patient's upper lid with the thumb or index finger of the opposite hand.
4. Move the contact lens close to the patient's eye. Instruct the patient to look straight ahead, and at the same instant, gently but quickly apply the lens to the central cornea (see Figure 6–18).
5. When the lens appears stable on the cornea, slowly release the lower lid.
6. Slowly release the upper lid. The lens should maintain centration on the cornea.
7. An inexperienced wearer may be bothered by lens edge awareness. If so, have him close his eyes or look downward. This will temporarily relieve some of the discomfort. Instruct the patient to blink normally.

Removal
1. Direct the patient's fixation straight ahead.
2. Place the tips of your index fingers or thumbs at the patient's lid margins at the 12:00 and 6:00 lens positions. Retract the lids until the lid margins are just outside the lens edge. Be sure not to allow either lid to evert, or the lens edge will slip under the lid.

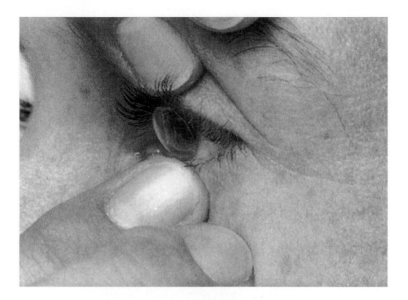

Figure 6–19. Removal of a gas permeable contact lens.

3. Gently press the lids against the globe. Move the lids toward each other to scissor the lens until one edge pops up from the corneal surface. Continue to move the lids toward each other until the lens is removed (see Figure 6–19).
4. Instruct the patient to close his eyes. The lens will often stay on the eyelashes where it can be easily retrieved.

Recentering

1. Locate the lens on the eye. You may have to direct the patient's gaze and pull the lids away from the eye to do this.
2. Instruct the patient to look in the direction opposite to where the lens is located.
3. With two index fingers placed at the lid margins, use the lids to gently guide the lens toward the cornea (see Figure 6–20). Never directly touch the lens itself with your fingers.
4. If the lens has suctioned onto the eye, use the eyelid to break the suction by pressing on the sclera just outside the lens edge.
5. When the lens is near the limbus and control of the lens is assumed, have the patient slowly look toward the lens. The lens should recenter onto the cornea.
   Note: Tips for handling gas permeable contact lenses are presented in Table 6–1.

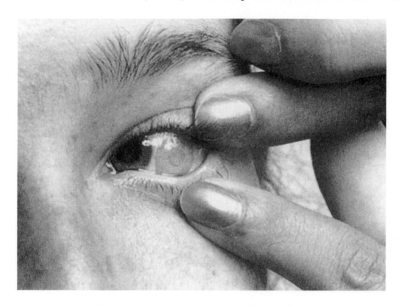

Figure 6–20. Recentering a gas permeable contact lens.

TABLE 6–1. HANDLING TIPS FOR GAS PERMEABLE CONTACT LENS

- **Dry your fingertips** to better grasp the patient's eyelids and for easier transfer of the lens to the cornea.
- **Control of the patient's eyelids** is essential.
- Always **direct the patient's fixation**.
- **Proper lens preparation** with appropriate wetting solutions will maximize the patient's initial comfort.
- **Quick, yet gentle,** lens insertion will improve success.
- **Maintain apposition** of the lid margin to the globe during removal to improve success.
- **Break suction,** almost to the point of removing the lens, to ease recentering.

Fit Assessment of Gas Permeable Contact Lenses: Biomicroscope

PURPOSE   To assess the fitting relationship of a gas permeable contact lens to the eye. The fitting relationship is crucial to the wearer's vision, comfort, and ocular surface health.

EQUIPMENT

- Biomicroscope.
- Yellow filter (Wratten #12 or #15). Although not necessary, the yellow filter enhances the quality of the fluorescein pattern.
- Fluorescein strips.

SET-UP

- Adjust the biomicroscope so that it is comfortable for the patient and examiner.
- Set the magnification to the lowest setting (6× or 10×).
- Insert the cobalt blue filter.
- Set the illumination arm to approximately 30° from the straight ahead position on the temporal side. Set the illumination level to medium to high, and open the slit beam fully.
- Place the yellow filter over the objective end of the biomicroscope. Do not place it over the cobalt blue light source.

STEP-BY-STEP PROCEDURE

1. Wet a fluorescein strip with a drop of sterile saline solution. Shake off the excess saline.
2. Instill a small amount of fluorescein into the inferior cul-de-sac or onto the superior bulbar conjunctiva. Have the patient blink two to three times to pump the fluorescein underneath the contact lens. The patient should be instructed to blink normally thereafter.
3. Instruct the patient to look straight ahead, toward the back of the exami-

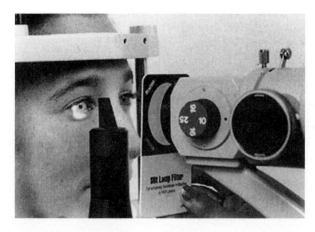

Figure 6–21. Gas permeable contact lens fit assessment using the biomicroscope. A yellow filter is held in front of the objective lens to enhance the fluorescein pattern.

nation room. Alternately, have the patient look at your ear. This will promote steady fixation in primary gaze.

4. View the contact lens through the biomicroscope (see Figure 6–21).

5. Observe static aspects of the fit: lens position and fluorescein pattern (see Table 6–2). The patient's lids may be used to manipulate the lens position or to pump fluorescein under the lens. The fluorescein pattern should be viewed first in the static position. If the lens is decentered, the pattern should also be viewed with the lens centered on the cornea to better assess the central fitting relationship.

6. Ask the patient to blink and observe dynamic aspects of the fit: movement and stability (see Table 6–2).

RECORDING

- Record the lens position, blink movement, stability, and fluorescein pattern observed for each eye.

TABLE 6–2. SUMMARY OF GAS PERMEABLE CONTACT LENS FIT CHARACTERISTICS

Fit Characteristic	Description
Lens position	Corneal location where the lens settles after the blink.
Blink movement	The amount of vertical excursion the lens makes across the cornea after the blink.
Stability	How well the lens maintains its static position between blinks.
Fluorescein pattern	The amount of fluorescein, and therefore tears, underneath the contact lens evaluated in the central, midperipheral, and peripheral zones of the lens. Darker areas indicate touch or bearing, while greenish-yellow areas indicate clearance or pooling of tears. Areas of alignment between the contact lens back surface and the cornea appear an even greenish-black.

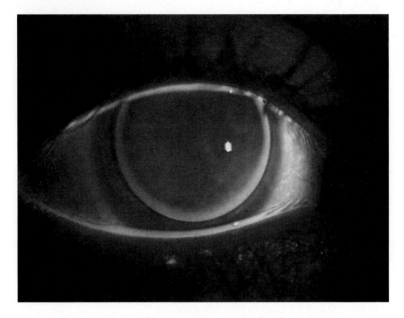

Figure 6–22. Acceptable gas permeable contact lens fit with central position.

EXAMPLES

- Acceptable fit (see Figure 6–22)
- Lens position: central
- Blink movement: good—approximately 2 mm
- Stability: good—remains central
- Fluorescein pattern: central alignment, midperipheral bearing, peripheral clearance
- Acceptable fit (see Figure 6–23)
- Lens position: superior central
- Blink movement: good—approximately 2 mm
- Stability: good—lid attachment
- Fluorescein pattern: central alignment, midperipheral alignment, and peripheral clearance
- Unacceptably steep fit (see Figure 6–24)
- Lens position: inferior-nasal
- Blink movement: poor—approximately 1 mm
- Stability: poor—drops between blinks
- Fluorescein pattern: excessive central clearance, midperipheral bearing, and minimal peripheral clearance
- Unacceptably flat fit (see Figure 6–25)

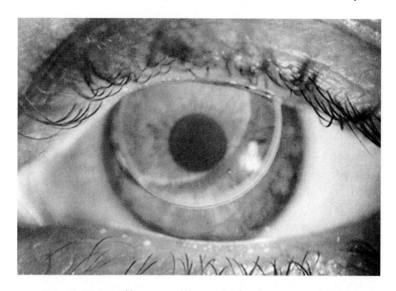

Figure 6–23. Acceptable gas permeable contact lens fit with superior central position.

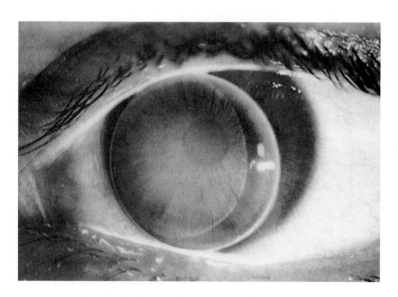

Figure 6–24. Unacceptably steep gas permeable contact lens fit.

- Lens position: inferior-central, crossing the limbus
- Blink movement: excessive—traverses past limbus
- Stability: poor—drops between blinks
- Fluorescein pattern: central touch, midperipheral clearance, and wide band of peripheral clearance with bubbles

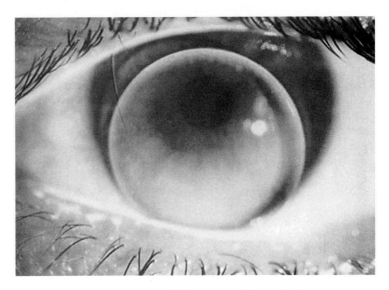

Figure 6–25. Unacceptably flat gas permeable contact lens fit.

GAS PERMEABLE CONTACT LENS FIT ASSESSMENT *at a glance*

FIT CHARACTERISTIC	EXPECTED FINDING
Lens position	Central to superior-central
Movement on blink	1 to 3 mm (vertically)
Stability	Remains in static position
Fluorescein pattern	Central alignment to minimal clearance Midperipheral alignment Peripheral clearance

Fit Assessment of Gas Permeable Contact Lenses: Burton (UV) Lamp

PURPOSE
To assess the fitting relationship of a gas permeable contact lens to the eye. The fitting relationship is crucial to the wearer's vision, comfort, and ocular surface health.

Note: The Burton lamp cannot be used to evaluate gas permeable lenses made of materials containing a UV blocker.

EQUIPMENT

- Burton (UV) lamp.
- Fluorescein strips.

SET-UP

- No specific set-up is required.

STEP-BY-STEP PROCEDURE

1. Wet a fluorescein strip with a drop of sterile saline solution. Shake off the excess saline.
2. Instill a moderate amount of fluorescein into the inferior cul-de-sac or onto the superior bulbar conjunctiva. Instruct the patient to blink two to three times to pump fluorescein underneath the contact lens. The patient should be instructed to blink normally thereafter.
3. Hold the Burton lamp in front of the patient and view the eyes and contact lenses through the rectangular magnifying lens. Instruct the patient to look through the magnifying lens toward you (see Figure 6–26).
4. Observe static aspects of the fit: lens position and fluorescein pattern (see Table 6–2). The patient's lids may be used to manipulate the lens position or to pump fluorescein under the lens. The fluorescein pattern should be viewed in the static position. If the lens is decentered, the pattern should

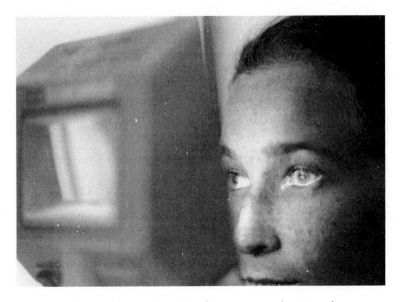

Figure 6–26. Gas permeable contact lens fit assessment using the Burton UV lamp.

also be viewed with the lens centered on the cornea to better assess the central fitting relationship pattern.

5. Ask the patient to blink and observe dynamic aspects of the fit: movement and stability (see Table 6–2).

RECORDING

- Record the lens position, blink movement, stability, and fluorescein pattern observed for each eye.

EXAMPLES

- See examples in previous section: Fit Assessment of Gas Permeable Contact Lenses: Biomicroscope

INSPECTION AND VERIFICATION OF SOFT CONTACT LENSES

PURPOSE   To verify the power of a soft contact lens. To inspect the surface of a soft contact lens to determine the type and degree of deposition of various organic and inorganic substances.

Back Vertex Power

EQUIPMENT

- Lensometer.
- Lint-free cloth or tissue.
- Contact lens tweezers.

SET-UP

- Use a daily cleaner to clean the surface of the contact lens. Rinse with sterile saline solution.
  Note: Tap water should never be used to rinse or store soft contact lenses.

STEP-BY-STEP PROCEDURE

1. Rotate the spring-loaded lens holder of the lensometer away from the lens stop. Clean any ink or debris from the lens stop with a tissue. Turn on the lensometer.
2. Place the wet lens on a lint-free cloth or tissue and gently blot excess fluid from the lens surface by folding the cloth over onto the lens. Alternately, hold the lens with contact lens tweezers, rinse the lens with saline solution, and wait for the excess fluid to evaporate. Moving the lens back and forth may speed up this process. For either method, do not allow the lens to dehydrate excessively. This will cause the lens optics to distort and the lens power to change slightly.
3. Center the lens on the lensometer so that the concave surface is against the stop. Drape the lens evenly so that there are no wrinkles or folds (see Figure 6–27).
4. Measure the lens power as for spectacles. When reading the power, the mires may not be as clear as when measuring a gas permeable lens, but a reasonably clear mire is obtainable. If a reasonably clear mire image is not obtained, rinse the lens with saline and repeat.

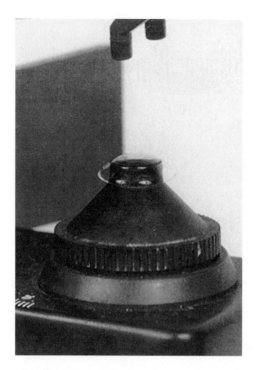

Figure 6–27. Positioning of a soft contact lens on the lensometer stop for back vertex power measurement.

INSPECTION AND VERIFICATION OF SOFT CONTACT LENSES
at a glance

PARAMETER	INSTRUMENT
Back vertex power	Lensometer

Lens surface
    Films and spots
    Discoloration
    Tears, nicks, and scratches
	Biomicroscope

Surface Inspection: Films and Spots

EQUIPMENT

- Biomicroscope.
- Contact lens tweezers.

SET-UP

- Clean the lens surface with a daily cleaner and rinse with sterile saline.
- Face the biomicroscope toward a dark background, such as a tangent screen.
- Move the slit lamp toward you as far as it can go. Open the slit to a wide beam, and move the illumination arm to the side (90° angle or more). Set the magnification to the lowest setting.

STEP-BY-STEP PROCEDURE

1. Hold the lens with contact lens tweezers. Rinse with sterile saline solution to remove any loose debris. Shake off any excess fluid.
2. Hold the lens in the path of the light beam (see Figure 6–28).
3. Move the lens back and forth until it comes into focus through the biomicroscope.
4. Observe any film, hazy regions, or spots on the lens surface. Increase the magnification, if needed.
5. Observe changes in the appearance of the surface as the lens dries. Milder deposits may not appear until the lens surface is dry.

RECORDING

- Draw and describe the appearance, size, location, and severity of the deposits (see Figure 6–29).

EXAMPLES

- *Protein film:* can range from a clear, transparent, thin film (mild deposition) to a semi-opaque, white, hazy film (severe deposition).

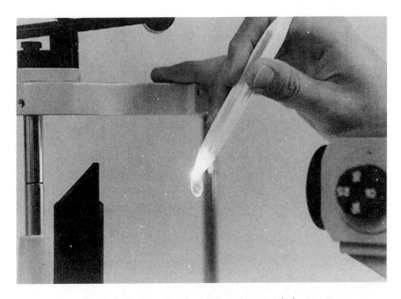

Figure 6–28. Surface inspection of a soft contact lens using the biomicroscope.

- *Lens calculi* (jelly bumps, mulberry spots): raised, birefringent spots on the anterior lens surface that penetrate into the lens matrix. Growth rings may be seen under higher magnification.
- *Lipid deposits:* greasy, shiny, smeary deposits that change by rubbing. Often in a fingerprint pattern, they are easily seen under low magnification.
- *Calcium deposits:* may form a whitish film or discrete chalk white deposits. Alternately, they can form milky white films with discrete borders within the lens matrix.
- *Fungi:* filamentary growths within the lens matrix in a variety of colors: black, gray, brown, orange, pink, or white.

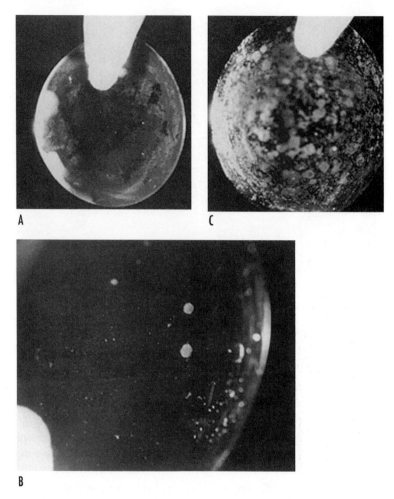

Figure 6–29. Examples of soft contact lens surface deposits. **A.** Protein film. **B.** Lens calculi. **C.** Lipid deposits.

Surface Inspection: Tears, Nicks, and Scratches

EQUIPMENT

- Biomicroscope.

SET-UP

- Set up the biomicroscope so that it is comfortable for the patient and the examiner.
- Use low magnification and a wide parallelepiped with the illumination arm at a 30° to 40° angle from the straight ahead position.

STEP-BY-STEP PROCEDURE

1. Instruct the patient to look straight ahead. Scan from temporal to nasal across the lens and inspect the surface for any physical defects.
2. Instruct the patient to look up and inspect the inferior region of the lens.
3. Instruct the patient to look down. Lift the patient's upper lid and inspect the superior region of the lens.

RECORDING

- Describe and draw any tears, nicks, scratches, or other surface defects you observe.

EXAMPLE (see Figure 6–30).

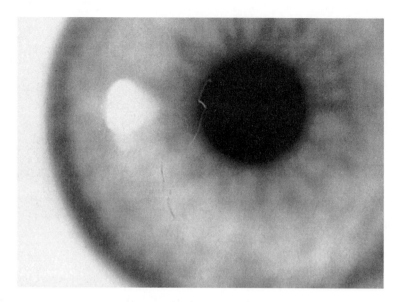

Figure 6–30. Surface fracture on a soft contact lens.

Insertion and Removal of Soft Contact Lenses

PURPOSE   To insert or remove a patient's soft contact lenses.

INDICATIONS

There are certain situations when the examiner must be able to insert and remove a patient's soft contact lenses. New contact lens patients will be unable to perform these tasks themselves. Patients with poor manual dexterity or new wearers who are still learning these skills will also have difficulty with these tasks.

EQUIPMENT

- Soft contact lens daily cleaner and saline solution.

SET-UP

- Prior to handling lenses, wash your hands with a soap that does not contain lotions or fragrances. Dry your hands with a lint-free towel.
- Make sure the lens is not inside out.
- Inspect the lens for surface debris, tears, or other surface defects. You may have to use daily cleaner and a saline rinse to remove any debris. It is a good habit to rinse the lens with sterile saline solution even if it is a new lens and appears clean.
- Avoid touching the ocular (concave) surface of the lens once you have cleaned and rinsed it.
- Dry the finger that you will use to insert the lens. A hydrophilic lens tends to stick to a wet finger more than to the patient's eye.
- For thin or low modulus lenses, it may help to allow the lens to air dry for several seconds on your finger before attempting to insert it.

STEP-BY-STEP PROCEDURE

Insertion

1. Place the lens on the tip of the index finger of your dominant hand.
2. Instruct the patient to look down. Place the index finger or thumb of your other hand at the lid margin of the patient's upper lid. Retract the upper lid and hold it firmly against the upper brow.
3. Instruct the patient to look up. Place the middle or fourth finger of your dominant hand at the lower lid margin and retract the lower lid.
4. Gently apply the lens to the eye in one of three ways:
   a. While the patient is looking up, place the lens on the inferior sclera (see Figure 6–31).
   b. Instruct the patient to look nasally and place the lens on the temporal sclera (see Figure 6–32).
   c. Instruct the patient to look straight ahead and place the lens directly on the cornea.
   The lens should adhere to the eye without excessive pressure.
5. While maintaining control of the lids, instruct the patient to slowly look into the lens. This should allow the lens to center on the cornea. If the lens still has not centered, or if air bubbles are present under the lens, instruct

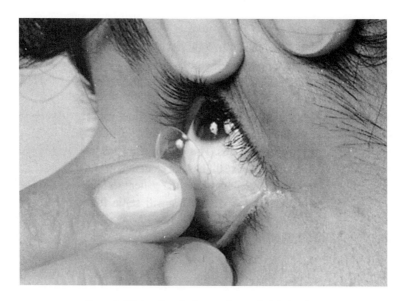

Figure 6–31. Insertion of soft contact lens on the inferior sclera.

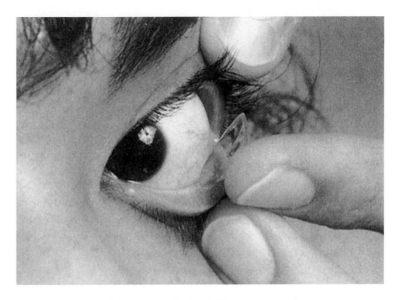

Figure 6–32. Insertion of soft contact lens on the temporal sclera.

the patient to look down, to the left, and then to the right. This will settle the lens onto the cornea.

6. Slowly release the lower lid, then the upper lid.
7. You can pat or massage the closed lid to help the lens further settle. You may also have the patient look left, right, up, and down while his eyes are closed.

Removal

1. Instruct the patient to look down. Hold the patient's upper lid against the upper brow with your nondominant hand.
2. Instruct the patient to look up. Retract the lower lid with your dominant hand's middle or fourth finger.
3. Place the index finger of your dominant hand on the inferior edge of the lens. Pull the lens down onto the sclera and in one continuous motion, gently pinch the lens off with your thumb and index finger (see Figure 6–33).
4. Alternately, instruct the patient to look nasally.
5. Place the index finger of your dominant hand at the temporal edge of the lens and slide it temporally. Continue to slide it temporally until the lens comes out or is bunched up at the lateral canthus (see Figure 6–34). Gently pinch the lens off. Table 6–3 provides tips for the eye care provider on handling hydrophilic contact lenses.

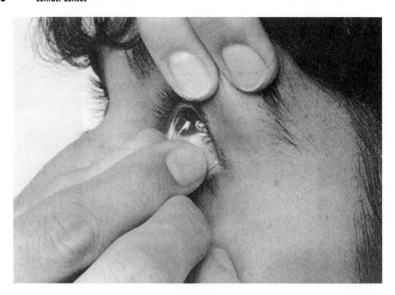

Figure 6–33. Removal of soft contact lens by pinching the inferior edge of the contact lens.

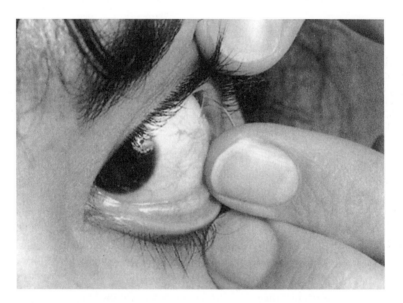

Figure 6–34. Removal of soft contact lens by sliding it off temporally.

TABLE 6–3. HANDLING TIPS FOR SOFT CONTACT LENS

- **Dry your fingertips** to enhance the transfer of the soft contact lens to the eye.
- **Place your fingers at the patient's lid margins** to allow maximum eye opening during insertion.
- If unable to insert the lens on the inferior sclera, **try the temporal sclera.**
- **Quick, yet gentle,** insertion and removal will increase success and patient confidence.

Fit Assessment of Soft Contact Lenses

PURPOSE   To determine whether a soft contact lens is fitting adequately so that vision and comfort are optimized, and contact lens–related anterior segment complications are minimized.

EQUIPMENT

• Biomicroscope.

SET-UP

• Adjust the biomicroscope so that it is comfortable for the patient.
• Set the magnification to the lowest setting (6× or 10×).
• Set the illumination arm to approximately 30° from the straight ahead position on the temporal side. Set the illumination level to medium to high. Open the slit beam to a medium parallelepiped.

STEP-BY-STEP PROCEDURE

1. Instruct the patient to look straight ahead, toward the back of the examination room. Alternately, you can instruct the patient to look at your right ear (see Figure 6–35). Focus on the patient's right contact lens.
2. Move the slit beam from temporal to nasal lens edge and observe the lens position and corneal coverage. If the lens position is difficult to determine due to a small palpebral aperture, try moving the patient's upper and lower lids away from the lens. However, be aware that lid manipulation can alter lens position.
3. Instruct the patient to blink once and observe the amount of lens movement induced. If you can see the lens edge at the 6:00 position, view the edge at this location. If not, view the lens edge adjacent to the lower lid on both nasal and temporal sides. Repeat two or three times.

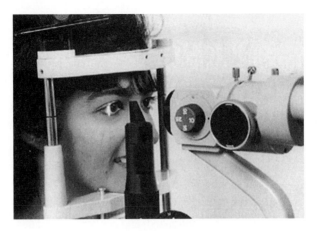

Figure 6–35. Appropriate positioning of the patient in the biomicroscope for soft contact lens fit assessment.

4. Instruct the patient to look straight up. Observe the amount of vertical lag demonstrated by the lens.

5. While the patient is looking up, instruct the patient to blink once. Observe the amount of lens movement induced. Repeat two to three times.

6. Instruct the patient to look straight ahead again. Then instruct the patient to look to his right. Observe the amount of lateral lag movement demonstrated by the lens. Instruct the patient to look to his left and repeat.

7. While the patient is looking straight ahead, perform the push-up test by using the patient's lower lid to push up on the inferior edge of the contact lens. Assess the ease or difficulty with which the lens moves upward (see Table 6–4).

8. If you are assessing a toric contact lens, you must make two additional observations, rotational orientation and stability (see Table 6–5).

9. While the patient is looking in primary gaze, locate the toric lens markings (see Figure 6–36). Measure or estimate the amount of rotation, in degrees, of the lens markings from their intended position. Also note the direction of this rotation. If the lower lid is covering lens markings at 6:00, gently pull down the lower lid until you are just able to see the markings. Be careful not to pull on the lid too much because this can cause the lens to rotate slightly. Do not have the patient look up because this can also cause the lens to rotate.

10. Instruct the patient to blink once. Observe the rotational stability of the lens markings. Repeat two or three times.

11. Repeat steps 2 to 10 for the left eye.

TABLE 6–4. SUMMARY OF SOFT CONTACT LENS FIT CHARACTERISTICS

Fit Characteristic	Description
Lens position	Position of the contact lens relative to the cornea, assessed by observing the amount of \ lens overlap onto the sclera. If this overlap is fairly equal around the lens, the lens is well centered.
Corneal coverage	The extent to which the contact lens covers the corneal surface.
Blink movement	The amount of vertical movement demonstrated by the lens when the patient blinks.
Lag movement	The amount by which the lens follows behind any eye excursion.
Push-up movement	The ease with which the lens moves upward when pushed by the lower lid.

TABLE 6–5. SUMMARY OF ADDITIONAL TORIC SOFT CONTACT LENS FIT CHARACTERISTICS

Fit Characteristic	Description
Rotational orientation	The static position of the lens markings in primary gaze. Refer to Figure 6–40 for examples of common toric lens markings.
Rotational stability	The amount of lens rotation demonstrated by the contact lens when the patient blinks.

RECORDING

- Record the lens position, corneal coverage, blink and lag movement, and push-up movement observed.
- If you are assessing a toric lens, also record the rotational orientation and stability observed.

EXAMPLES

- Well-fitting spherical soft lens
- Lens position and coverage: central and full
- Blink movement: 1 mm in primary gaze, 1.5 mm in upgaze
- Lag movement: 1.5 mm in upgaze and lateral gaze
- Push-up movement: optimal
- Unacceptably tight-fitting soft lens
- Lens position and coverage: central and full
- Blink movement: less than 0.5 mm in primary and upgaze
- Lag movement: less than 0.5 mm in upgaze and lateral gaze
- Push-up movement: difficult
- Well-fitting soft toric lens
- Lens position and coverage: central and full
- Blink movement: 1 mm in primary gaze, 1.5 mm in upgaze
- Lag movement: 1.5 mm in upgaze and lateral gaze

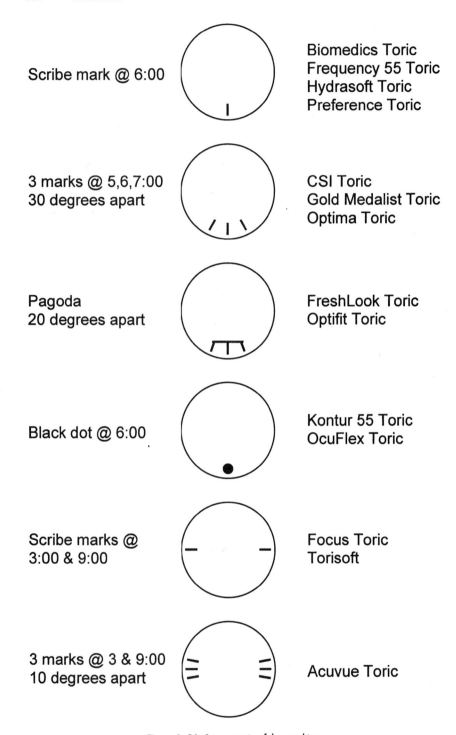

Scribe mark @ 6:00 — Biomedics Toric / Frequency 55 Toric / Hydrasoft Toric / Preference Toric

3 marks @ 5,6,7:00 / 30 degrees apart — CSI Toric / Gold Medalist Toric / Optima Toric

Pagoda / 20 degrees apart — FreshLook Toric / Optifit Toric

Black dot @ 6:00 — Kontur 55 Toric / OcuFlex Toric

Scribe marks @ / 3:00 & 9:00 — Focus Toric / Torisoft

3 marks @ 3 & 9:00 / 10 degrees apart — Acuvue Toric

Figure 6–36. Common toric soft lens markings.

- Push-up movement: optimal
- Rotational orientation: 5° clockwise
- Rotational stability: no rotation on blink
- Unacceptable toric soft lens fit
- Lens position and coverage: superior temporal, inadequate coverage inferior nasally
- Blink movement: 2 mm in primary and upgaze
- Lag movement: 3 mm in upgaze and lateral gaze
- Push-up movement: easy
- Rotational orientation: 25° counterclockwise
- Rotational stability: rotates 10° on the blink, requires several seconds to return to original position

SOFT CONTACT LENS FIT ASSESSMENT *at a glance*

FIT CHARACTERISTIC	EXPECTED FINDING
Lens position	Centered, or slightly decentered but maintaining full coverage
Corneal coverage	The contact lens should cover the entire cornea and overlap the limbus by 1 to 2 mm around the entire cornea. If you note any area of corneal exposure, there is inadequate corneal coverage
Blink movement	0.5–2.0 mm
Lag movement	0.5–2.0 mm
Push-up movement	The lens should move easily and freely when pushed by the lower lid
Rotational orientation	Not more than 20° from intended position
Rotational stability	No rotation on the blink, or slight rotation with rapid return to original position

Over-Refraction: Phoropter

PURPOSE
To determine the final contact lens power required by the patient during diagnostic fitting. To determine whether a patient's contact lenses are providing the optimal power and vision during follow-up visits. *Note*: This procedure assumes that the examiner is familiar with refraction procedures presented in Chapter 3.

EQUIPMENT

- Phoropter.
- VA chart.
- Retinoscope.

SET-UP

- Set up the patient behind the phoropter as indicated for retinoscopy. Perform static retinoscopy.

STEP-BY-STEP PROCEDURE

Spherical Over-Refraction

In most cases, a spherical over-refraction is sufficient to determine whether the contact lens is the appropriate power.

1. Remove any cylinder power you obtained during retinoscopy.
2. Occlude the patient's left eye.
3. Measure the patient's VA.
4. Fog the right eye with +0.75 D or to 20/40 and obtain monocular MP-MVA.
5. Occlude the patient's right eye and repeat steps 1 to 4 for the left eye.
6. Unocclude both eyes. Perform a binocular balance.
7. Fog both eyes with +0.75 D or to 20/40 and obtain binocular MPMVA.
8. Record the spherical over-refraction and endpoint VA for each eye.

Sphero-Cylindrical Over-Refraction

This can be performed when a spherical over-refraction does not provide adequate VA. This may occur in cases of moderate residual cylinder or with toric contact lenses.

1. Occlude the left eye and perform a monocular refraction with JCC test on the right eye.
2. Fog with +0.75 D or to 20/40 and obtain monocular MPMVA.
3. Occlude the right eye and repeat steps 1 and 2 for the left eye.
4. Unocclude both eyes. Perform a binocular balance.
5. Fog both eyes with +0.75 D or to 20/40 and obtain binocular MPMVA.
6. Record the sphero-cylindrical over-refraction and endpoint VA for each eye.

RECORDING

- Record the power in the phoropter and the endpoint VA obtained for each eye. The power in the phoropter is the over-refraction.

EXAMPLES

- Spherical over-refraction
  OD −0.50 sphere   20/20
  OS −0.75 sphere   20/25
- Sphero-cylindrical over-refraction
  OD + 0.25 − 0.75 × 165 20/20
  OS + 0.50 − 1.25 × 045 20/20

EXPECTED FINDINGS

If the contact lens power is appropriate for the patient, a spherical equivalent of plano to + 0.50 is expected.

Over-Refraction: Spectacle Trial Lenses

PURPOSE To quickly determine whether a patient's contact lenses are providing the optimal power without the use of the phoropter.

EQUIPMENT

- Spectacle trial lenses.
- VA chart.
- Occluder.

SET-UP

- With patient in the examination chair, project a full VA chart so that the patient's best corrected VA is the bottom line.

STEP-BY-STEP PROCEDURE

1. Occlude the patient's left eye with a hand held occluder.
2. Instruct the patient to view the lowest line he can read.
3. Place the + 0.50 D trial lens in front of the right eye (see Figure 6–37).
4. If this plus lens does not blur the bottom line, or if the line becomes clearer, use a +0.75 D trial lens and repeat. Continue to increase the plus power in +0.25 D steps until the patient reports blur. The last lens that did not cause blur is the over-refraction endpoint.
6. If the +0.50 D trial lens causes the bottom line to blur, continue with minus lenses.
7. Place the −0.50 D trial lens in front of the right eye.
8. If this lens causes blur, or if the letters become smaller or darker, the over-refraction endpoint is plano.
9. If −0.50 D lens causes the bottom line to become clearer, obtain a −0.75 D trial lens and repeat. Continue to increase the minus power in −0.25 D steps until the MPMVA is reached. This is the over-refraction endpoint.

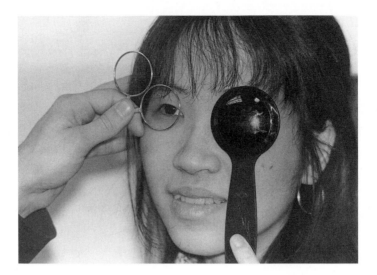

Figure 6–37. Monocular over-refraction using spectacle trial lenses.

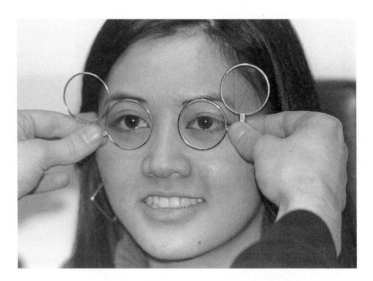

Figure 6–38. Binocular over-refraction using spectacle trial lenses.

10. Occlude the patient's right eye. Repeat steps 2 to 9 for the left eye.
11. Place the endpoint lenses in front of the eyes binocularly (see Figure 6–38). To ensure binocular MPMVA, obtain trial lenses with +0.25 D more plus for each eye and place in front of the eyes. If there is no loss in clarity, this is your binocular over-refraction endpoint.

RECORDING

• Record the power of the endpoint trial lenses and the endpoint VA for each eye.

EXAMPLE

• Over-refraction
  OD: plano   20/20
  OS: −0.50   20/20

EXPECTED FINDINGS

• If the contact lens power is appropriate for the patient, a spherical equivalent of plano to +0.50 is expected.
• Table 6–6 provides tips on using loose lenses for contact lens over-refraction.

TABLE 6–6. LOOSE LENS OVER-REFRACTION TIPS

• If ±0.50 D does not improve visual acuity, the lens power is optimal.
• Binocular MPMVA often results in 0.25 D more plus than monocular MPMVA.
• Loose lens over-refraction is quicker and less constrained than with the phoropter.
• Loose lens over-refraction is more appropriate for monovision or bifocal contact lenses.

Evaluation of the Monovision Patient

PURPOSE   To measure visual acuity and perform an over-refraction to improve vision for presbyopic patients wearing one lens for distance vision and the other for near vision.

EQUIPMENT

- Phoropter or loose trial lenses.
- VA chart.
- Near point card.

SET-UP

- Set up the patient in front of the distance VA chart to measure distance visual acuity.
- Give the patient a near point card to measure near visual acuity.
- Set up the patient behind the phoropter or use loose spectacle trial lenses to perform the over-refraction.

STEP-BY-STEP PROCEDURE

Distance and Near Visual Acuity

Measure the distance and near visual acuity using the same procedure for entering visual acuity.

RECORDING

- Record visual acuity at distance for each eye and both eyes together.
- Record visual acuity at near for each eye and both eyes together.

EXAMPLE

- Distance VA: OD 20/20, OS 20/100, OU 20/20
- Near VA: OD 20/100, OS 20/20, OU 20/20

EXPECTED FINDINGS

Because the monovision patient wears one contact lens that is prescribed for distance vision and the other for near vision, the two eyes will have different acuities at distance and near.

The eye corrected with the distance contact lens should have good visual acuity at distance, but poor visual acuity at near.

The eye corrected with the near contact lens should have good visual acuity at near, but poor visual acuity at distance.

Visual acuity at both distance and near should be good with both eyes together.

STEP-BY-STEP PROCEDURE

Distance Over-Refraction

1. Using either the phoropter or spectacle trial lenses, perform a spherical over-refraction at distance for each eye.
2. Unocclude both eyes and perform a binocular balance.
3. Fog both eyes with +0.75 D or to 20/40 and obtain binocular MPMVA.
4. Record the spherical over-refraction and endpoint VA for each eye.

RECORDING

• Record the distance over-refraction and the endpoint VA obtained for each eye.

EXAMPLE

• Distance over-refraction
  OD   plano sphere   20/20
  OS   −1.50 sphere   20/20

EXPECTED FINDINGS

• The distance eye should have a distance over-refraction between plano and +0.50 D.
• The near eye should have a distance over-refraction that is equal to the amount of add power the lens is providing, but in minus power. For example, if the over-refraction is −1.50 D, the lens is giving the patient a +1.50 add.

STEP-BY-STEP PROCEDURE

Near Over-Refraction

1. Have the patient hold the near point card at the appropriate working distance.
2. Keep both eyes unoccluded.
3. Using loose trial lenses, place lenses with powers ±0.25 and ±0.50 D over the eye corrected with the near contact lens (see Figure 6–39).
4. Determine the least-plus lens power that provides the best near visual acuity.
5. Have the patient view the distance VA chart with and without the over-refraction lens over the near eye.
   a. If the over-refraction lens does not decrease distance VA, record the near over-refraction lens power and endpoint near VA.
   b. If the over-refraction lens decreases distance VA, decrease the plus power in the over-refraction lens in +0.25 D steps until the distance VA is not decreased or you have reached plano. Record the final near over-refraction lens power and endpoint near VA.

RECORDING

• Record the near over-refraction and the endpoint VA obtained OU.

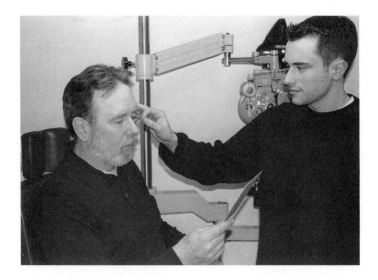

Figure 6–39. Over-refraction over near eye for monovision patient.

EXAMPLE

- Near over-refraction
  OS   +0.25 sphere   20/20

EXPECTED FINDINGS

- The near eye should have a near over-refraction that is within 0.25 D of plano.

7

SYSTEMIC HEALTH SCREENING

Robert C. Capone, OD

CHAPTER AT A GLANCE

INTRODUCTION TO SYSTEMIC HEALTH SCREENING

Primary eye care practitioners frequently encounter the manifestations of systemic disease. A number of systemic diseases, particularly those of infectious or inflammatory nature, affect the eyes as well as other organs or tissues within the body. Other systemic conditions may cause symptoms that the patient associates with the eyes, such as headaches or blurred vision. Occasionally, ocular signs present that may suggest the presence of a potentially life-threatening condition such as a space-occupying lesion in the brain, severe hypertension, or carotid artery disease. Many of these conditions can be detected by carefully listening to the patient's symptoms and the use of the problem-specific procedures described on the following pages. The patient is then referred to the appropriate provider in a timely manner.

The procedures included in this chapter are generally not considered part of the core ocular examination. Rather they are problem-specific tests that are employed when indicated by the patient's symptoms, case history, or abnormal test results noted during other procedures. Most of the techniques in this chapter will be used more frequently in examining elderly patients because they are at higher risk for many systemic diseases. Practitioners with a predominantly elderly patient population may choose to include some of these techniques in their core examination. Blood pressure measurement is sometimes performed routinely as an initial screening procedure, especially in offices that utilize ancillary personnel. All of these techniques may be used with any age group, when indicated.

Throughout this section, reference is made to universal health precautions whenever the examiner touches the patient. These standards are essential in the prevention of the spread of infection. Vigorous hand-washing with soap and water or a germicidal hand-washing solution is appropriate before and after every patient encounter. Disposable surgical gloves may also be used but should not substitute for hand-washing.

Blood Pressure Evaluation (Sphygmomanometry)

PURPOSE   To determine the pressure in the arteries at the height of ventricular contraction (systolic pressure) and ventricular relaxation (diastolic pressure).

EQUIPMENT

- Stethoscope with a two-sided head (bell and diaphragm).
- Blood pressure cuff with an aneroid or mercury column manometer. It is best to have a pediatric, adult, and large adult size cuff available.

SET-UP

- The patient is placed in a quiet setting for at least 5 minutes.
- The patient should not have consumed any caffeine-containing products, exercised, or smoked within 30 minutes before a reading is taken.
- The patient is seated with his arm free of clothing. The arm should be flexed and rest with the palm upward on the arm of a chair or table. Be sure that a rolled-up sleeve does not excessively constrict the upper arm.
- The examiner uses universal health precautions before touching the patient.
- The examiner is seated in front of or to the side of the arm being tested.

STEP-BY-STEP PROCEDURE

1. Inform the patient that you will be checking his blood pressure by wrapping a cuff around his arm and inflating the cuff with air. Advise the patient that he will feel pressure around his arm as you inflate the cuff, but that he should not experience any pain.
2. Palpate the patient's right brachial artery by placing your index and middle finger just below the bend of the elbow (antecubital crease) (see Figure 7–1).
3. Center the bladder of the cuff (indicated by an arrow or other marking on the cuff) on the patient's upper right arm overlying the brachial artery.

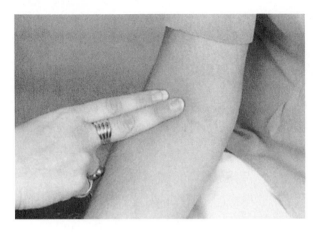

Figure 7–1. Examiner palpating the patient's brachial arterial pulse.

4. Adjust the cuff so that its lower edge is about 1 inch above the antecubital crease.
5. Secure the cuff at this location and determine that it is snug. The examiner should be able to slip only one finger between the patient's arm and the cuff edge (see Figure 7–2). If more of a gap is present, the cuff is too loose. If less of a gap is present, the cuff is too tight.
6. Determine the palpable systolic pressure to avoid discrepancies produced by an auscultatory gap:
   a. Use the index and middle finger on one of your hands to gently palpate the radial pulse on the patient's right wrist closest to the side of his thumb.
   b. Lock the air valve and inflate the cuff to 30 mm Hg above the level at which the radial pulse disappears.
   c. Unlock the air valve, then smoothly and slowly (2 to 3 mm Hg/sec) release the air from the cuff until the radial pulse is felt again. Make a mental note of the manometer reading when the pulse reappears. Deflate the cuff completely.
7. Position the earpieces of the stethoscope in your ears so they are comfortable.
8. Place the stethoscope head, with the diaphragm "clicked" into place, so that it gently rests over the brachial artery between the antecubital crease and the lower edge of the cuff (see Figure 7–3).
9. Lock the air valve and inflate the cuff 20 to 30 mm Hg above the palpated systolic pressure value determined in step 6c.
10. Unlock the air valve. Smoothly and slowly (2 to 3 mm Hg/sec) release the air from the cuff, listening for the Korotkoff sounds (see Table 7–1). Make a mental note of the manometer reading when phase I sounds oc-

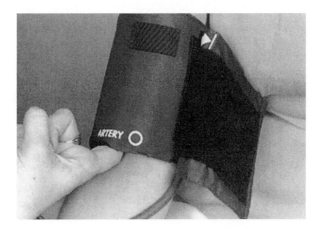

Figure 7–2. Examiner checking the fit of the blood pressure cuff.

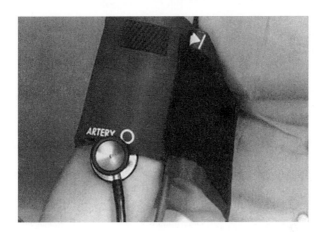

Figure 7–3. Proper positioning of the cuff and stethoscope head.

cur. Continue to slowly release air from the cuff and note the manometer reading when the phase V sounds occur.

11. Listen for an additional 10 to 20 mm Hg to confirm that all sounds have disappeared. Then completely deflate the cuff.
12. Repeat steps 2 to 11 on the left arm.

RECORDING

Record the following:

- Systolic pressure/diastolic pressure: recorded to the nearest whole number.
- Right arm or left arm.

TABLE 7–1. THE KOROTKOFF SOUNDS

- Phase I: The sudden appearance of regular tapping sounds—indicates the systolic pressure reading
- Phase II: A swishing, softening of sounds
- Phase III: Crisper sounds, increasing in intensity
- Phase IV: An abrupt muffling of sounds (diastolic pressure I)
- Phase V: The complete cessation of sounds (diastolic pressure II)—indicates the diastolic pressure reading

- Posture: sitting, standing, or lying down.
- Time of the day.
- Cuff size—if other than regular size.

EXAMPLES

- 120/80, right arm, sitting, @ 1:30 PM, large adult cuff
- 110/70, left arm, sitting, @ 10:00 AM, pediatric cuff
- 150/95, left arm, sitting, @ 9:00 AM

EXPECTED FINDINGS

- See Table 7–2.
- Diurnal variations in blood pressure are normal. Blood pressure is usually highest in the mid-morning and lowest during sleep.
- A 5 to 10 mm Hg discrepancy between the two arms is considered normal. Differences of greater than 10 to 15 mm Hg are abnormal and could be indicative of

TABLE 7–2. INTERPRETING SPHYGMOMANOMETRY VALUES

Blood Pressure (mm Hg)	Classification	Management Strategy
Diastolic Pressure		
<80	Normal	Recheck in 1 year
80–89	Pre-hypertension	Confirm within 2 months
90–99	Stage 1 hypertension	Confirm or refer within 1 month
≥100	Stage 2 hypertension	Immediate referral
Systolic Pressure		
<120	Normal	Recheck within 1 year
120–139	Pre-hypertension	Confirm within 2 months
140–159	Stage 1 hypertension	Confirm or refer within 1 month
≥160	Stage 2 hypertension	Immediate referral

Modified from the 2003 report of the Joint National Committee on Prevention, Detection, Evaluation, and Treatment of High Blood Pressure. *JAMA*, 2003; 289:2560–2571.

atherosclerotic narrowing of the subclavian or brachiocephalic arteries or part of subclavian steal syndrome.

- False low blood pressure readings may occur as the result of:
  1. The blood pressure cuff being too wide.
  2. The patient's arm being above heart level.
  3. Deflating the cuff too rapidly (affects the systolic reading).
  4. An auscultatory gap.
- False high blood pressure readings may occur as the result of:
  1. Patient anxiety or fear ("white coat syndrome").
  2. The blood pressure cuff being too loose or narrow.
  3. Deflating the cuff too slowly (affects the diastolic reading).
  4. The patient's arm being below heart level.
  5. Very rigid, calcified arteries, as seen in the elderly.

Carotid Artery Evaluation

PURPOSE   To assess the carotid arterial system for occlusive vascular disease.

INDICATIONS

This evaluation is indicated for any patient who presents with signs or symptoms of atherosclerotic plaque formation within the cerebrovascular arterial system.

EQUIPMENT

• Stethoscope with two-sided head (bell and diaphragm).

SET-UP

• The patient sits comfortably in front of the examiner.
• The patient should be relaxed and the room should be quiet.

STEP-BY-STEP PROCEDURE

PALPATION OF THE CAROTID PULSES

1. Perform a gross inspection of the patient's neck looking for any significant prominent pulsations.
2. Inform the patient that you will be placing your fingers on his neck to check his pulse.
3. To palpate the patient's right carotid pulse:
   a. Stand to the right of the patient and instruct the patient to turn his head to the left and tilt his chin slightly upward.
   b. Using the tips of the index and middle finger of your right hand, gently palpate the patient's neck in the groove located lateral to the trachea and medial to the sternocleidomastoid muscle, feeling for the pulse of the right common carotid artery (see Figure 7–4).
   c. Feel the pulse for 10 to 15 seconds, noting its amplitude, any variations of the beat, or variations with respiration.
4. To palpate the patient's left carotid pulse, repeat step 3, only this time stand to the left of the patient. Instruct the patient to turn his head to the

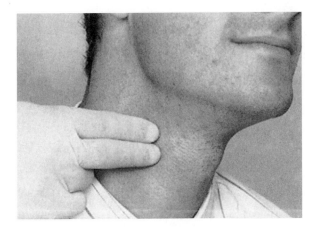

Figure 7–4. Examiner palpating the right carotid pulse.

right and tilt his chin slightly upward. Use the tips of the index and middle finger of your left hand to gently palpate for the pulse of the left common carotid artery.

Note:

- Do not apply excess pressure on the carotid artery during palpation.
- Never palpate the right and left carotid arteries at the same time. Excessive carotid massage can cause slowing of the pulse or a drop in blood pressure.

Auscultation of the Carotid Arteries

1. Inform the patient that you will be placing a stethoscope on his neck to check the circulation through the blood vessels.
2. Be sure the room is quiet.
3. To auscultate the patient's right carotid artery stand to the right of the patient. Instruct the patient to turn his head to the left and tilt his chin slightly upward.
4. Turn the head of the stethoscope so that the bell is "clicked" into position.
5. Place the bell of the stethoscope at the base of the patient's neck approximately 1 inch above the clavicle. This position allows you to listen to the common carotid area (see Figure 7–5).
6. Instruct the patient to hold his breath and listen for the presence of vascular turbulence (a bruit), described as a "whooshing" sound.
7. Instruct the patient to exhale. Reposition the bell of the stethoscope further up the neck. This position allows you to listen to the carotid bifurcation area. Repeat step 6.

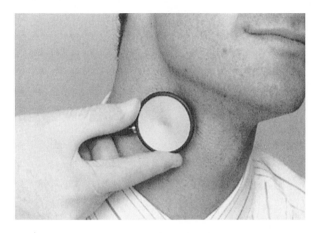

Figure 7–5. Examiner auscultating the right carotid artery.

8. Instruct the patient to exhale. Reposition the bell of the stethoscope further up the neck at the angle of the jaw. This position allows you to listen to the internal carotid artery. Repeat step 6.
9. To auscultate the patient's left carotid artery stand to the left of the patient. Instruct the patient to turn his head to the right and tilt his chin slightly upward.
10. Repeat steps 5 to 8 on the left carotid artery.

RECORDING

- Palpation of the carotid pulses
  1. Grade the pulse amplitude
     0 = no palpable pulse
     1+ = detectable but faint pulse
     2+ = stronger pulse, but slightly decreased intensity
     3+ = normal pulse
     4+ = bounding pulse
  2. Evaluate the symmetry between the right and left sides.
- Auscultation of the carotid arteries
  1. Note the presence or absence of a bruit on the right and left side.
  2. If a bruit is present, describe it:
     a. Soft, early systolic bruit: results from an artery that is occluded by 50%.
     b. Systolic and early diastolic bruit: results from an artery occluded by 70% to 80%.

EXAMPLES

- Palpation of carotid pulses: R: 3+ L: 3+
  Auscultation of carotid arteries: R: no bruits L: no bruits
- Palpation of carotid pulses: R: 2+ L: 1+
  Auscultation of carotid arteries: R: no bruits L: soft systolic bruit

EXPECTED FINDINGS

- Normal
  Palpation of carotid pulses: 2+ to 3+ pulses without asymmetry
  Auscultation of carotid arteries: no bruits on the right or left sides.
- Abnormal
  Palpation of carotid pulses: decreased pulse amplitudes or asymmetry
  Auscultation of carotid arteries: the presence of a bruit.
  Note:
- Not all carotid bruits are due to atherosclerotic occlusion. Some may be the result of:
  a. transmitted murmurs from valvular aortic stenosis, severe aortic regurgitation, or a damaged mitral valve.
  b. vigorous left ventricular ejection (more common in children).
- The absence of a bruit does not rule out atherosclerotic plaque formation because a totally occluded artery will not have an associated bruit.

Orbital Auscultation

PURPOSE   To aid in the differential diagnosis of orbital congestion.

EQUIPMENT

• Stethoscope with a two-sided head (bell and diaphragm).

SET-UP

• The patient sits comfortably in front of the examiner.
• The patient should be relaxed and the room should be quiet.

STEP-BY-STEP PROCEDURE

1. Inform the patient that you will be placing your stethoscope over his closed eyes and on his head to listen for any abnormal sounds. Tell the patient that he should experience no pain or discomfort.
2. To evaluate the patient's right orbit, stand or sit on the patient's right side.
3. Turn the head of the stethoscope so that the bell is "clicked" into position.
4. Ask the patient to close his eyes and hold his breath. The patient is told not to move his eyes under his closed eyelids, because these movements can be heard with the stethoscope.
5. Gently place the bell of the stethoscope over the closed eyelid of the right eye (see Figure 7–6). Listen carefully (10 to 15 seconds) for a "whooshing" sound (orbital bruit) synchronous with the heartbeat. Instruct the patient to exhale.
6. Reposition the bell of the stethoscope and listen for a bruit above the bridge of the nose (mid-line), above the right brow, and over the right temple (see Figures 7–7, 7–8, and 7–9). Instruct the patient to hold his breath while you are listening over each anatomical site.
7. Stand or sit on the patient's left side and repeat steps 3 to 6 on the left orbit.
   Note: Use extreme caution when examining a patient who has an eye that has suffered blunt trauma or recent intraocular surgery.

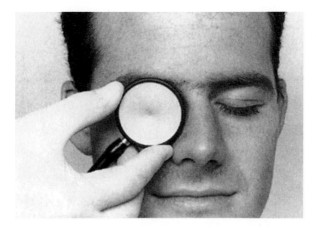

Figure 7–6. Examiner auscultating for bruits over the closed eye.

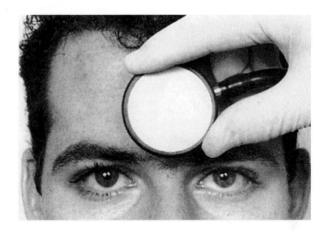

Figure 7–7. Examiner auscultating for bruits at the mid-line position.

RECORDING

• Note the presence or absence of a bruit in the right or left orbit.

EXAMPLES

• R-orbit: no bruits
  L-orbit: no bruits
• R-orbit: bruit present, best heard over the right temple
  L-orbit: no bruit

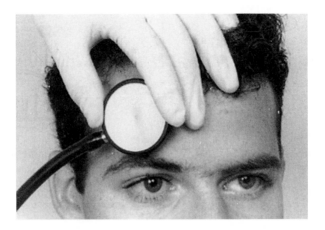

Figure 7–8. Examiner auscultating for bruits above the brow.

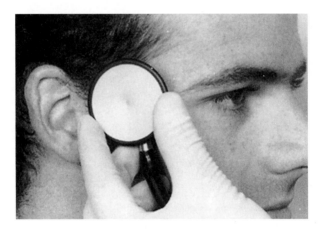

Figure 7–9. Examiner auscultating for bruits over the right temple.

EXPECTED FINDINGS

- *Normal:* No bruits present.
- *Abnormal:* bruit present.
- Unilateral orbital bruits may result from:
    1. Carotid cavernous fistulas: congenital, traumatic, or atherosclerotic.
    2. Arteriovenous (AV) malformations.
    3. Thrombosis of the ipsilateral internal carotid artery (ICA).
    4. Atherosclerotic or mechanical narrowing of the ICA.
- Bilateral orbital bruits may result from anemias or hyperthyroidism.
- The presence of a carotid bruit and a simultaneous orbital bruit is indicative of a significant atheromatous lesion at the carotid bifurcation.

Lymph Node Evaluation

PURPOSE   To determine the presence of lymphadenopathy, providing information about the differential diagnosis of a red eye.

EQUIPMENT

• No specific equipment is called for.

SET-UP

• The patient sits comfortably in a chair with his chin slightly elevated, facing the examiner.
• The examiner sits or stands in front of the patient.
• The examiner uses universal health precautions before touching the patient.

STEP-BY-STEP PROCEDURE

Palpating the Preauricular Lymph Nodes

1. Place your hands on the patient's face so that the index and middle fingers of each hand are positioned in front of the patient's external ear.
2. Applying minimal pressure, locate the bony structures of the temporomandibular joint (TMJ).
3. Slowly move your fingers in a circular motion to slide the patient's skin over the overlying bony structures. Search for a depression of the joint (normal) or an elevated nodular lesion (swollen lymph node indicating lymphadenopathy) (see Figure 7–10). A swollen preauricular node will feel like a pebble or bean under the patient's skin.
4. Compare the right and left sides noting the presence or absence of palpable nodes. If a swollen node is present, note its size, whether or not it is mobile, and if there is warmth overlying or surrounding the node. Ask the patient if the area is tender when touched.

Palpating the Cervical, Submaxillary, and Submental Lymph Nodes

1. Place the fleshy tips of your index, middle, and ring fingers of each hand on the patient's neck.

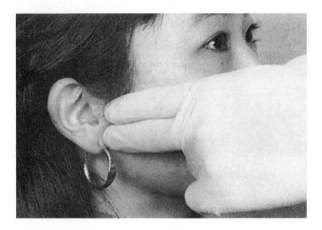

Figure 7–10. Examiner palpating the preauricular nodes.

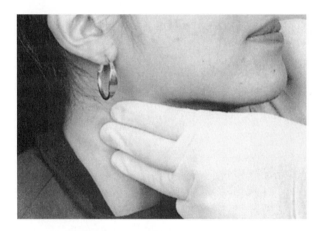

Figure 7–11. Examiner palpating the cervical nodes.

2. To palpate the cervical nodes, begin at the angle of the jaw. Gently rotate the patient's skin between your fingers and the underlying sternocleidomastoid muscle. Slowly move your fingers down, continuing to palpate, following the sternocleidomastoid muscle to the base of the neck (see Figure 7–11).
3. Compare the right and left sides, noting the presence or absence of palpable nodes. If a swollen node is present, note its size, whether or not it is mobile, and if there is warmth overlying or surrounding the node. Ask the patient if the area is tender when touched.
4. To palpate the submaxillary nodes, place your finger tips along (but under) the edge of the jaw bone, and massage the patient's skin between your fingers and the underlying tissue (see Figure 7–12).

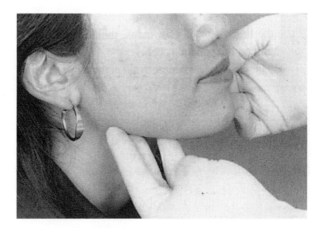

Figure 7–12. Examiner palpating the submaxillary nodes.

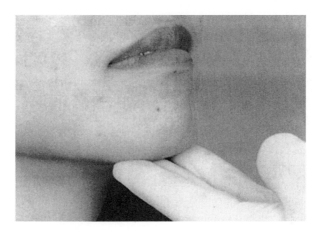

Figure 7–13. Examiner palpating the submental nodes.

5. To palpate the submental lymph nodes, place your finger tips under the tip of the chin and massage the patient's skin between the fingers and the underlying tissue (see Figure 7–13).
6. If a swollen node is present, note its size, whether or not it is mobile, and if there is warmth overlying or surrounding the node. Ask the patient if the area is tender when touched.

RECORDING

- Record if nodes are palpable (positive finding) or not (negative finding).
- If nodes are palpable characterize them by:

Laterality: unilateral or bilateral
Tenderness: tender or nontender
Mobility: mobile or nonmobile
Size: small or large
Warmth: presence or absence

EXAMPLES

- No palpable preauricular, cervical, submaxillary, or submental lymph nodes.
- Positive right preauricular node. Approximately 1 cm in size, mobile, tender, with no overlying warmth. No palpable cervical, submaxillary, or submental lymph nodes.

EXPECTED FINDINGS

- *Normal:* No palpable lymph nodes.
- *Abnormal:* Palpable lymph nodes (lymphadenopathy) are commonly seen in the following conditions:
  1. Viral conjunctivitis: preauricular lymphadenopathy often greater on the side of the more involved eye.
  2. Severe bacterial lid conditions such as preseptal cellulitis or infection in the medial canthal region: preauricular or submental lymphadenopathy.
  3. Parinaud's oculoglandular conjunctivitis: preauricular lymphadenopathy.
  4. Following the resolution of an ocular infection.
  5. Upper respiratory infection: cervical and submaxillary lymphadenopathy.

Paranasal Sinus Evaluation

PURPOSE   To aid in the diagnosis of acute frontal or maxillary sinusitis.

INDICATIONS

Indicated when the patient presents with pressure or pain in or behind one or both eyes.

EQUIPMENT

- Transilluminator.

SET-UP

- The patient sits comfortably in front of the examiner.
- The examiner sits comfortably in front of the patient.
- The examiner uses universal health precautions before touching the patient.

STEP-BY-STEP PROCEDURE

Palpation of the Frontal and Maxillary Sinuses

1. Instruct the patient to look straight ahead and inform him that you will be touching his brow and cheek to examine his sinuses for swelling.
2. To palpate the patient's frontal sinus, use your thumb to gently press upward under the bony brow on each side of the patient's nose. Use your left thumb on the patient's right brow and your right thumb on the patient's left brow (see Figure 7–14).
3. To palpate the patient's maxillary sinus, use your thumb to gently press upward along the zygomatic processes (the patient's cheek bones) (see Figure 7–15).
4. Note any swelling over the soft tissue. Ask the patient to report any tenderness as the area is touched.

Percussion of the Frontal and Maxillary Sinuses

1. Inform the patient that you will be tapping his brow and cheek with your finger. Ask the patient to report any pain or discomfort during the procedure.

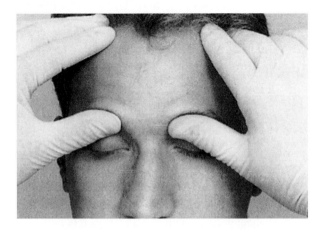

Figure 7–14. Examiner palpating the frontal sinuses.

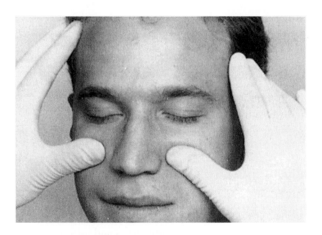

Figure 7–15. Examiner palpating the maxillary sinuses.

2. Perform percussion of the frontal sinuses:
   a. With the index or middle finger of your dominant hand, lightly tap directly over the patient's right brow, using your wrist to produce the force behind your finger (see Figure 7–16).
   b. Repeat step 2a over the patient's left brow.
   c. Note any swelling, tenderness, or pain over the sinuses.
3. Perform percussion of the maxillary sinuses:
   a. With the index or middle finger of your dominant hand, lightly tap directly over and along the patient's right cheek bone, using your wrist to produce the force behind your finger (see Figure 7–17).

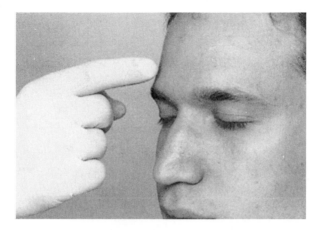

Figure 7–16. Examiner percussing the frontal sinuses.

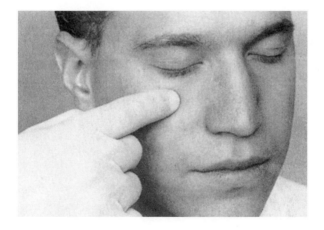

Figure 7–17. Examiner percussing the maxillary sinuses.

　　b. Repeat step 3a over the patient's left cheek bone.
　　c. Note any swelling, tenderness, or pain over the sinuses.

Transillumination of the Frontal and Maxillary Sinuses

1. Inform the patient that you will be looking at his sinuses with a bright light and that he should experience no discomfort.
2. Turn the transilluminator on to its highest rheostat setting.
3. Turn off all room illumination.
4. Perform transillumination of the frontal sinuses:
　　a. Place the tip of the transilluminator against the medial aspect of the patient's right supraorbital rim to assess the right frontal sinus (see Figure 7–18).

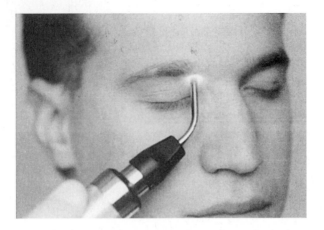

Figure 7–18. Examiner transilluminating the frontal sinus.

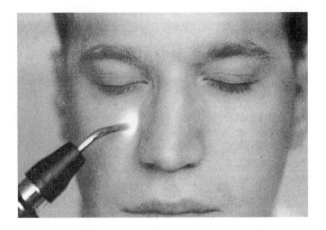

Figure 7–19. Examiner transilluminating the maxillary sinus.

    b. Look for a dim red glow as the light is transmitted just above the eyebrow.

    c. Repeat steps 4a and 4b on the patient's left frontal sinus.

  5. Perform transillumination of the maxillary sinuses:

    a. Place the tip of the transilluminator against the patient's skin just lateral to the nose and beneath the medial aspect of the patient's right eye (see Figure 7–19).

    b. Instruct the patient to open his mouth wide. Observe the roof of his open mouth for a dim red glow through the hard palate (see Figure 7–20).

    c. Repeat steps 5a and 5b on the patient's left maxillary sinus.

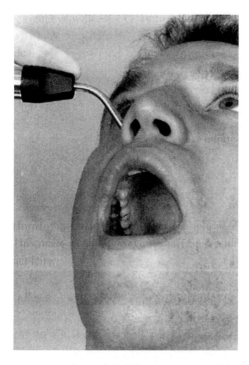

Figure 7–20. Examiner observes the hard palate through the patient's open mouth for the presence or absence of a dim glow when transilluminating the maxillary sinus.

RECORDING

- Palpation—record the presence or absence of swelling or tenderness.
- Percussion—record the presence or absence of swelling or tenderness.
- Transillumination—record your observation:
  normal = normal light transmission
  dull = reduced light transmission
  opaque = no light transmission
- Compare one side of the face to the other.

EXAMPLES

- Paranasal sinus evaluation: No swelling or tenderness with palpation or percussion. Normal frontal and maxillary sinus transillumination.
- Paranasal sinus evaluation: No swelling but tenderness experienced with palpation and percussion of the right and left maxillary sinus. Opaque transillumination of the right and left maxillary sinus.

EXPECTED FINDINGS

* Normal
Palpation and percussion: no swelling or tenderness.
Transillumination: normal.
* Abnormal
Palpation and percussion: swelling or tenderness may indicate infection or obstruction of sinus drainage.
Transillumination: dull or opaque. The absence of a dim glow indicates that the sinus is either filled with secretions or that the sinus never fully developed. Dull transillumination is a frequent finding that is unreliable in predicting whether a sinus is normal or diseased.
Note: The ethmoid or sphenoid sinuses cannot be assessed by transillumination. Transillumination also does not appear to be sensitive or specific for detecting mucosal thickening.

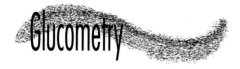

Glucometry

PURPOSE To determine the blood glucose level of a patient who may present with signs or symptoms of hypo- or hyperglycemia. This procedure is also helpful in the differential diagnosis of the patient with a shift in refractive error.

EQUIPMENT

- Glucose monitor (Glucometer).
- Test strips.
- Calibration device.
- Disposable lancets.
- Lancing device.
- Alcohol swabs.
- Disposable rubber gloves.
- Sharps container.
- Biohazard container.

SET-UP

- The patient sits comfortably in front of the examiner.
- The patient should be relaxed.
- The glucose monitor and test strips should be kept at room temperature.

STEP-BY-STEP PROCEDURE

1. Calibrate the monitor.
   a. Calibration is the process of programming the monitor for each new box of test strips.
   b. Follow the directions outlined in the owner's manual of your particular model of glucometer to calibrate the instrument.
   c. Be certain that all calibration devices and test strips are not past their labeled expiration dates.
2. Prepare the patient.
   a. Instruct the patient to wash his hands with soap and water or use an alcohol swab to clean his finger tip.

    b. Explain the purpose and procedure of the test to the patient to de-
crease any anxiety he may have.

3. Wash your hands with soap and water, thoroughly dry them, and then put on a pair of sterile rubber gloves.

4. Turn the glucometer on and insert a fresh test strip.

5. Wait for the monitor to prompt you to apply a sample of blood to the test strip.

6. Insert a sterile lancet into the lancing device and activate the spring-loaded tension device.

7. Place the lancing device firmly along the side of the patient's finger (see Figure 7–21)

8. Press the lancing device's release button, which will cause the lancet to penetrate the patient's skin surface.

9. You may massage the patient's finger tip to create a well-formed drop of blood.

10. Touch the drop of blood to the target area of the test strip (see Figure 7–22).

11. Once the target area is adequately covered with blood, the monitor will begin a countdown and then display a number.

12. Record the number in milligrams per deciliter (mg/dL) (see Figure 7–23).

13. Dispose of used lancets in a sharps container.

14. Dispose of used alcohol swabs, used test strips, and used rubber gloves in a biohazard container for appropriate removal.

15. Turn off the glucometer.

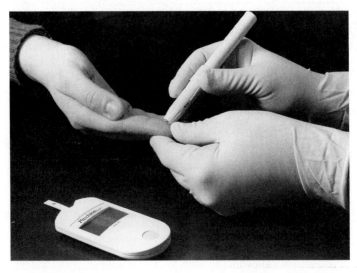

Figure 7–21. Examiner places the lancing device in position to acquire a sample of blood.

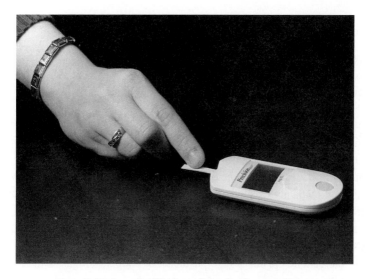

Figure 7–22. A sample of blood is applied to the glucometer test strip.

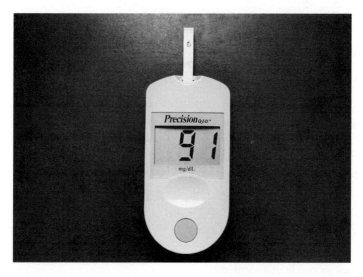

Figure 7–23. Digital readout showing results of glucometry, recorded in milligrams per deciliter (mg/dL).

RECORDING

- Glucometry (list brand of instrument).
- Record the number displayed in mg/dL.
- Date and time of sample.
- Time of last meal (if known).
- Any other comments.

EXAMPLES

- Glucometry (Precision QID): 100 mg/dL; 12/27/01 @ 4 PM.
- Glucometry (One-Touch II): 40 mg/dL; 12/28/01 @ 10 AM. 2 hr postprandial; patient light headed.

EXPECTED FINDINGS

- See Table 7–3.
- Findings vary depending on the time since last meal. Findings may also vary depending on medications used, the presence of blood dyscrasias, and grossly elevated triglycerides or cholesterol.
- Refer to the owner's manual of the instrument you are using for the normal ranges of that given instrument.
- Notify the patient's primary care physician or endocrinologist with any abnormal results.

TABLE 7–3. GUIDELINES FOR INTERPRETING GLUCOMETER RESULTS

Normal	
Fasting	70–130 mg/dL
Postprandial (1 hr)	100–180 mg/dL
Postprandial (2 hr)	80–150 mg/dL
Abnormal	
Hypoglycemia	<70 mg/dL
Hyperglycemia	>highest range for the above categories

TABLE 7–4. SYSTEMIC HEALTH SCREENING NORMS

- Blood pressure evaluation:<120/<80 (see Table 7–2)
- Carotid artery evaluation
    Palpation of the carotid pulses: 2+ to 3+ pulses without assymmetry
    Auscultation of the carotid arteries: No bruits
- Orbital auscultation: No bruits
- Lymph node evaluation: No palpable lymph nodes
- Paranasal sinus evaluation
    Palpation: No swelling or tenderness
    Percussion: No swelling or tenderness
    Transillumination: Normal
- Glucometry
    Fasting 70–130 mg/dl
    Postprandial (1 hr) 100–180 mg/dL
    Postprandial (2 hr) 80–150 mg/dl

CRANIAL NERVE SCREENING

Daniel Kurtz, OD, PhD

CHAPTER AT A GLANCE

INTRODUCTION TO CRANIAL NERVE SCREENING

Many patients with neurological problems seek the professional services of an optometrist because their condition produces symptoms that they associate with their eyes. Such symptoms include double vision, blurry vision, reduced peripheral vision, headaches, and dizziness.

Consequently, optometrists need to be able to detect neurological disease in their patients. Optometrists also need to be able to determine if their patient's condition warrants monitoring or treatment. If monitoring is called for, the optometrist must be confident that no harm will come to the patient while he waits and watches the patient over an extended period of time.

If treatment is required and falls within the scope of practice of the optometrist, he needs to refine his diagnosis in order to prescribe the appropriate therapy. If the treatment falls outside the optometrist's scope of practice, he needs to decide the type of specialist the patient will need to see and how soon therapy must begin. To make these decisions, the optometrist uses data about the neurological status of the patient. Such information is not gathered during the routine ocular examination, but is obtained by problem-specific testing.

A thorough exposition of the general neurological examination is beyond the scope of this text and can be found in other sources (see References for Chapter 8). This chapter is limited to problem-specific procedures for assessing the functions of the cranial nerves. Ocular or visual symptoms that are likely to motivate a patient to see an eye care specialist are likely to affect the functions of the cranial nerves. The reader should remember that many of the routinely performed entrance tests also assess the function of certain cranial nerves. In particular, tests of visual acuity, color vision, visual fields, and ophthalmoscopy test the optic nerve. The standard EOM testing, cover test, pupillary testing, and Maddox rod technique test the oculomotor, trochlear, and/or abducens nerves.

The techniques described here are easy to perform and use equipment and supplies that are readily available at the doctor's office.

CRANIAL NERVE SCREENING *at a glance*

EQUIPMENT	USE
Penlight	• Hirschberg test • Extraocular motilities (EOMs) • Pupils • Muscle field with red lens, ductions, and saccades • Test for a paretic horizontal muscle • Park's 3-step method
Occluder with red lens at one end	• Muscle field with red lens, ductions, and saccades • Test for a paretic horizontal muscle • Park's 3-step method
Direct ophthalmoscope	• Dim–bright pupillary test
Slit lamp biomicroscope	• Pupil cycle time
Distant fixation target	• Pupils • Dim–bright pupillary test • Accommodative response of the pupil
Pupil gauge	• Dim–bright pupillary test • Pharmacologic tests of the pupil
Small ruler marked in millimeters	• Dim–bright pupillary test • Facial nerve function test
Near accommodative target	• Accommodative response of the pupil

CRANIAL NERVE SCREENING *at a glance (cont.)*

EQUIPMENT	USE
Various pharmacologic agents	• Pharmacologic tests of the pupil
Two or three vials containing different aromatic substances	• Screening test for cranial nerve I
A ticking watch	• Screening test for cranial nerve VIII
Two sterile cotton-tipped applicators	• Trigeminal nerve function test • Facial nerve function test
Table salt	• Facial nerve function test
Glass of clean water	• Facial nerve function test
Equipment for a Schirmer #1 test	• Facial nerve function test
Piece of lint-free tissue	• Trigeminal nerve function test
Safety pin	• Trigeminal nerve function test
Standard alcohol preparation pad	• Test the olfactory nerve (CN I)

Muscle Field With Red Lens, Ductions, and Saccades

PURPOSE   To determine if the patient has a comitant or an incomitant deviation. To obtain additional diagnostic information about the function of his extraocular muscles.

INDICATIONS

Indicated if the patient experiences diplopia or the examiner detects a misalignment of the eyes at any point during ocular motility testing.

EQUIPMENT

- Penlight.
- Occluder with red lens at one end.

SET-UP

- The patient removes his spectacles and covers his right eye with the red lens.
- The examiner holds the penlight.

STEP-BY-STEP PROCEDURE

1. Perform steps 1 through 4 of the extraocular motilities procedure (see Chapter 2). Modify the instructions as follows: tell the patient not only to tell you when he sees two lights, one of which will be white and the other red, but also to report where the lights are located relative to one another. Ask him to report if the lights stay about the same distance apart in all positions or if they get closer or further apart in different directions of gaze. This is known as *comitancy testing*.
2. Based on the patient's responses, note if the diplopia is horizontal (red and white lights are always side by side) or if there is a vertical component to the deviation (red and white lights are not on the same horizontal level).

Note: Many vertical deviations contain a horizontal component as well, but they are nevertheless classified as vertical deviations.

3. Remove the red lens and occlude the patient's left eye. Have the patient follow the light with his open eye without moving his head. Test all nine positions of gaze (see Figure 2–7), observing whether or not the eye can follow the light extensively to all nine locations.

4. Repeat step 3 with the right eye occluded and the left eye open.
   Note: Steps 3 and 4 test ductions for each eye.

5. If the patient's ocular deviation is incomitant, identify the paretic muscle or muscles as follows. If the deviation is purely horizontal, perform the *test for a paretic horizontal muscle*. If the deviation has a vertical component, perform *Park's 3-step method*.

6. Test for voluntary saccades by having the patient look from position 1 to position 6 and back to position 1 of Figure 2–7. Repeat for rapid shifts of gaze between positions 1 and 2, 1 and 5, and 1 and 8.
   Note: Step 1 of muscle field testing (comitancy testing) can also be done with the cover test procedure, rather than with a red lens and a penlight, by performing the cover test in the nine positions of gaze shown in Figure 2–7.

RECORDING

- If the patient's ocular deviation is the same size in all directions of gaze, record "comitant deviation" and indicate the direction of deviation.
- If the deviation is *incomitant* (is not the same size in all directions of gaze), indicate the directions of gaze that have the greatest deviation and the smallest deviation. Then record as instructed in the procedures for identifying the paretic muscle(s).
- If only one eye is abnormal, be sure to identify it.

EXAMPLES

- Comitant deviation: exo in all positions
- Diplopia on up right gaze, OD lagging. Fusion in other positions.
- Diplopia in all positions, greatest on up left gaze, least on down right gaze.
- Fusion in some positions, diplopia in others (see Figure 8–1).

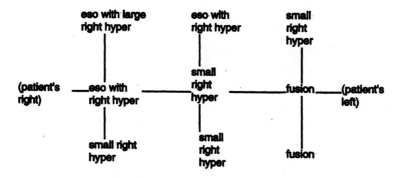

Figure 8–1. Example of a diagram used to record the results of muscle field testing.

Test for a Paretic Horizontal Muscle

PURPOSE To identify the paretic muscle in a purely horizontal incomitant deviation. This is a continuation of the muscle field with red lens test and
uses the same equipment and set-up.

STEP-BY-STEP PROCEDURE

1. Determine the direction of deviation. If the patient experiences crossed
   diplopia, he has an exo deviation. If he experiences uncrossed diplopia he
   has an eso deviation.
2. Instruct the patient to follow the light to the left and to the right. Determine if the deviation is greater on left gaze or on right gaze. If this is difficult to determine, ask the patient when the separation between the two
   lights is greatest.
3. Trace through the flowchart in Figure 8–2 to identify the paretic muscle.

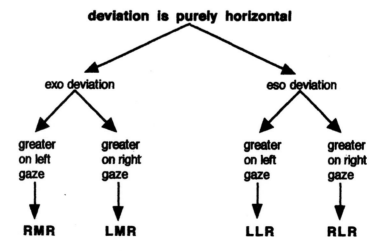

Figure 8–2. Flowchart for identifying the paretic muscle in cases of horizontal incomitant deviations.

RECORDING

- Record the type of deviation (eso or exo) and the direction of gaze in which the deviation is greater.
- Record the identity of the paretic muscle.

EXAMPLE

Eso deviation > on left gaze: paretic LLR.

Park's 3-Step Method

PURPOSE To identify the paretic muscle in an incomitant deviation with a vertical component. This is a continuation of the muscle field with red lens test and uses the same equipment and set-up.

STEP-BY-STEP PROCEDURE

1. Determine which is the hyperdeviated eye. The target seen by the hyperdeviated eye will appear lower than the image seen by the other eye.
2. Instruct the patient to follow the light to the left and to the right without moving his head. Determine if the deviation is greater on left gaze or on right gaze. If this is difficult to determine, ask the patient when the separation between the two lights is greatest.
3. With the patient looking straight ahead at the light, determine if the deviation is greater on tilting the head toward the left or toward the right shoulder.
4. Trace through the flowchart (Figure 8–3) to identify the paretic muscle.

RECORDING

- Write "Park's 3-step" followed by the identity of any paretic muscle or muscles.

EXAMPLES

- Park's 3-step: paretic LIO
- Park's 3-step: paretic RSO

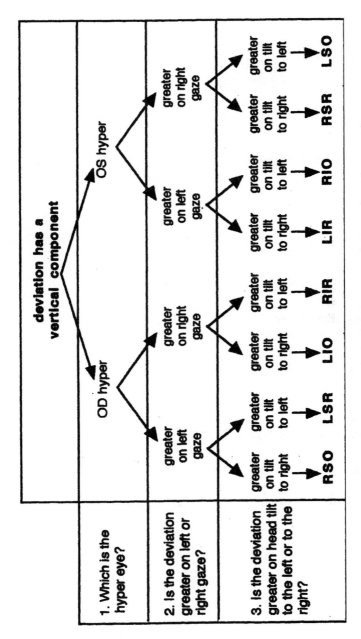

1. Which is the hyper eye?	OD hyper				OS hyper			
2. Is the deviation greater on left or right gaze?	greater on left gaze		greater on right gaze		greater on left gaze		greater on right gaze	
3. Is the deviation greater on head tilt to the left or to the right?	greater on tilt to right	greater on tilt to left	greater on tilt to right	greater on tilt to left	greater on tilt to right	greater on tilt to left	greater on tilt to right	greater on tilt to left
	RSO	**LSR**	**LIO**	**RIR**	**LIR**	**RIO**	**RSR**	**LSO**

deviation has a vertical component

Figure 8–3. Flowchart for Park's 3-step method for identifying the paretic muscle in cases of vertical incomitant deviations.

433

Dim–Bright Pupillary Test

PURPOSE To provide additional diagnostic information about the efferent neurological pathways responsible for pupillary and eyelid function.

INDICATIONS

Indicated when the pupils appear to be unequal in size during the pupillary entrance tests.

EQUIPMENT

- Direct ophthalmoscope.
- Distance fixation target (e.g., projected 20/400 E).
- Pupil gauge.
- Small ruler marked in millimeters (PD ruler).

SET-UP

- Position yourself directly in front of the patient and slightly below his line of sight.
- Darken the room completely so that the only available light is that reflected from the fixation target.
- Turn on the ophthalmoscope to full intensity and set it to the largest available beam. Set the ophthalmoscope to +1.0.

STEP-BY-STEP PROCEDURE

1. Instruct the patient to look at the distant target and not at you or your light.
2. From a distance of about 1 m, shine the ophthalmoscope beam onto the patient's face so that both pupils are illuminated at the same time. Look through the aperture of the ophthalmoscope at the patient's pupils. Within each pupil you will see orange-red reflexes due to the reflection of light from the patient's retina. Observing these red pupillary reflexes will enhance your ability to detect small differences in the sizes of the pupils.

3. Observe the relative diameter of each pupil, noting which eye has the larger pupil and estimating the amount of the difference in millimeters. This is the "bright" condition.

4. Gradually reduce the illumination level of the ophthalmoscope while observing the red reflexes and comparing the sizes of the pupils. Continue to reduce the illumination until the red reflexes are barely visible.

5. Observe the diameter of each pupil, estimating the amount of the difference in millimeters. This is the "dim" condition.

6. Repeat steps 2 through 5 one or two times to confirm your observations. Note also the dynamic rates of changes of the pupils to see if they dilate and constrict in unison or if one pupil responds more briskly than the other.

7. If no difference in anisocoria is observed, end the test and record "anisocoria equal in dim or bright." If a difference in anisocoria is detected, the amount of anisocoria is quantified as follows:

   a. Decrease the room illumination until you are just able to see the pupils with your unaided eyes. Using the pupil gauge, measure the diameter of each pupil. The difference in diameter is the amount of anisocoria in dim illumination.

   b. Increase the room illumination to its maximum amount. Using the pupil gauge, measure the diameter of each pupil. The difference in diameter is the amount of anisocoria in bright illumination.

8. With the patient looking straight ahead at the fixation target, use the PD ruler to measure the size of each palpebral aperture in millimeters. Note the position of the upper and the lower lid of each eye relative to the limbus and the cornea.

9. Instruct the patient to fixate on your finger and have him follow it gradually into up gaze. While he is doing this, compare the intersections of the lower lids with each limbus, noting which lid clears the limbus first or if they clear the limbus simultaneously. Once again, measure the size of the palpebral aperture in millimeters.

RECORDING

- Record the difference in pupillary diameters (amount of anisocoria) under bright conditions. You may also elect to record the sizes of each pupil.
- Record the difference in pupillary diameters (amount of anisocoria) under dim conditions. You may also elect to record the sizes of each pupil.
- If the difference in pupil diameters is the same under dim and bright conditions, record "anisocoria equal in dim and bright." Record the size of the difference in millimeters.
- Record the size of each palpebral aperture in millimeters in straight ahead gaze and in up gaze. If the apertures were equal, and both intersect the limbus in the

normal position approximately 2 mm below its top, record "no ptosis of the upper lid."

- If the lower lids cleared the limbus at the same time when the patient looked upward, record "no ptosis of lower lid." If one lid cleared the limbus sooner than the other, it indicates a ptosis of the more elevated lower lid. Record "ptosis of the lower lid" and indicate the eye whose lid cleared second.

EXAMPLES

- Pupils: OD > OS by 0.5 mm in dim and bright, no ptosis of upper or lower lid. Palp. aper: 9 mm OD & OS
- Pupils: in bright OD = 3.5 mm, OS = 3.0 mm/in dim OD = 7.0 mm, OS = 4.5 mm / + ptosis upper and lower lids OS

EXPECTED FINDINGS

- Anisocoria of equal amounts under dim and bright conditions and in the absence of ptosis characterizes physiological (also known as simple or essential) anisocoria. It can frequently be observed in old photographs of the patient (the FAI or "family album imaging" test).
- Anisocoria more pronounced under dim conditions, with a mild ptosis of the upper and lower lid in the eye with the smaller pupil, is characteristic of oculosympathetic paresis (Horner's syndrome).
- Anisocoria more pronounced under bright conditions is characteristic of dysfunction in the parasympathetic control of the pupil. If there is a ptosis in the eye with the larger pupil, a lesion of the oculomotor nerve (CN III) should be suspected.

Near (Accommodative) Response of the Pupil

PURPOSE To test the responsiveness of the pupil to near viewing (accommodation and convergence).

INDICATIONS

Indicated when the light response of either or both pupils is or is suspected of being sluggish.

EQUIPMENT

- Distance fixation target (e.g., 20/400 E).
- Near accommodative target (containing fine visual detail).

STEP-BY-STEP PROCEDURE

1. Tell the patient to maintain distance fixation while you hold up a target containing fine visual detail at 10 to 40 cm from the patient. If the patient is myopic, it is necessary to hold the target close to his eyes, preferably well within his far point, to stimulate accommodation.
2. Instruct the patient to look at the near target. The examiner should look for pupillary constriction. This is known as the *near* or *accommodative response* of the pupil.
3. Instruct the patient to return his gaze to the distance target. The examiner looks for dilation of the pupil to confirm that it had constricted during near viewing.
4. Repeat steps 1 to 3 if necessary to confirm your observations.
5. Compare the magnitude and briskness of the near response to the magnitude and briskness of the light response of the pupils.

RECORDING

- If all pupillary functions are within normal limits, add the letter "A" after the "PERRL" when recording the results of pupillary testing.
- If the abbreviation "PERRL" does not apply to your patient, write "pupils constrict to near" or "pupils unresponsive to near," or "near response brisker than light response," whichever applies.

EXAMPLES

- PERRLA no APD
- OD unresponsive to light direct or consensual; both pupils constrict to near; OS responds to light D & C.

Pupil Cycle Time

PURPOSE   To assess the conduction velocity of the optic nerve–pupillary light response reflex arc by observing the responsiveness of the pupil to cyclical light stimulation

EQUIPMENT

- Distance fixation target (e.g., 20/400 E).
- Stop watch accurate to the second.
- Slit lamp biomicroscope, set to medium magnification and high intensity.

STEP-BY-STEP PROCEDURE

1. Tell the patient to maintain distance fixation on the distance target while you focus a horizontal 0.50-mm wide parallelepiped on the inferior iris adjacent to the pupil of the eye in question.
2. Start the stopwatch as you rapidly move the beam 1.0 mm into the pupillary opening. The pupil should constrict such that most or all of the incident beam is blocked from entering the pupil by the iris. Once the beam is blocked from the pupil due to pupillary contraction, it is expected that the pupil will redilate, readmitting the beam of light through the pupil, whereupon the pupil should constrict once again.
   One full cycle of the pupil is defined as a combination of one contraction combined with one redilation.
3. Measure the time it takes for 30 full cycles.
4. Calculate the mean cycle time by dividing the total elapsed time in seconds by 30.

RECORDING

- Write "pupil cycles" and the eye that was tested.

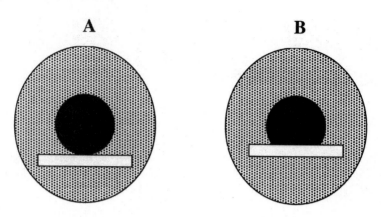

Figure 8–4. A. Placement of the slit beam at the set-up of pupil cycle time testing. **B.** Placement of the beam to begin stimulation of the pupillary response.

- Write down the mean cycle time in seconds, or write down the total elapsed time needed to complete 30 full cycles.

EXAMPLES

- Pupil cycles OD—32 sec for 30 cycles
- pupil cycles OD—0.9 sec/cycle
- pupil cycles OS—1.5 sec/cycle

EXPECTED FINDINGS

- A pupil cycle time of 1.1 sec/cycle or faster is considered a sign of health in the pupillary reflex arc. A pupil cycle time of slower than 1.1 sec/cycle suggests a reduced conduction time in the optic nerve of the affected eye.
- If both eyes are tested, their mean pupil cycle times should be within 0.1 sec/cycle of one another.

Pharmacological Tests of the Pupil

PURPOSES Topical pharmaceuticals play several roles in assessing the patient with anisocoria (unequal pupil sizes). They can help to distinguish pathological from nonpathological causes of anisocoria. In cases of pathological etiologies, they can help to localize the pathology within the postganglionic, preganglionic, or central compartments of the neurological circuitry for control of the pupillary responses.

INDICATIONS

Indicated when the patient has anisocoria but clinical signs do not clearly distinguish physiological from pathological etiologies or clinical signs do not clearly pinpoint the location of the pathology.

EQUIPMENT

- Slit lamp.
- Penlight or transilluminator.
- Pupil gauge.
- Time piece accurate to the minute.
- The particular pharmaceutical test agent to be used (see Table 8–1 below).
- Camera equipped to take close-up photographs of the face showing both eyes including the pupils, if available.

SET-UP

- Prior to instilling the test agent, perform and record a complete assessment of pupillary responses without pharmaceutical agents (see Pupils, Chapter 2, and Dim–Bright Pupillary Test, Chapter 8). Check for the presence of a ptosis and measure and record the widths of the palpebral apertures.
- Perform a thorough biomicroscopic examination of both eyes, paying particular attention to the cornea and iris.
- Make certain that neither eye is at risk for angle closure should the agent have the potential to cause pupillary dilation.
- If a camera is available, take a pretest baseline picture of the face showing the pupils of both eyes.

STEP-BY-STEP PROCEDURE

1. Seat the patient comfortably with head reclined.
2. Instill one drop of the test agent in each eye with as little interval as possible between medicating the two eyes (see Installation of Drops, Chapter 5). Record the time of instillation (see note 1 and 2).
3. Monitor the state of the pupils at the earliest interval indicated in Table 8–1, comparing the sizes of the pupils in the two eyes.
4. Continue comparing the responses and sizes of the pupils in the two eyes until a definitive difference in pupillary behavior is observed or until the longest time indicated in Table 8–1 has elapsed.
5. Use the Table 8–1 to assist in interpretation of the findings.

RECORDING

- Record the agent used and the time of its instillation.
- If a camera is available, take a picture of the face showing the pupils of both eyes at the end of the test.
- Record the final response of each pupil (e.g., full dilation, minimal dilation, miosis, depending on the agent used) and the time of observation.

EXAMPLES

- Instill cocaine 4% OD & OS 3:30 PM. dilation OD, no dilation OS 4:05 PM
- Instill Paredr. 1% 11:10 OD & OS. OD pupil = 7 mm, OS pupil = 4 to 5 mm, 11:40 AM

EXPECTED FINDINGS

See Table 8–1 for the response of a nonpathological pupil and the response of a compromised pupil, for each pharmaceutical test agent.

NOTES

1. Alexander, Skorin, and Bartlett recommend instillation of two drops of each test agent separated by a few minutes.
2. Instillation of test agent in both eyes is indicated except in cases of suspected bilateral pharmacological block; in such cases, place the test agent in only one eye.

TABLE 8–1. SUMMARY OF PHARMACOLOGIC TESTS OF THE PUPIL

Indication: Primary Purpose of the Test	Drug and Concentration	Check In (min)	Nonpathological Response	Response of Compromised Pupil	Mode of Action (Basis of Test)
To confirm or rule out oculosympathetic paresis (Horner's syndrome), regardless of the location of the pathology	Cocaine 4–10% (do nothing to disrupt corneal epithelium prior to test)	30–60	Dilation	Reduced dilation for all lesion locations: central, preganglionic, or postganglionic.	Blocks reuptake of norepinephrine.
To distinguish postganglionic from preganglionic or central locations of pathology in oculosympathetic paresis	Hydroxyamphetamine (Paredrine) 1.0%	40–60	Dilation	Reduced dilation if the lesion is postganglionic. Normal dilation if the lesion is preganglionic or central.	Directly stimulates the release of norepinephrine from nerve endings.
To distinguish postganglionic from preganglionic or central locations of pathology in oculosympathetic paresis	Epinephrine 0.1%	20–30	No dilation	Dilation if the lesion is postganglionic. Normal dilation if the lesion is preganglionic or central.	Denervation supersensitivity.
To distinguish postganglionic from preganglionic or central locations of pathology in oculosympathetic paresis	Phenylephrine 1.0%	30	Slight dilation	Dramatic dilation if the lesion is postganglionic. Slight dilation if the lesion is preganglionic or central.	Denervation supersensitivity.
To confirm or rule out Adie's tonic pupil	Pilocarpine 0.125 or 0.063%	30	No miosis	Miosis only if there is a postganglionic parasympathetic lesion, such as in Adie's pupil	Denervation supersensitivity.
To confirm or rule out pharmacologic block of the sphincter of the pupil	Pilocarpine 2.0 % or 4.0%	30–40	Miosis	No miosis if the cholinergic receptors of the sphincter are pharmacologically blocked.	Direct acting cholinergic agonist.

Trigeminal Nerve Function Test

To test the functional integrity of the trigeminal nerve, CN V.

EQUIPMENT

- Two sterile cotton-tipped applicators with a small amount of cotton pulled out to form a point.
- Piece of lint-free tissue.
- Safety pin.

SET-UP

- Have the patient seated and looking straight ahead initially. No other set-up is necessary.

STEP-BY-STEP PROCEDURE

1. Show the patient the lint-free tissue and say that this is what you will be using to touch him. Then have him close his eyes.
2. Instruct the patient to tell you when he feels you touch his face and to compare the strength of the touch on the left and right sides of his face.
3. Test the patient's light touch sensation with the tissue at each of the six locations diagrammed in Figure 8–5: the left and right forehead, the left and right cheek near the upper lip, and the left and right chin or lower lip. These locations allow sampling of areas innervated by each of the main branches of the trigeminal nerve. The points of touch should be symmetrical with respect to the midline of the patient's face.

   An alternative to step 3 is to simultaneously touch the face with equal pressure in two mirror image locations. Have the patient report if the touches are equal or if one is stronger than the other.
4. Drag the tip of the tissue across the patient's forehead from left to right and then from right to left. Instruct the patient to tell you if the sensations are approximately equal on both sides of his forehead or if he notices a change when the tissue moves from one side to the other.

   If you intend to conduct only a minimal, rapid test of trigeminal nerve

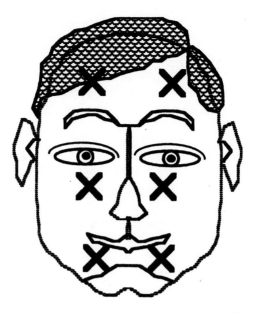

Figure 8–5. Diagram of points on the face to test when assessing trigeminal nerve function.

function, stop here and record your findings. If your patient requires a more thorough evaluation of the nerve, proceed to step 5.

5. Next tell the patient that you will be touching his face very gently with part of a safety pin. Ask him to report whether he has been touched with the "sharp" or the "dull" part of the pin.

6. Touch him with the sharp or dull part of the pin in approximately the same six locations as tested in step 3. Vary the order so the patient cannot easily predict which part of the pin you will use next. As in step 3, the tested points should be symmetrical with respect to the midline of the patient's face.

7. Pick up the cotton tipped applicators. Hold one in each hand. Use different applicators to test the two eyes.

8. Have the patient open his eyes and look up and to the left. Approach him in such a way that he cannot see your hand. Touch his right cornea near the limbus with the wisp of cotton at the end of the cotton-tipped applicator. Observe the strength of the reflex blink response in this eye.

9. Have the patient look up and to the right. Using the second cotton-tipped applicator, approach the patient in such a way that he cannot see your hand. Touch his left cornea near the limbus with the wisp of cotton at the end. Observe the strength of the reflex blink response in this eye. *Note:* During steps 8 and 9 be sure to avoid touching the eyelashes of either eye.

10. Compare the strength of the blink responses elicited by touching the right and the left corneas.
11. With both your hands, gently grab the patient's lower jaw. Instruct him to try to keep his mouth closed as you gently but firmly try to force it open. Compare the relative strength of both sides of the patient's jaw. Check carefully for a deviation of the jaw toward one side of the face.

RECORDING

- If all functions of the trigeminal nerve are normal and both sides of the face are equally sensitive and equally strong, record "trigeminal nerves intact" or "trigeminal nerves symmetrical."
- If the patient has reduced sensitivity to the tissue, record "fine touch reduced" and indicate the part of the face that is affected.
- If the patient has reduced sensitivity to the sharp part of the safety pin, record "pain sensation reduced" and indicate the part of the face that is affected.
- If the jaw muscles are equally strong, record "trigeminal motor division intact" or "motor divisions symmetrical." If one side of the jaw appears to be weaker than the other, indicate the weaker side.

EXAMPLES

- Trigeminal: sensory and motor divisions intact.
- Trigeminal: reduced light touch sensitivity upper left forehead. Other sensory divisions intact. Motor divisions symmetrical.
- Trigeminal nerve: reduced light touch and pain sensation in lower left jaw. Muscles weaker on left. Other divisions intact.

Facial Nerve Function Test

PURPOSE   To assess the functional integrity of the somatic motor, taste, and parasympathetic divisions of the facial nerve, CN VII, and its supranuclear control pathways.

EQUIPMENT

- Table salt and/or sugar.
- Glass of clean water.
- Two sterile cotton-tipped applicators with a small amount of cotton pulled out to form a point.
- Equipment for a Schirmer #1 test.
- Small ruler marked in millimeters.

SET-UP

- The patient should be seated upright in normal room illumination.

STEP-BY-STEP PROCEDURE

1. Carefully examine the patient's face, comparing the left and right sides, looking for asymmetries. In particular, look for a loss of facial wrinkles or of the nasolabial fold on one side of the face when the patient relaxes his facial muscles. Look separately for asymmetries in the upper and the lower face.
2. Place all four fingers of both your hands over the patient's eyebrows. As you pull down gently, instruct the patient to attempt to raise both eyebrows together. Compare the strength with which he can elevate his right and left eyebrows against the resistance of your fingers. Look for left versus right asymmetries in the amount of wrinkling of the skin of the forehead.
3. Instruct the patient to "knit his brow," or to pull his eyebrows together. Look for asymmetry in his ability to pull the left and right brow together.
4. Measure in millimeters the size of the palpebral apertures of each eye. Compare the pattern of folds in the upper lids of the two eyes.

5. Instruct the patient to close his eyes tightly. Look at the lids and lashes of both eyes. The base of the lashes should be hidden by lid tissue. Compare the left and right eyes.

6. Instruct the patient to close his eyes tightly while you attempt to pull his eyes open. Be careful to avoid applying pressure directly on either globe. Compare the ability of the right and left orbicularis oculi muscles to resist the forced opening of the eyes. Look for a Bell's phenomenon (upward and sometimes outward rolling of the eyes on attempted eyelid closure).

7. Instruct the patient to inflate or "blow out" both cheeks simultaneously. Instruct him to attempt to smile, then to frown. Finally, have the patient purse his lips or attempt to whistle. Look for asymmetries in the size and tightness of the left and right cheeks.

8. Measure the distance between each outer canthus and the ipsilateral corner of the mouth.

9. Instruct the patient to rinse out his mouth with clean water and stick out his tongue. Sprinkle a small quantity of salt on one side near the front of the tongue and have the patient report what he tastes. Have him rinse out his mouth again and sprinkle salt on the other side of the tongue. Instruct the patient to compare his taste sensation on the two presentations to the best of his ability.

   As an alternative, sprinkle salt and sugar on his tongue and ask him to identify what he is tasting.

10. Test the blink reflex by touching the right and then the left cornea near the limbus with a cotton wisp. Compare the blink response of the two eyes. This is the same as steps 7 to 9 for testing the trigeminal nerve.

11. Perform a Schirmer #1 test (see Chapter 5) to assess lacrimal gland functioning.

RECORDING

- If all CN VII functions are within normal limits, record "all facial muscles symmetrical, taste WNL," and record the results of the Schirmer #1 test per the instructions for that test.
- Describe any facial asymmetry or functional abnormality observed.

EXAMPLES

- All facial muscles symmetrical, taste WNL, Schirmer #1: >25 mm OD and OS in 5 min.
- Weakness of upper and lower muscles on left face; taste intact; Schirmer #1: >25 mm OD and 7 mm OS/5 min.

Screening Tests for Cranial Nerves I, VIII, XI, and XII

PURPOSE To test rapidly and superficially the functions of the cranial nerves not closely associated with ocular functions. The glossopharyngeal and vagus nerves are not included in this screening regimen because they are rarely compromised.

EQUIPMENT

- Two or three vials containing different aromatic substances such as coffee, vanilla, chocolate powder, soap, or oil of wintergreen, or standard 70% isopropyl alcohol preparation pad.
  Note: Avoid noxious chemicals.
- Optional: a ticking watch.

SET-UP

- The patient should be seated comfortably in the examination chair under bright illumination.
- The patient closes his eyes.

STEP-BY-STEP PROCEDURE

1. Test the olfactory nerve (CN I).
   a. Have the patient occlude his left nostril. Hold one of the vials containing an aromatic substance beneath his right nostril and have him inhale. Ask him if he smells anything. If he reports that he does, ask him to identify it.
   b. Have the patient occlude his right nostril. Hold another of the vials containing an aromatic substance beneath his left nostril and have him inhale. Ask him if he smells anything. If he reports that he does, ask him to identify it.

c. Ask the patient to report any differences he may have noticed in his sense of smell in the right and left nostril.

d. As an alternative, have the patient occlude his left nostril and hold the alcohol pad 30 cm from his nose. Gradually bring it toward the patient until he detects the odor and measure this distance. Repeat with the right nostril occluded.

2. Test the vestibulocochlear nerve (CN VIII).

a. Tell the patient that you will be making a sound on either side of his head near his ears. Instruct him to tell you when he first hears the sound and to point to the ear in which he hears it.

b. Hold your hand approximately 50 cm away from the patient's right ear and rub your index finger and thumb together gently to produce a soft sound. Slowly move your hand toward the patient's right ear until he reports that he hears the sound. Note the distance at which this takes place.

c. Repeat step 2b for the patient's left ear and compare the distance at which each ear first heard the fingers rubbing together.

d. Instruct the patient to hum. Ask him if his voice sounds louder in one ear or the other or if it sounds equally loud.

Note: A ticking watch can be used as an alternative to rubbing fingers.

3. Test the accessory nerve (CN XI).

a. Observe the relative height of the patient's shoulders.

b. Have the patient shrug both shoulders simultaneously. Compare the elevation of the left and right shoulder during the shrug.

c. Place both hands on the patient's shoulders and push down gently.

d. Have the patient shrug both shoulders and compare the force with which the left and right shoulders push against the resistance of your pressing them down.

4. Test the hypoglossal nerve (CN XII).

a. Instruct the patient to stick his tongue straight out.

b. Note whether the tongue lies straight along the patient's midline or if it deviates to one side or the other.

RECORDING

• For each nerve describe the patient's response to the test.

EXAMPLES

• CN I: correctly identified coffee and chocolate in left and right nostril
• CN VIII: heard fingers @ 35 cm right ear/@ 5 cm left ear. Hum sounded louder in right ear.
• CN XI: left shoulder lower than right/right shoulder elevates more during shrug

- CN XII: tongue protrudes on midline
- CN I: correctly identified coffee and chocolate in left nostril, barely able to smell in right nostril/failed to ID coffee or chocolate.
- CN VIII: heard fingers @ 35 cm right ear/@ 35 cm left ear. Hum sounded equal in both ears
- CN XI: shoulders at equal height during rest and during shrug
- CN XII: tongue protrudes to the left

TABLE 8–2. SUMMARY OF CRANIAL NERVE ASSESSMENT TESTS

Cranial Nerve Number	Name	Procedures That Assess the Functions of This Nerve
I	Olfactory	Screening tests*
II	Optic	Visual acuity (Snellen and LogMAR) Pinhole visual acuity Color vision Screening visual fields Finger counting visual fields Amsler grid Tangent screen Pupil cycle time
III	Oculomotor	Cover test Extraocular motilities (EOMs) Pupils Muscle field with red lens, ductions, and saccades Test for a paretic horizontal muscle Park's 3-step method Dim–bright pupillary test Pupil cycle time Pharmacological tests of the pupil
IV	Trochlear	Cover test EOMs Muscle field with red lens, ductions, and saccades Park's 3-step method
V	Trigeminal	Trigeminal nerve function test
VI	Abducens	Cover test EOMs Muscle field with red lens, ductions, and saccades Test for a paretic horizontal muscle
VII	Facial	Facial nerve function test Tear break-up time Schirmer tests
VIII, XI, and XII	Vestibulocochlear, accessory, hypoglossal	Screening tests*

*Screening tests for CNs I, VIII, XI, and XII are treated in one section.

Atchinson DA, Claydon CA, Irwin SE. Amplitude of accommodation for different head positions and different directions of eye gaze. *Optom Vis Sci.* 1994;71:339–345.

Daum K. Accommodative insufficiency. *Am J Optom Physiol Opt.* 1983;60:352–359.

Sun F, Stark L, Nguyen A, et al. Changes in accommodation with age: static and dynamic. *Am J Optom Physiol Opt.* 1988;65:492–498.

Color Vision

Adams A. Color vision testing in optometric practice. *J Am Optom Assoc.* 1974;45:35–42

Chen A, O'Leary DJ. Validity and repeatability of the modified push-up method for measuring the amplitude of accommodation. *Clin Exp Optom.* 1998;81:63–71.

Chioran G, Sheedy J. Pseudoisochromatic plate design—Macbeth or tungsten illumination? *Am J Optom Physiol Opt.* 1983;60:204–215.

Diez MA, Luque MJ, Capilla P, et al. Detection and assessment of color vision anomalies and deficiencies in children. *J Pediatr Ophthalmol Strab.* 2001;38;195–205.

Genco L. Fundamentals of color vision, part I. *Optom Monthly* 1978;69:959–963.

Genco L. Fundamentals of color vision, part II. *Optom Monthly.* 1978;69:1050–1054.

Graham BV. Mechanisms of color vision—A review. *J Am Optom Assoc.* 1974;45: 25–29.

Grosvenor T. The preliminary examination, Part II. Color vision testing. *Optom Weekly.* 1978; (Feb):149–155.

Ishihara S. *The Series of Plates Designed as a Test for Colour-Blindness Instructional Manual.* Tokyo: Kanehara, 1980.

Marlowe S. Federal color vision requirements. *J Am Optom Assoc.* 1974;45:78.

Rodgin S. Acquired color vision defects. *N Engl J Optom.* 1986;38:11–24.

Somerfield M, Long J, et al. Effects of viewing conditions on standard measures of acquired and congenital color defects. *Optom Vis Sci.* 1989;66:29–33.

Cover Test

Daum KM. Heterophoria and heterotropia. In Eskridge JB, Amos JF, Bartlett JD, eds. *Clinical Procedures in Optometry.* Philadelphia: Lippincott, 1991.

Eskridge J. The complete cover test. *J Am Optom Assoc.* 1973;44:602–609.

Newell FW. *Ophthalmology: Principles and Concepts.* 7th ed. St. Louis: Mosby Year Book, 1992.

Rainey BB, Schroeder TL, Goss DA, Grosvenor TP. Reliability of and comparisons among three variations of the alternating cover test. *Ophthalmol Physiol Optom.* 1998;18:430–437.

Scheiman M, Wick B. *Clinical Management of Binocular Vision: Heterophoric, Accommodative and Eye Movement Disorders.* Philadelphia: Lippincott, 1994.

Sheedy JE, Saladin JJ. Exophoria at near in presbyopia. *Am J Optom Physiol Opt.* 1975;52:474–481.

Sloan P. The cover test in clinical practice. *Am J Optom Arch Am Acad Optom.* 1954;31:3–11.

Worth 4 Dot

Gcala PE. When the patient can't see 20/20. *Rev Optom.* 1984;(Aug):42.

Stereopsis

Cooper J, Feldman J. Assessing the Frisby stereo test under monocular viewing conditions. *J Am Optom Assoc.* 1979;50:807.

Cooper J, Feldman K, Medlin D. Comparing stereoscopic performance of children using the Titmus, TNO, and Randot stereo tests. *J Am Optom Assoc.* 1979;50:821.

Hinchliffe HA. Clinical evaluation of stereopsis. *Br Orthopt J.* 1978;35:46.

Lang JI, Lang T. Eye screening with the Lang stereotest. *Am Orthopt J.* 1988;38:48.

Parks M. Single Binocular Vision. In Duane T, ed. *Duane's Clinical Ophthalmology.* 1971, pp 1–13.

Randot Stereotests. *Instructional Manual.* Chicago: Stereo Optical Co, 1988.

Reading RW. *Binocular Vision Foundations and Applications.* Boston: Butterworth, 1983.

Near Point of Convergence

Amos JF. *Diagnosis and Management in Vision Care*. Boston: Butterworth, 1987.

Capobianco NM. The subjective measurement of the nearpoint of convergence and its significance in the diagnosis of convergence insufficiency. *Am Orthopt J*. 1952;2:40.

Scheiman M, Gallaway M, Franta KA, Peters RJ, Hatch S, Cuff M, and Mitchel GL. Nearpoint of convergence: Test procedure, target selection, and normative data. Optom Vis Sci. 2003;80:214–225.

Hirschberg Test

Eskridge JB, Wick B, Perrigin D. The Hirschberg test: A double-masked clinical evaluation. *Am J Optom Physiol Opt*. 1988;65:745–750.

Griffin JR. *Binocular Anomalies Procedures for Vision Therapy*. Chicago: Professional Press, 1982.

Scheiman M. Hirschberg, Krimsky, Brückner Tests. In Eskridge JB, Amos JF, Bartlett JD, eds. *Clinical Procedures in Optometry*. Philadelphia: Lippincott, 1991.

Brückner Test

Caloroso EE, Rouse MW, Cotter SA. *Clinical Management of Strabismus*. Boston: Butterworth-Heinemann, 1993.

Griffin JR, Cotter SA. The Brückner test: Evaluation of clinical usefulness. *Am J Optom Physiol Opt*. 1986;63:957.

Roe LD, Gutyon DL. The light that leaks: Brückner and the red reflex. *Surv Ophthalmol*. 1984;28:665.

Tongue AC, Cibis GW. Brückner test. *J Am Acad Ophthalmol*. 1981;88:1041.

EOMs

Eskridge J. Evaluation and diagnosis of incomitant ocular deviations. *J Am Optom Assoc*. 1989;60:375–388.

Eskridge J, Wick B, Perrigin D. The Hirschberg test: A double-masked clinical evaluation. *Am J Optom Physiol Opt*. 1988;65:745–750.

Genco L. Ocular motility, part I. *Optom Monthly*. 1979;70:37–41.

Genco L. Ocular motility, part II. *Optom Monthly*. 1979;70:101–105.

Genco L. Ocular motility, part III. *Optom Monthly*. 1979;70:185–189.

Genco L. Testing extraocular muscles and visual skills. *Optom Monthly*. 1979; 70: 261–266.

Gray L. Doctor I see double. *Rev Optom*. 1985;(Mar):41–49.

Grosvenor T. The preliminary examination, Part 5. Motility tests. *Optom Weekly*. 1977;(Dec 15):33–35.

Rush JA, Younge BR. Paralysis of Cranial III, IV, and VI. Cause and prognosis in 1000 cases. *Arch Ophthalmol*. 1981;99:76–79.

Sheni D, Remole A. Variation of convergence limits with change in direction of gaze. *Am J Optom Physiol Opt*. 1988;65:76–83.

Pupils

Carter J. Diagnosis of pupillary anomalies. *J Am Optom Assoc*. 1979;50:671–680.

Genco L. The pupillary reflex pathway. *Optom Monthly*. 1978;69:774–778.

Gray L. The five-step pupil evaluation. *Rev Optom*. 1981;(Feb):38–44.

Higgins JD. Pupil. In Barresi BJ, ed. *Ocular Assessment: The Manual of Diagnosis for Office Practice*. Boston: Butterworth, 1984, pp 189–199.

Nyman J, Nyman N. Pupillary examination. *J Am Optom Assoc*. 1977;48:1375–1380.

Slamovits TL, Glaser JS. The pupils and accommodation. In Glaser JS, ed. *Neuro-ophthalmology*. Philadelphia: Lippincott, 1990, pp 459–486.

Thompson HS. Pupillary signs in the diagnosis of optic nerve disease. *Trans Ophthalmol Soc UK*. 1976;96:377–381.

Thompson HS, Pilley SF. Unequal pupils. A flowchart for sorting out the anisocorias. *Surv Ophthalmol*. 1976;21:45–48.

Walsh TJ. Pupillary abnormalities. In Walsh TJ, ed. *Neuro-ophthalmology: Clinical Signs and Symptoms.* Philadelphia: Lea & Febiger, 1992.

Zinn K. *The Pupil.* Springfield, IL: Thomas, 1972.

Screening Fields

Berman R. Classification of visual field defects. *Rev Optom.* 1978;115:57–60.

Genco L. Visual losses and perimetry. *Optom Monthly.* 1979;70:621–626.

Goodlaw E. A case in point extended. *J Am Optom Assoc.* 1985;56:564–565.

Grosvenor T. The preliminary examination, part 10. Visual field screening. *Optom Weekly.* 1978;64:111–116.

Reader A, Harper D. Confrontation visual-field testing. *JAMA.* 1976;236:250.

Trobe JD, Acosta PC, Krischer JP, et al. Confrontation visual field techniques in the detection of anterior visual pathway lesions. *Ann Neurol.* 1981;10:28–34.

Wirtschafter J, Hard-Boberg A, Coffman S. Evaluating the usefulness in neuro-ophthalmology of visual field examinations peripheral to 30 degrees *Trans Am Ophthalmol Soc.* 1984;82:329–357.

CHAPTER THREE: REFRACTION

General References

Amos JF. *Diagnosis and Management in Vision Care.* Boston: Butterworth, 1988.

Bannon RE. Binocular refraction—A survey of various techniques. *Optom Weekly.* 1965:(August 5):25–31.

Bartlett, JD, Jaanus SD, eds. *Clinical Ocular Pharmacology.* 4th ed. Boston: Butterworth-Heinemann, 2001.

Benjamin WJ, ed. *Borish's Clinical Refraction.* Philadelphia: Saunders, 1998.

Borish IM. *Clinical Refraction.* 3rd ed. Chicago: Professional Press, 1975.

Duke-Elder S. *The Practice of Refraction.* St. Louis: Mosby, 1969.

Edwards K, Llewellyn R. *Optometry.* Boston: Butterworth, 1988.

Grosvenor T. *Primary Care Optometry: A Clinical Manual.* 2nd ed. Chicago: Professional Press, 1989

Kurtz, D. The Perfect Eye: A novel model for teaching the theory of refraction. *J Optom Ed.* 1999;24:91–95.

Michaels D. *Visual Optics and Refraction: A Clinical Approach.* 3rd ed. St. Louis: Mosby, 1985.

Michaels DD. *Basic Refraction Techniques.* New York: Raven, 1988.

Sloane AE. *Manual of Refraction.* 3rd ed. Boston: Little, Brown, 1979.

Zadnik K, ed. *The Ocular Examination.* Philadelphia: Saunders, 1997.

Technique-Specific References

Lensometry

Fannin TE, Grosvenor T. *Clinical Optics.* Boston: Butterworth, 1987.

Kozol F. *Clinical Optics.* Boston: New England College of Optometry, 1980, pp 24–30, 66–69.

Rubin M. *Optics for Clinicians.* 2nd ed. Gainesville: Triad, 1974, pp 310–319.

Retinoscopy

Corboy JM. *The Retinoscopy Book.* Thorofare, NJ: Slack, 1989.

Duke-Elder S. *System of Ophthalmology,* vol, 5. *Ophthalmic Optics and Refraction.* St. Louis: Mosby, 1970, p 391.

Jones R. Physiological pseudomyopia. *Optom Vis Sci.* 1990;67:610.

Mutti DO, Zadnik K. Refractive error. Chapter 4 in Zadnik K, ed. *The Ocular Examination*. Philadelphia: Saunders, 1997, pp 64–74.

Roorda A, Bobier WR. Geometrical technique to determine the influence of monochromatic aberrations of retinoscopy. *J Opt Soc Am.* 1996;13:3–11.

Subjective Refraction

Abel CA. *Outline of Refracting Procedure*. Southern California College of Optometry (no date).

American Academy of Ophthalmology. *Ophthalmology Basic and Clinical Science Course*, section 2. *Optics, Refraction, and Contact Lenses*. San Francisco: American Academy of Ophthalmology, 1984.

Atchison DA, Charman WN, Woods RL. Subjective depth-of-focus of the eye. *Optom Vis Sci.* 1997:74:511–520.

Bannon RE. *Clinical Manual on Refraction with the AO Ultramatic Rx Master Phoropter*. Buffalo, NY: American Optical Corporation, 1975.

Grosvenor T. The refractive examination, part 3. Subjective testing. *Optom Monthly.* 1978: (Jul);74–83.

Johnson BL, Edwards JS, Goss DA, et al. A comparison of three subjective tests for astigmatism and their interexaminer reliabilities. *J Am Optom Assoc.* 1996;67:590–598.

Marcos S, Moreno E, Navarro R. The depth-of-field of the human eye from objective and subjective measurements. *Vision Res.* 1999;39:2039–2049.

Milder B, Rubin ML. *The Fine Art of Prescribing Glasses Without Making a Spectacle of Yourself.* 2nd ed. Gainesville: Triad Scientific, 1991.

Miller AD, Kris MJ, Griffiths AC. Effect of small focal errors on vision. *Optom Vis Sci.* 1997;74:521–526.

Mutti DO, Zadnik K. Refractive error. Chapter 4 in Zadnik, K. *The Ocular Examination*. Philadelphia: Saunders, 1997; pp 74–81.

Reinecke RD, Herm RJ. *Refraction: A Programmed Text*. 2nd ed. New York: Appleton-Century-Crofts, 1976.

Rosenfield M, Chiu NN. Repeatability of subjective and objective refraction. *Optom Vis Sci.* 1995: 72:577–579.

Ward PA, Charman WN. An objective assessment of the effect of fogging on accommodation. *Am J Optom Physiol Opt.* 1987;64:762–767.

Jackson Cross Cylinder

Brookman, KE. The Jackson crossed cylinder: historical perspective. *Optom Vis Sci.* 1993; 64:329–331.

Del Priore L, Guyton D. The Jackson cross cylinder. A reappraisal. *Ophthalmology.* 1966; 93:1461–1465.

Frank H. An experimental study on the cross-cylinder technique. *Am J Optom Arch Am Acad Optom.* 1950;27:572–575.

O'Leary D, Yang PH, Yeo CH. Effect of cross cylinder power on cylinder axis sensitivity. *Am J Optom Physiol Opt.* 1987;64:367–369.

Binocular Balance

Gentsch L, Goodwin H. A comparison of methods for the determination of binocular refractive balance. *Am J Optom Arch Am Acad Optom.* Oct, 1966.

Grosvenor T. Determining the binocular balance. *Optom Weekly.* 1976;67:33–35.

Layton A. A supplementary technique for balancing refraction. *Am J Optom Physiol Opt.* 1975;52:125–127.

Determining the Add for the Presbyope

Blystone PA. Relationship between age and presbyopic addition using a sample of 3,645 examinations from a single private practice. *J Am Optom Assoc.* 1999;70:505–508.

Carter JH. Determining the nearpoint addition. *N Engl J Optom.* 1985;37:4–13

Kurtz D. Presbyopia. In Brookman KE, ed. *Refractive Management of Ametropia.* Boston: Butterworth-Heinemann, 1996, pp 145–179.

Pointer JS. The presbyopic add. I. Magnitude and distribution in a historical context. *Ophthalmol Physiol Optom.* 1995;15:235–240.

Pointer JS. The presbyopic add. III. Influence of the distance refractive type. *Ophthalmol Physiol Optom.* 1995;15:249–253.

Trial Frame Refraction

Bailey I. Refracting low-vision patients. *Optom Monthly.* 1978;(May):131–135.

Margach C. Trial frame examinations: Back to basics. *Opt J Rev Optom.* 1976;(Oct):52–58.

Newman J. *A Guide to the Care of Low Vision Patients.* St. Louis: AOA, 1974, pp 67–99.

Stenopaic Slit Refraction

Long W. Stenopaic slit refraction. *Optom Weekly.* 1975;(Nov 6):33–36.

Cycloplegic Refraction

Amos D. Cycloplegic refraction. In Bartlett J, Janus S, eds. *Ocular Pharmacology.* Boston: Butterworth, 1984, pp 469–482.

Chung I. Topical ophthalmic drugs and the pediatric patient. *Optometry* 2000;71:511–518.

Kleinstein RN, Mutti DO, Manny RE, et al. Cycloplegia in African-American children. *Optom Vis Sci.* 1999;76:102–107.

Lahdes KK, Huupponen RK, Kaila RJ. Ocular effects and systemic absorption of cyclopentolate eyedrops after canthal and conventional application. *Acta Ophthalmol.* 1994;72:698–702.

Manny RE, Fern KD, Zervas HJ, et al. 1% cyclopentolate hydrochloride: another look at the time course of cycloplegia using an objective measure of the accommodative response. *Optom Vis Sci.* 1993;70:651–665.

Manny RE, Scheiman M, Kurtz D, et al and The COMET Study Group. Tropicamide 1%: An effective cycloplegic agent for myopic children. *Invest Ophthalmol Vis Sci.* 2001;42:1728–1735.

Mutti DO, Zadnik K. Refractive error. Chapter 4 in Zadnik K, ed. *The Ocular Examination.* Philadelphia: Saunders, 1997, pp 82–84.

Nelson LB. *Pediatric Ophthalmology.* Philadelphia: Saunders, 1984.

Delayed Subjective Refraction

Grosvenor T. How to keep your patient from accommodating. *Optom Weekly.* 1976;(June 24):44–46.

Binocular Refraction: Vectographic and Humphriss Immediate Contrast Technique

Bannon R. Binocular refraction: a survey of various techniques. *Optom Weekly.* 1965;56:25–31.

Chiu NN, Rosenfield M, Wong LC. Effect of contralateral fog during refractive error assessment. *J Am Optom Assoc* 1997;68:305–308.

Grolman B. Binocular refraction: a new system. *N Engl J Optom.* 1966;17:118–129.

Humphriss D, Woodruff E. Refraction by immediate contrast. *Optom Weekly.* 1962;53:2171–2175.

Mohindra's Near Retinoscopy

Mohindra I. Comparison of near retinoscopy and subjective refraction in adults. *Am J Optom Physiol Opt.* 1977;54:319–322.

Mohindra I. A non-cycloplegic refraction technique for infants and young children. *J Am Optom Assoc.* 1977;48:518–523.

Mohindra I. Physiological basis for near retinoscopy. *Optom Monthly.* 1980; 71:43–45.

Saunders KJ, Westall CA. Comparison between near retinoscopy and cycloplegic retinoscopy in the refraction of infants and children. *Optom Vis Sci.* 1992;69:615–622.

Twelker JD, Mutti DO. Retinoscopy in infants using a near noncycloplegic technique, cycloplegia with tropicamide 1%, and cycloplegia with cyclopentolate 1%. *Optom Vis Sci.* 2001;78:215–222.

Wesson MD, Mann KR, Bray NW. A comparison of cycloplegic refraction to the near retinoscopy technique for refractive error determination. *J Am Optom Assoc* 1990;61:680–684.

Septum Near Balance

Morgan MW. The Turville infinity binocular balance test. *J Am Optom Assoc* 1960;(January): 447–450.

CHAPTER 4: FUNCTIONAL TESTS

General References

Amos JF. *Diagnosis and Management in Vision Care*. Boston: Butterworth, 1987.

Benjamin WJ. *Borish's Clinical Refraction*. Philadelphia: Saunders, 1998.

Borish IM. *Clinical Refraction*. 3rd ed. Chicago: Professional Press, 1975.

Edwards K, Llewellyn R. *Optometry*. Boston: Butterworth, 1988.

Griffith JR. *Binocular Anomalies: Procedures for Vision Therapy*. 2nd ed. Chicago: Professional Press, 1982.

Grosvenor T. *Primary Care Optometry*. 4th ed Boston: Butterworth Heinemann, 2002.

Scheiman M, Wick B. *Clinical Management of Binocular Vision: Heterophoric, Accommodative and Eye Movement Disorders*. 2nd ed. Philadelphia: Lippincott, Williams & Williams, 2002.

Schor CM, Ciuffreda KJ. *Vergence Eye Movements: Basic and Clinical Aspects*. Boston: Butterworth, 1983.

Technique-Specific References

Lateral and Vertical Phorias

Calvin H, Rupnow P, Grosvenor T. How good is the estimated cover test at predicting the von Graefe phoria measurement? *Optom Vis Sci.* 1996;73:701–706.

Kromeier M, Schmitt C, Bach M, Kommereli G. Heterophoria measured with white, dark-grey and dark-red Maddox rods. *Graefes Arch Clin Exp Ophthalmol* 2001;239:937–940.

Robertson KM. Symptoms, signs, and diagnostic testing of vertical misalignment. *Prob Optom.* 1992;4:541–555.

Saladin JJ, Sheedy JE. Population study of fixation disparity, heterophoria, and vergence. *Am J Optom Physiol Opt.* 1978;55:744–750.

Schroeder TL, Rainey BB, Goss DA, Grosvenor TP. Reliability of and comparisons among methods of measuring dissociated phoria. *Optom Vis Sci.* 1996;73:389–397.

Walline JJ, Mutti DO, Zadnik K, Jones L. Development of phoria in children. *Optom Vis Sci.* 1998;75:605–610.

Horizontal and Vertical Vergences

Feldman J, Cooper J, Carniglia P, et al. Comparison of fusional ranges measured by Risley prisms, vectograms, and computer orthopter. *Optom Vis Sci.* 1989;66:375–382.

Fry G. An analysis of the relationships between phoria, blur, break and recovery findings at the near point. *Am J Optom Arch Am Acad Optom.* 1941;18:393–402.

Gall R, Wick B, Bedell H. Vergence facility: establishing clinical utility. *Optom Vis Sci* 1998; 75:731–742.

Goss DA. Effect of test sequence on fusional vergence ranges. *N Engl J Optom.* 1995;47:39–42.

Jackson TW, Goss DA. Variation and correlation of standard clinical phoropter tests of phorias, vergence ranges, and relative accommodation. *J Am Optom Assoc.* 1991;62:540–547.

Morgan MW. Analysis of clinic data. *Am J Optom Arch Am Acad Optom.* 1944;21:477–491.

Penisten DK, Hofstetter HW, Goss DA. Reliability of rotary prism fusional vergence ranges. *Optometry.* 2001;72:117–122.

Saladin JJ, Sheedy JE. Population study of fixation disparity, heterophoria, and vergence. *Am J Optom Physiol Opt.* 1978;55:744–750.

Scheiman M, Herzberg H, Frantz K, et al. A normative study of step vergences in elementary schoolchildren. *J Am Optom Assoc.* 1989;60:276–280.

Sheedy JE, Saladin JJ. Association of symptoms with measures of oculomotor deficiencies. *Am J Physiol Opt.* 1978;55:670–676.

Tuff LC, Firth AY, Griffiths HJ. Prism vergence measurements following adaptation to a base out prism. *Brit Orthop J.* 2000;57:42–44.

Accommodative Facility

Eskridge J. Clinical objective assessment of the accommodative response. *J Am Optom Assoc.* 1989;60:272–274.

McKenzie K, Kerr S, Rouse M. Study of accommodative facility testing reliability. *Am J Optom Physiol Opt.* 1987;64:186–194.

Pica M, Redmond MS, Zost M. Polarized versus anaglyphic materials. *J Behav Optom.* 1996; 7:43–45.

Rouse M, Deland P, Chous R, et al. Monocular accommodative facility testing reliability. *Optom Vis Sci.* 1989;66:72–77.

Rouse M, Hutter R. A normative study of the accommodative lag in elementary school children. *Am J Optom Physiol Opt.* 1984;61:693–697.

Scheiman M, Herzberg H, Frantz K, et al. Normative study of accommodative facility in elementary schoolchildren. *Am J Optom Physiol Opt.* 1988;65:127–134.

Siderov J, Johnston AW. The importance of the test parameters in the clinical assessment of accommodative facility. *Optom Vis Sci.* 1990;67:551–557.

Zellers JA, Alpert TL, Rouse MW. A review of the literature and a normative study of accommodative facility. *J Am Optom Assoc.* 1984;55:31–37.

Dynamic Retinoscopy

Apell R. Clinical application of bell retinoscopy. *J Am Optom Assoc.* 1975;46:1023–1027.

Bieber J. Why nearpoint retinoscopy with children? *Optom Weekly.* 1974;(Jan 17):23–26.

Haynes H. Clinical approaches to near point lens power determination. *Am J Optom Physiol Opt.* 1985;62:375–385.

Locke LC, Somers W. A comparison study of dynamic retinoscopy techniques. *Optom Vis Sci* 1989;66:540–544.

Rouse M, Hutter R. A normative study of the accommodative lag in elementary school children. *Am J Optom Physiol Opt.* 1984;61:693–697.

Rouse M, London R, Allen D. An evaluation of the monocular estimate method of dynamic retinoscopy. *Am J Optom Physiol Opt.* 1982;59:234–239.

Streff J, Claussen V. Retinoscopy measurement differences as a variable of technique. *Am J Optom Arch Am Acad Optom.* 1971;48:671–676.

Associated Phoria

Borish I. The Borish nearpoint chart. *J Am Optom Assoc.* 1978;49:41–44.

Carter D. Fixation disparity and heterophoria following prolonged wearing of prisms. *Am J Optom Arch Am Acad Optom.* 1965;42:141–152.

Eskridge JB. Adaptation to vertical prism. *Am J Optom Physiol Opt.* 1988; 65:371–376.

Pickwell LD, Yekta AA, Jenkins TC. Effect of reading in low illumination on fixation disparity. *Am J Optom Physiol Opt.* 1987;64:513–518.

Rutstein R, Eskridge J. Clinical evaluation of fixation disparity, part one. *Am J Optom Physiol Opt.* 1983;60:688–693.

Rutstein R, Eskridge J. Studies in vertical fixation disparity. *Am J Optom Physiol Opt.* 1986; 63:639–644.

Sheedy JE. Analysis of near oculomotor balance. *Rev Optom* 1979;(July):44–45.

Sheedy JE. Actual measurement of fixation disparity and its use in diagnosis and treatment. *J Am Optom Assoc* 1980;51:1079–1084.

Minus Lens to Blur

Edwards K, Llewellyn R. *Optometry*. Boston: Butterworth, 1988.

Rosenfield M, Cohen AS. Repeatability of clinical measurement of the amplitude of accommodation. *Ophthalmol Physiol Opt.* 1996;16:247–249.

4Δ Base Out Test

Frantz KA, Cotter SA, Wick B. Re-evaluation of the four prism diopter base-out test. *Optom Vis Sci.* 1992;69:777–786.

CHAPTER 5: OCULAR HEALTH ASSESSMENT

General References

Alexander LJ. *Primary Care of the Posterior Segment*. 2nd ed. Norwalk, CT: Appleton & Lange, 1994.

Bartlett JD, Jaanus SD. *Clinical Ocular Pharmacology*. Boston: Butterworth, 1989.

Brandreth R. *Clinical Slit Lamp Biomicroscopy*. San Leandro: Blaco Printers, 1978.

Budenz DL, McSoley J. Evaluating patients for glaucoma: A history- and examination-driven method. *Practical Optometry* 2002;13:6–12.

Casser L, Fingeret M, Woodcome HT. *Atlas of Primary Eyecare Procedures*. 2nd ed. Norwalk, CT: Appleton & Lange, 1997.

Catania L. *Primary Care of the Anterior Segment*. 2nd ed. Norwalk, CT: Appleton & Lange, 1994.

Duane T. *Clinical Ophthalmology*. Philadelphia: Lippincott, 1988.

Eskridge JB, Amos JF, Bartlett JD. *Clinical Procedures in Optometry*. Philadelphia: Lippincott, 1991.

Havener W. *Synopsis of Ophthalmology*. 5th ed. St. Louis: Mosby, 1979.

Pavan-Langston D. *Manual of Ocular Diagnosis and Therapy*. Boston: Little, Brown, 1980.

Terry J. *Ocular Disease Detection, Diagnosis and Treatment*. Boston: Butterworth, 1984.

Thomann KH, Marks ES, Adamczyk DT. *Primary Eyecare in Systemic Disease*. 2nd ed. New York: McGraw-Hill, 2001.

Technique-Specific References

Introduction

AIDS Task Force. Policy Statement. Section of Public Health and Occupation Vision of the American Academy of Optometry. *Am J Optom Physiol Opt.* 1988;65:599–601.

Whitmer L. To see or not to see: routine pupillary dilation. *J Am Optom Assoc.* 1989;60:496–499.

Biomicroscopy

Chaong R, Simpson T, Fonn D. The repeatability of discrete and continuous anterior segment grading scales. *Optom Vis Sci.* 2000;77:244–251.

Garston M. Turn up the light Part II. How to see more with your slit lamp. *Rev Optom.* 2002;(Sept 15):75–78.

Polse K. Technique for estimating the angle of the anterior chamber with the slit lamp. *Optom Weekly.* 1975;(June 12):13–16.

Van Herick W, Shaffer R, Schwartz A. Estimation of width of angle of anterior chamber. *Am J Ophthalmol.* 1969;68:626–629.

Walker R. Fundamentals of biomicroscopy. *OJRO.* 1977;(Jan):60–74.

Walker R. Biomicroscopic examination of the normal eye. *OJRO.* 1977;(May):59–64.

Instillation of Drops

Lahdes KK, Huupponen RK, Kaila RJ. Ocular effects and systemic absorption of cyclopentolate eyedrops after canthal and conventional application. *Acta Ophthalmologica.* 1994;72:698–702.

Smith SE. Eyedrop instillation for reluctant children. *Br J Ophthalmol.* 1991;75:480–481.

Gonioscopy

Cockburn D. A new method for gonioscopic grading of the anterior chamber angle. *Am J Optom Physiol Opt.* 1980;57:258–261

Fisch BM. *Gonioscopy and the Glaucomas.* 1993. Boston: Butterworth-Heinemann.

Fisch BM, Scott C. Gonioscopy in optometric practice: How to perform the examination, what to look for. *Contemp Optom.* 1987;6:27–34.

Gray L. Fundamentals of gonioscopy. *Rev Optom.* 1977;(Oct):51–60.

Gray L. Fundamentals of gonioscopy, part 2. *Rev Optom.* 1978;(Jul):47–55.

Penisten, D. Get a better angle on the gonio exam. *Rev Optom.* 1998;(Nov 15):62–66.

Prokopich CL, Flanagan JG. Gonioscopy: evaluation of the anterior chamber angle. Part I. *Ophthalmic Physiol Opt.* 1996;16:S39–S42.

Prokopich CL, Flanagan JG. Gonioscopy: evaluation of the anterior chamber angle. Part II. *Ophthalmic Physiol Opt.* 1997;17:S9–S13.

Williams KC, Barnebey HS. Meeting the challenge of secondary glaucomas. *Rev Optom.* 1998;(July 15):74–91.

Lacrimal/Tear Integrity Testing/Tear Break-up Time

Bron AJ. Diagnosis of dry eye. *Surv Ophthalmol.* 2001;45(2):S221–S226.

Campbell H, et al. A simple test for lacrimal obstruction. *Am J Ophthalmol.* 1962;53:611–613.

Cho P, Yap M. Schirmer Test 1. A Review. *Optom Vis Sci.* 1993;70:152–156.

Clompus R. When the patient complains of excessive tearing. *Rev Optom.* 1983;120:51–55.

Dundas M, Walker A, Woods RL. Clinical grading of corneal staining of non-contact lens wearers. *Ophthalmol Physiol Opt.* 2001;21:30–35.

Flachs A. The fluorescein appearance test for lacrimal obstruction. *Ann Ophthalmol.* 1979;(Feb): 237–242

Guzek JP, Yoon PS, Stephenson CB, et al. Lacrimal testing: the dye disappearance test & the Jones test. *An Ophthalmol* 1996;28:357–363.

Holly FJ, Lemp MA. Tear physiology and dry eyes. *Surv Ophthalmol.* 1977;22:69–87.

Jaanus S. Managing the Dry Eye. *Clin Eye Vis Care.* 1990;2:38–44.

Jones L, Linn M. The diagnosis of the causes of epiphora. *Am J Ophthalmol.* 1969;67:751–754.

Korb DR. Survey of preferred tests for the diagnosis of the tear film and dry eye. *Cornea.* 2000; 19:483–486.

Korb DR, Greiner JV, Herman J. Comparison of fluorescein break-up time measurement reproducibility using standard fluorescein strips versus the Dry Eye Test (DET) method. *Cornea.* 2001;20:811–815.

Manning FJ, Wehrly SR, Foulks GN. Patient tolerance and ocular surface staining characteristics of lissamine green versus rose Bengal. *Ophthalmology.* 1995;102:1953–1957.

Norn MS. Desiccation of the precorneal film. I: Corneal wetting time. *Acta Ophthalmol (Copenh).* 1969;47:865–880.

Pflugfelder SC, Scheffer CG, Tseng SC, et al. Evaluation of subjective assessments and objective diagnostic tests for diagnosing tear-film disorders known to cause ocular irritation. *Cornea.* 1998;17:38–56.

Putterman A. Evaluation of the lacrimal system. *Eye Ear Nose Throat Mon.* 1972;51:31–39.

Tsubota K, Kaido M, Yagi Y, et al. Diseases associated with ocular surface abnormalities: the importance of reflex tearing. *Br J Ophthalmol.* 1999;83:89–91.

Veirs E. *Lacrimal Disorders Diagnosis and Treatment.* St. Louis: Mosby, 1976, pp 15–30.

Yokoi N, Kinoshita S, Bron AJ, et al. Tear meniscus changes during cotton thread and Schirmer testing. *Invest Ophthalmol Vis Sci.* 2000;41:3748–3753.

Direct Ophthalmoscopy

Bass S. Examining the retina. *Rev Optom.* 1986;123:64–70.

Grosvenor T. The preliminary examination, part 9. Ophthalmoscopy. *Optom Weekly.* 1978;(Jan 19):29–33.

Raasch T. Funduscopic systems: a comparison of magnification. *Am J Optom Physiol Opt.* 1982; 59:595–601.

Binocular Indirect Ophthalmoscopy

Alexander A. Peripheral retinal examination in optometric practice. *Rev Optom.* 1978;(Dec):27–30.

Bass, S. How to achieve a greater appreciation of retinal scenery. *Rev Optom.* 1995;(Feb 15):89–97.

Cavallerano A, Garston M. Examination of the peripheral ocular fundus. *Rev Optom.* 1979; (May):43–49.

Cavallerano A, Gutner R, Garston M. Indirect biomicroscopy techniques. *J Am Optom Assoc.* 1986;57:755–758.

Chung I. Topical ophthalmic drugs and the pediatric patient. *Optometry.* 2000;71:511–518.

Denial A, Hanley M. Safe exposure times for slit lamp fundus biomicroscopy with high plus lenses. *Optometry.* 2000;72:45–51.

Garston M. Turn up the light on your diagnosis: part 1. *Rev Optom.* 2002;(Aug 14):71–74.

Patorgis CJ, Augeri PA. Binocular indirect ophthalmology: diagnostic applications, examination techniques. *Contemp Optom.* 1987;6:23–31.

Potter J, Semes L, Cavallerano A, et al. *Binocular Indirect Ophthalmoscopy.* Boston: Butterworth, 1988.

Rutnin U. Fundus appearance in normal eyes. *Am J Ophthalmol.* 1967;64:821–839.

Semes L. Sharpen your retinal exam skills. *Rev Optom.* 1989;(May):57–60.

Fundus Biomicroscopy

Barker F. Vitreoretinal biomicroscopy: A comparison of techniques. *J Am Optom Assoc.* 1987; 58:985–992.

Besada E. Examination of retinal lesions using binocular indirect ophthalmoscopy and non-contact lens biomicroscopy. *Practical Optometry.* 2002;13:162–174.

Cavallerano A, Gutner R, Garston M. Indirect biomicroscopy techniques. *J Am Optom Assoc.* 1986;57:755–758.

Houston G. Fundus photography using the Volk 90 diopter lens. *So J Optom.* 1988;6:23–26.

Jackson J, Fisher M. Evaluation of the posterior pole with a 90D lens and the slit-lamp biomicroscope. *So J Optom.* 1987;5:80–83.

Tanner V, Williamson TH. Watzke-Allen slit beam test in macular holes confirmed by optical coherence tomography. *Arch Ophthalmol.* 2000;118:1059–1063.

Volk Optical/Tech Optics, Inc. *Volk Double Aspheric 90D BIO Lens Instruction Manual.* Mentor, OH: Volk Tech Optics, 1985.

Watzke RC, Allen L. Subjective slitbeam sign for macular disease. *Am J Ophthalmol.* 1969; 68:449–453.

Wing J, Barker F. Wide field fundus biomicroscopy lenses—a comparative study. *J Am Optom Assoc.* 1990;61:544–547.

Goldmann 3-Mirror Lens

Barker F. Vitreoretinal biomicroscopy: a comparison of techniques. *J Am Optom Assoc.* 1987; 58:985–992.

Bock W. Fundus contact lens and Hruby lens. *J Am Optom Assoc.* 1977;48: 1425–1429.

Siegel D. Beyond binocular indirect. *Rev Optom.* 1990;(Jan):64–71.

Tonometry

Agudelo LM, Molina CA, Alvarez DL. Changes in intraocular pressure after laser in situ keratomileusis for myopia, hyperopia, and astigmatism. *J Refract Surg.* 2002;18:472–474.

Blumenthal EZ. Aligning the Goldmann tonometer tip by means of the "precontact whitish rings." *Surv Ophthalmol.* 1999;44:171–172.

Burvenich H, Sallet G, DeClercq J. The correlation between IOP measurement, central corneal thickness and corneal curvature. *Bull Soc Belge Ophthalmol.* 2000;276:23–26.

Doughty MJ, Zamen ML. Human corneal thickness and its impact on intraocular pressure measures: A review and meta-analysis approach. *Surv Ophthalmol.* 2000;44:367–408.

Faucher A, Gregoire J, Blondeau P. Accuracy of Goldmann tonometry after refractive surgery. *J Cataract Refract Surg.* 1997;23:832–838.

Gimeno JA, Munoz LA, Valenzuela LA, et al. Influence of refraction on tonometric readings after photorefractive keratectomy and laser assisted in situ keratomileusis. *Cornea.* 2000;19:512–516.

Gloster J. Tonometry and tonography. *Int Ophthalmol Clin.* 1965;15:990–1005.

Holladay J, Allison M, Prager T. Goldmann applanation tonometry in patients with regular corneal astigmatism. *Am J Ophthalmol.* 1983;96:90–93.

Moses R. The Goldmann applanation tonometer. *Am J Ophthalmol.* 1958;46:865–869.

Motolko MA, Feldman F, Hyde M, Hudy D. Sources of variability in the results of applanation tonometry. *Can J Ophthalmol.* 1982;17:93–95.

Rosenthal J, Werner D. *Tonometry and Glaucoma Detection.* Chicago: Professional Press; 1969, pp 111–113.

Amsler Grid

Marmor MF. A brief history of Macular grids: from Thomas Reid to Edvard Munch and Marc Amsler. *Surv Ophthalmol.* 2000;44:343–353.

Saito Y, Hirata Y, Hayashi A, et al. The visual performance and metaqmorphopsia of patients with macular holes. *Arch Ophthalmol.* 2000;118:41–46.

Red Desaturation

Liu GT, Volpe NJ, Galetta SL. *Neuro-Ophthalmology: Diagnosis and Management.* Philadelphia: Saunders, 2001, pp 7–40.

Modica PA. *Neuro-ophthalmic System: Clinical procedures.* Boston: Butterworth-Heinemann, 1999, pp 139–140.

Skarf B, Glaser JS, Trick GL, et al. Neuro-ophthalmic examination: the visual system. In Glaser JS, ed. *Neuro-ophthalmology.* 3rd ed. Philadelphia: Lippincott, Williams & Wilkins, 1999, pp 7–4.

Skarf B, Glaser JS, Trick GL, et al. Neuro-ophthalmologic examination: the visual sensory system. In Tasman W, Jaeger EA, eds. *Duanes' Clinical Ophthalmology.* Philadelphia: Lippincott, Williams & Wilkins, 2000, Vol 2, Ch 2, pp 1–46.

Townsend JC. Brightness and color comparison. In Eskridge JB, et al, eds. *Clinical Procedures in Optometry.* Philadelphia: Lippincott, 1991, pp 493–497.

Exophthalmometry

Chang AA, Bank A, Francis IC, Kappagoda MB. Clinical exophthalmometry: a comparative study of the Luedde and Hertel exophthalmometers. *Aust NZ J Ophthalomol* 1995;23:315–318.

Drews LC. Exophthalmometery. *Am J Ophthalmol.* 1957;43:37–58.

Luedde WH. An improved transparent exophthalmometer. *Am J Ophthalmol.* 1938;21:426.

Migliori ME, Gladstone GJ. Determination of the normal range of exophthalmometric values for black and white adults. *Am J Opthalmol.* 1984;98:438.

CHAPTER 6: CONTACT LENSES

General References

Bennett ES, Henry VA. *Clinical Manual of Contact Lenses.* Philadelphia: Lippincott Williams & Wilkins, 2000.

Bennett ES, Weissman BA, eds. *Clinical Contact Lens Practice.* 2nd ed. Philadelphia: Lippincott, 1992.

Hom MM. *Manual of Contact Lens Prescribing and Fitting.* 2nd ed. Boston: Butterworth-Heinemann, 2000.

Mandell RB. *Contact Lens Practice.* 4th ed. Springfield, IL: Thomas, 1988.

Phillips AJ, Speedwell L. *Contact Lenses.* 4th ed. Oxford: Butterworth-Heinemann, 1997.

Ruben M, Guillon M, eds. *Contact Lens Practice.* London: Chapman & Hall, 1994.

Veys J, Meyler J, Davies I. *Essential Contact Lens Practice.* Oxford: Butterworth-Heinemann, 2002.

Technique-Specific References

Contact Lens Case History

Bennett ES, Watanabe RK. Preliminary evaluation. In Bennett ES, Henry VA, eds. *Clinical Manual of Contact Lenses.* Philadelphia: Lippincott Williams & Wilkins, 2000, pp 3–5.

Veys J, Meyler J, Davies I. Patient selection and pre-screening for contact lens wear. In Veys J, Meyler J, Davies I, eds. *Essential Contact Lens Practice.* Oxford: Butterworth-Heinemann, 2002, pp 2–4.

Contact Lens External Examination

Bennett ES, Watanabe RK. Preliminary evaluation. In Bennett ES, Henry VA, eds. *Clinical Manual of Contact Lenses.* Philadelphia: Lippincott Williams & Wilkins, 2000, pp 5–33.

Guillon JP, Guillon M. Tear film examination of the contact lens patient. *Optician.* 1993;5421:21–29.

Guillon M, Weissman BA. Preliminary examination. In Ruben M, Guillon M, eds. *Contact Lens Practice.* London: Chapman & Hall, 1994, pp 517–528.

Josephson JE. Examination of the anterior ocular surface and tear film. In Stein H, Slatt B, Stein R, eds. *Fitting Guide for Rigid and Soft Contact Lenses.* 3rd ed. St. Louis: Mosby, 1990, pp 39–50.

Veys J, Meyler J, Davies I. Patient selection and pre-screening for contact lens wear. In Veys J, Meyler J, Davies I, eds. *Essential Contact Lens Practice.* Oxford: Butterworth-Heinemann, 2002, pp 1–7.

White PF, Gilman EL. Preliminary evaluation. In Bennett ES, Weissman BA, eds. *Clinical Contact Lens Practice.* 2nd ed. Philadelphia: Lippincott, 1992, pp 1–18.

Inspection and Verification of Gas Permeable Contact Lenses

Grohe RM, Caroline PJ. Surface deposits on contact lenses. In Bennett ES, Weissman BA, eds. *Clinical Contact Lens Practice.* 2nd ed. Philadelphia: Lippincott, 1992, pp 1–12.

Henry VA. Verification of rigid lenses. In Bennett ES, Henry VA, eds. *Clinical Manual of Contact Lenses.* Philadelphia: Lippincott Williams & Wilkins, 2000, pp 160–180.

Pearson RM. Quality control of rigid lenses in clinical practice. In Ruben M, Guillon M, eds. *Contact Lens Practice.* London: Chapman & Hall, 1994, pp 149–166.

Insertion, Removal, and Recentering of Gas Permeable Contact Lenses

Bennett ES. Lens care and patient education. In Bennett ES, Henry VA, eds. *Clinical Manual of Contact Lenses.* Philadelphia: Lippincott Williams & Wilkins, 2000, pp 132–137.

Mandell RB. Clinical procedures. In Mandell RB, ed. *Contact Lens Practice*. 4th ed. Springfield, IL: Thomas, 1988, pp 310–325.

Fit Assessment of Gas Permeable Contact Lenses

Bennett ES, Sorbara L. Lens design, fitting, and evaluation. In Bennett ES, Henry VA, eds. *Clinical Manual of Contact Lenses*. Philadelphia: Lippincott Williams & Wilkins, 2000, pp 83–90.

Fonn D. Progress evaluation procedures. In Bennett ES, Weissman BA, eds. *Clinical Contact Lens Practice*. 2nd ed. Philadelphia: Lippincott, 1992.

Guillon M. Basic contact lens fitting. In Ruben M, Guillon M, eds. *Contact Lens Practice*. London: Chapman & Hall, 1994, pp 602–622.

Veys J, Meyler J, Davies I. Rigid contact lens fitting. In Veys J, Meyler J, Davies I, eds. *Essential Contact Lens Practice*. Oxford: Butterworth-Heinemann, 2002, pp 37–45.

Inspection and Verification of Soft Contact Lenses

Biddle SP, Janoff LE. Verification of hydrogel lenses. In Bennett ES, Henry VA, eds. *Clinical Manual of Contact Lenses*. Philadelphia: Lippincott Williams & Wilkins, 2000, pp 303–312.

Jones WJJ. Contact lens deposits: their causes and control. *Contact Lens J*. 1992;20:6–12.

Kleist FD. Appearance and nature of hydrophilic contact lens deposits, 1. Protein and other organic deposits. *Int Contact Lens Clin*. 1979;6:49–58.

Kleist FD. Appearance and nature of hydrophilic contact lens deposits, 2. Inorganic deposits. *Int Contact Lens Clin*. 1979;6:177–186.

Port MJA. The verification of soft lenses in clinical practice. In Ruben M, Guillon M, eds. *Contact Lens Practice*. London: Chapman & Hall, 1994, pp 167–181.

Insertion and Removal of Soft Contact Lenses

Henry VA. Lens care and patient education. In Bennett ES, Henry VA, eds. *Clinical Manual of Contact Lenses*. Philadelphia: Lippincott Williams & Wilkins, 2000, pp 291–296.

Mandell RB. Lens handling, care and storage. In Mandell RB, ed. *Contact Lens Practice*. 4th ed. Springfield, IL: Thomas, 1988, pp 568–597.

Fit Assessment of Soft Contact Lenses

Guillon M. Basic contact lens fitting. In Ruben M, Guillon M, eds. *Contact Lens Practice*. London: Chapman & Hall, 1994, pp 587–601.

Henry VA. Fitting and evaluation. In Bennett ES, Henry VA, eds. *Clinical Manual of Contact Lenses*. Philadelphia: Lippincott Williams & Wilkins, 2000, pp 259–273.

Kame RT, Hayashida JK. Lens evaluation procedures and problem solving. In Bennett ES, Weissman BA, eds. *Clinical Contact Lens Practice*. 2nd ed. Philadelphia: Lippincott, 1992, pp 1–10.

Veys J, Meyler J, Davies I. Soft contact lens fitting. In Veys J, Meyler J, Davies I, eds. *Essential Contact Lens Practice*. Oxford: Butterworth-Heinemann, 2002, pp 29–36.

Assessment of the Monovision Patient

Bennett ES, Jurkus JM, Schwartz CA. Bifocal contact lenses. In Bennett ES, Henry VA, eds. *Clinical Manual of Contact Lenses*. Philadelphia: Lippincott Williams & Wilkins, 2000, pp 437–442.

deCarle JT. Bifocal and multifocal contact lenses. In Phillips AJ, Speedwell L, eds. *Contact Lenses*. 4th ed. Oxford: Butterworth-Heinemann, 1997, pp 547–548.

Hom MM. Monovision and bifocals. In Hom MM, ed. *Manual of Contact Lens Prescribing and Fitting*. 2nd ed. Boston: Butterworth-Heinemann, 2000, pp 327–329.

Mandell RB. Presbyopia. In Mandell RB. *Contact Lens Practice*. 4th ed. Springfield, IL: Thomas, 1988, pp 787–790.

CHAPTER 7: SYSTEMIC HEALTH SCREENING

Blood Pressure Evaluation

Bickley LS, Hoelelman RA. The Cardiovascular System. In *Bates' Guide to Physical Examination and History Taking*. Philadelphia: Lippincott, Williams & Wilkins, 1999, pp 277–332

Chobanian AV, et al. The Seventh report of the Joint National Committee on Prevention, Detection, Evaluation, and Treatment of High Blood Pressure. JAMA. 2003;289:2560–2571.

De Gaudemaris R, Chau NP, Mallon JM. Home blood pressure: variability, comparison with office readings and proposal for reference values. *J Hypertens*. 1994;12:831–838.

Fingeret M, Casser L, Woodcome HT. *Atlas of Primary Eyecare Procedures*. Norwalk, CT: Appleton & Lange, 1990.

Frolich ED. Blood pressure measurement. *Can J Cardiol*. 1995;11(suppl H):35–37.

Garcia-Vera MP, Sanz J. How many self-measurement blood pressure readings are needed to estimate hypertensive patients' true blood pressure. *J Behav Med*. 1999;22:93–113

Good GW, Augsburger AR. Role of optometrists in combating high blood pressure. *J Am Optom Assoc*. 1989;60:352–355.

Imai Y, Poncelet P, DeBuyzere M, et al. Prognostic significance of self-measurements of blood pressure. *Blood Press Monit*. 2000;5:137–143.

Krumholz DM.. Patient assessment. In Thomann KH, Marks ES, Adamczyk DT, eds. *Primary Eyecare in Systemic Disease*. 2nd ed. New York: McGraw-Hill, 2001.

Locke LC. Sphygmomanometry. In Eskridge JB, Amos JF, Bartlett JD, eds. *Clinical Procedures in Optometry*. Philadelphia: Lippincott, 1991.

Luft FC. Recent clinical trial highlights in hypertension. *Curr Hypertens Rep*. 2001;3:133–138.

Mancia G, Zanchetti A, Agabiti-Rosei E, et al. Ambulatory blood pressure is superior to clinic blood pressure in predicting treatment induced regression of left ventricular hypertrophy. *Circulation*. 1997;95:1464–1470.

Park MK, Menard SW, Yuan C. Comparison of auscultatory and oscillometric blood pressures. *Arch Pediatric Adolesc Med*. 2001;155:50–53.

Perloff D, Grim C, Flack J, et al. Human blood pressure determination by sphygmomanometry. *Circulation*. 1993;88:2460–2470

Seidel HM, Ball JW, Dains JE, Benedict GW. *Mosby's Guide to Physical Examination*. 3rd ed. St. Louis: Mosby-Yearbook, 1995.

Wasloski EJ. How to take the doubt out of blood pressure screening. *Rev Optom*. 1999;136:58–60.

Carotid/Orbital Evaluation

Abramson DI. Vascular disorders of the extremities, part 1. Clinical assessment and differential diagnosis of chronic occlusive arterial disease. *Pract Cardiol*. 1980;6:133–151

Alexander LJ. *Primary Care of the Posterior Segment*. 2nd ed. Norwalk, CT: Appleton & Lange, 1994.

Bickley LS, Hoelelmann RA. The cardiovascular system. In *Bates' Guide to Physical Examination and History Taking*. Philadelphia: Lippincott, Williams & Wilkins, 1999, pp 277–332.

Carter SA. Arterial auscultation in peripheral vascular disease. *JAMA*. 1981;246:1682–1686.

Casser L, Fingeret M, Woodcome HT. *Atlas of Primary Eyecare Procedures*. 2nd ed. Norwalk, CT: Appleton & Lange, 1997.

Cohen JH, Muller S. Eyeball bruits. *N Engl J Med*. 1956;255:459–464.

Harvey J. Introduction to orbital disease. In Tasman W, Jaegar EA, eds. *Duane's Clinical Ophthalmology*. Philadelphia: Lippincott, 1992, pp 2–8.

Hurst JW, Hopkins LS, Smith RB. Noises in the neck. *N Engl J Med*. 1980;302:862.

Jennings BJ. Carotid artery assessment. In Eskridge JB, Amos JF, Bartlett JD, eds. *Clinical Procedures in Optometry.* Philadelphia: Lippincott, 1991.

Kurtchner MM, McRae LP. Auscultation for carotid bruits in cerebrovascular insufficiency. *JAMA.* 1969;210:494–497.

Mathias A, Newton W. Risk of stroke in patients with carotid bruits. *J Fam Pract.* 1998;46:453–454.

Nabel EG. Essential features of the cardiac history and physical examination. In Humes HD, ed. *Kelley's Textbook of Internal Medicine.* 4th ed. Philadelphia: Lippincott, Williams & Wilkins, 2000, pp 360–367.

Seidel HM, Ball JW, Dains JE, Benedict GW. *Mosby's Guide to Physical Examination.* 3rd ed. St. Louis: Mosby, 1995.

Lymph Node Evaluation

Bates B. *A Guide to Physical Examination.* 5th ed. Philadelphia: Lippincott, 1990.

Bickley LS, Hoelelman RA. The head and neck. In *Bates' Guide to Physical Examination and History Taking.* Philadelphia: Lippincott, Williams & Wilkins, 1999, pp 163–244.

Casser L, Fingeret M, Woodcome HT. *Atlas of Primary Eyecare Procedures.* 2nd ed. Norwalk, CT: Appleton & Lange, 1997.

Edwards CRW. The general examination and external features of disease. In MacLeod J, Munro J, eds. *Clinical Examination.* 7th ed. Edinburgh: Churchill Livingstone, 1986.

Ghirardelli ML, Jemos V, Gobbi PG. Diagnostic approach to lymph node enlargement. *Haematologica.* 1999;84:242–247.

Krumholz DM. Patient assessment. In Thomann KH, Marks ES, Adamczyk DT, eds. *Primary Eyecare in Systemic Disease.* 2nd ed. New York: McGraw-Hill, 2001.

May LA. The physical examination. In Muchnick BG, ed. *Clinical Medicine in Optometric Practice.* St. Louis: Mosby-Yearbook, 1994.

Seidel HM, Ball JW, Dains JE, Benedict GW. *Mosby's Guide to Physical Examination.* 3rd ed. St. Louis: Mosby, 1995.

Vaughn DJ. Approach to the patient with lymphadenopathy. In Humes HD, ed. *Kelley's Textbook of Internal Medicine.* 4th ed. Philadelphia: Lippincott, Williams & Wilkins, 2000, pp 1522–1530.

Paranasal Sinus Evaluation

Ausband JR. *Ear, Nose and Throat Disorders.* 2nd ed. New Hyde Park, NY: Medical Examination Publishing, 1982.

Ballenger JJ. *Diseases of the Nose, Throat, Ear, Head, and Neck.* 14th ed. Philadelphia: Lea & Febiger, 1992.

Bickley LS, Hoelelman RA. The head and neck. In *Bates' Guide to Physical Examination and History Taking.* Philadelphia: Lippincott, Williams & Wilkins, 1999: 163–244

Corren J. Making the diagnosis of sinusitis—sinusitis in primary care. *Clin Focus Symposium.* 1993;Dec (suppl):10–17.

Donald PJ, Gluckman JL, Rice DH. *The Sinuses.* New York: Raven, 1995.

Ferguson BJ. Acute and chronic sinusitis. How to ease symptoms and locate the cause. *Postgrad Med.* 1995;97:45–48.

Friedman M, Landsberg R, Tanyeri H. Intraoperative and post-operative assessment of frontal sinus patency by transillumination. *Laryngoscope.* 2000;110:683–684.

Maltinski G. Nasal disorders and sinusitis. *Primary Care.* 1998;25:663–683.

Seidel HM, Ball JW, Dains JE, Benedict GW. *Mosby's Guide to Physical Examination.* 3rd ed. St. Louis: Mosby, 1995.

Thaler ER, Kennedy DW. Medical Otolaryngology. In Humes HD, ed. *Kelley's Textbook of Internal Medicine.* 4th ed. Philadelphia: Lippincott, Williams & Wilkins, 2000, pp 291–299.

Williams JW, Simel DL, Roberts L, Samsa GP. Clinical evaluation for sinusitis—making the diagnosis by history and physical examination. *Ann Intern Med.* 1992;117:705–710.

Williams JW Jr, Simel DL. Does this patient have sinusitis? Diagnosing acute sinusitis by history and physical examination. *JAMA.* 1993;270:1242–1246.

Glucometry

Bode BW, Sabbah H, Davidson PC. What's ahead in glucose monitoring? New techniques hold promise for improved ease and accuracy. *Postgrad Med.* 2001;109:41–44; 47–49.

Faas A, Schellevis FG, Van Eijk JT. The efficacy of self-monitoring of blood glucose in NIDDM subjects—a criteria-based literature review. *Diabetes Care.* 1997;20:1482–1486.

Gifford-Jorgensen RA, Borchert J, Hassanein R, et al. Comparison of five glucose meters for self-monitoring of blood glucose by diabetic patients. *Diabetes Care.* 1986;9:70–76.

Glasmacher AG, Brennermann W, Hahn C, et al. Evaluation of five devices for self-monitoring of blood glucose in the normoglycemic range. *Exp Clin Endocrinol Diabetes.* 1998;106:360–364.

Hoskins PL, Alford JB, Handelsman DJ, et al. Comparison of different models of diabetes care on compliance with self-monitoring of blood glucose by memory glucometer. *Diabetes Care.* 1998; 11:719–724.

Karter AJ, Ferrara A, Darbinian JA, et al. Self-monitoring of blood glucose—language and financial barriers in a managed care population with diabetes. *Diabetes Care.* 2000;23:477–483.

Lask I. Screening blood glucose levels—a pilot project for optometrists. *Optometry Today (UK).* 1997;37:29.

The National Steering Committee for Quality Assurance in Capillary Blood Glucose Monitoring. Proposed strategies for reducing user error in capillary blood glucose monitoring. *Diabetes Care.* 1993;16:493–498.

Poirier JY, LePrieur N, Campiom L, et al. Clinical and statistical evaluation of self-monitoring blood glucose meters. *Diabetes Care.* 1998;21:1919–1924.

Petersen KA, Petersen AM, Corbett V. Comparison of home glucose monitoring with the oral glucose tolerance test to detect gestational glucose intolerance. *J Fam Pract.* 1994;39:558–563.

Portable blood glucose monitors. *Health devices.* 2000;29:201–232.

Swanson MW. In-office laboratory testing for diabetes mellitus. *Optom Clin.* 1992;2:117–129.

CHAPTER 8: CRANIAL NERVE SCREENING

General References

Broadway DC, Tufail A, Khaw PT. *Ophthalmology Examination Techniques, Questions, and Answers.* Oxford: Butterworth-Heinemann, 1999, pp 19–32.

Burde RM, Savino PJ, Trobe JD. *Clinical Decisions in Neuro-ophthalmology.* St. Louis: Mosby, 1992

Fite JD. *The Neuro-ophthalmological examination* (video recording). Leonia, NJ: S/T Videocassette Duplicating, 1978.

Friedman NJ, Pineda R II, Kaiser PK. *The Massachusetts Eye and Ear Infirmary Illustrated Manual of Ophthalmology.* Philadelphia: Saunders, 1998.

Glaser JS. *Neuro-ophthalmology.* Philadelphia: Lippincott, 1990.

Goldberg S. *The 4-Minute Neurologic Exam.* Miami: Medmaster, 1987.

Hart WM, ed. *Adler's Physiology of the Eye.* 9th ed. St. Louis: Mosby, 1992.

Miller NR, Newman NJ. *The Essentials: Walsh & Hoyt's Clinical Neuro-Ophthalmology.* Philadelphia: Lippincott, Williams & Wilkins. 1999.

Netter FH. *CIBA Collection of Medical Illustrations.* Vol. 1, *Nervous System.* West Caldwell, NJ: Ciba Pharmaceutical, 1983.

Newman NM. *Neuro-ophthalmology: A Practical Text.* Norwalk, CT: Appleton & Lange, 1992.

Sendrowski DP. *Cranial Nerve Evaluation of an Optometric Patient.* Class handout. Southern California College of Optometry, 1989.

Skorin L, Muchnick BG. Neuro-ophthalmic disorders. Chapter 22 in Bartlett JD, Jaanus SD, eds. *Clinical Ocular Pharmacology*. 4th ed. Boston: Butterworth-Heinemann, 2001.

Walls LL. *The Screening Neurological Examination* (video recording). Beaverton, OR: Pro Vid 20/20, 1994.

Walsh TJ. *Clinical Neuro-ophthalmology: Clinical Signs and Symptoms*. Philadelphia: Lea & Febiger, 1992.

Willard FH, Perl DP. Medical Neuroanatomy: *A Problem-oriented Manual with Annotated Atlas*. Philadelphia: Lippincott, 1993.

Technique-Specific References

Pupil Cycle Time

Day RT. Pupil cycle time in the long-term neurologic assessment of divers. *Undersea & Hyperbaric Medicine*. 1994;21:31–41.

Martyn CN, Ewing DJ. Pupil cycle time: a simple way of measuring an autonomic reflex. *J Neurol Neurosurg Psychiatry*. 1986;49:771–774.

Miller SD, Thompson HS. Edge-light pupil cycle time. *Brit J Ophthalmol*. 1978;62:495–500.

Pharmacological Tests of the Pupil

Alexander LJ, Skorin L Jr, Bartlett JD. Neuro-ophthalmic disorders. Chapter 23 in *Clinical Ocular Pharmacology*. Bartlett JD, Jaanus SD, eds. Boston: Butterworth-Heinemann, 2001, pp 521–532.

Friedman NE. The pupil. Chapter 3 in Zadnik K, ed. *The Ocular Examination*. Philadelphia: Saunders, 1997, pp 45–49.

Jacobson DM, Vierkant RA. Comparison of cholinergic supersensitivity in third nerve palsy and Adie's syndrome. *J Neuro-Ophthalmol*. 1998;18:171–175.

Leavitt JA, Wayman LL, Hodge DO, Brubaker RF. Pupillary response to four concentrations of pilocarpine in normal subjects: application to testing for Adie tonic pupil. *Am J Ophthalmol*. 2002; 133:333–336.

Miller NR, Newman NJ. Examination of the pupils, accommodation, and lacrimation. Chapter 14 in *Walsh & Hoyt's Clinical Neuro-Ophthalmology, The Essentials*. 5th ed. Miller NR, Newman NJ, eds. Philadelphia: Lippincott, Williams & Wilkins, 1999, pp 422.

Morales J, Brown SM, Abdul-Rahim AX, Crosson CE. Ocular effects of apraclonidine in Horner syndrome. *Arch Ophthalmol*. 2000;118:951–954.

Trigeminal Nerve Function Test

Posnick JC, Grossman JA. Facial sensibility testing: a clinical update. *Plast Reconstr Surg*. 2000; 106:892–894.

Screening Tests for Cranial Nerves I, VIII, XI, and XII

Davidson TM, Freed C, Healy MP, Murphy C. Rapid clinical evaluation of anosmia in children: the alcohol sniff test. *Ann NY Acad Sci*. 1998;855:787–792.

Davidson TM, Murphy C. Rapid clinical evaluation of anosmia. *Arch Otolaryngol Head Neck Surg*. 1997;123:591–594.

INDEX

Page numbers followed by *f* refer to figures; those followed by *t* refer to tables.